The Vaccine Handbook:
A Practical Guide for Clinicians

Third Edition

Gary S. Marshall, MD

Professor of Pediatrics
Chief, Division of Pediatric Infectious Diseases
University of Louisville School of Medicine

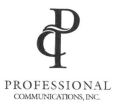

PROFESSIONAL
COMMUNICATIONS, INC.

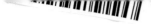

Copyright 2010
Gary S. Marshall, MD

Professional Communications, Inc.
A Medical Publishing & Communications Company

400 Center Bay Drive	PO Box 10
West Islip, NY 11795	Caddo, OK 74729-0010
(t) 631/661-2852	(t) 580/367-9838
(f) 631/661-2167	(f) 580/367-9989

For orders only, please call
1-800-337-9838
or visit our website at
www.pcibooks.com

ISBN: 978-1-932610-64-2

Printed in the United States of America

DISCLAIMER

The opinions expressed in this publication reflect those of the author. However, the author makes no warranty regarding the contents of the publication. The protocols described herein are general and may not apply to a specific patient. Any product mentioned in this publication should be taken in accordance with the prescribing information provided by the manufacturer.

This text is printed on recycled paper.

TABLE OF CONTENTS

General Principles of Vaccinology and Vaccine Practice	Introduction to Vaccinology	1
	Vaccine Infrastructure in the United States	2
	Standards, Principles, and Regulations	3
	Vaccine Practice	4
	General Recommendations	5
	Vaccination in Special Circumstances	6
	Addressing Concerns About Vaccines	7
	Schedules	8
Diseases and Vaccines	Anthrax	9
	Diphtheria, Tetanus, Pertussis	10
	Haemophilus influenzae type b	11
	Hepatitis A	12
	Hepatitis B	13
	Human Papillomavirus	14
	Influenza	15
	Japanese Encephalitis	16
	Measles, Mumps, Rubella	17
	Neisseria meningitidis	18
	Polio	19
	Rabies	20
	Rotavirus	21
	Smallpox	22
	Streptococcus pneumoniae	23
	Typhoid Fever	24
	Varicella	25
	Yellow Fever	26
	Zoster	27
	Combination Vaccines	28
Appendix		29
Index		30

Preface

In 1982, children in the United States received one shot series (5 DTPs followed by a Td booster), one oral vaccination series (4 or 5 OPVs), and one MMR by 18 years of age...7 injections, a few sugar cubes, and 7 diseases prevented. By 2010, children and adolescents routinely received 11 or 12 vaccination series—HepB, RV, DTaP, Hib, PCV, IPV, yearly influenza vaccine, MMR, VAR, HepA, MCV, and HPV vaccine (for girls)—as many as 53 doses (50 for boys) and 16 dreadful diseases prevented! There's no question about it—vaccination is one of the greatest public health achievements of the 20th century. We enjoy a freedom from contagious diseases that is unprecedented in human history and could not have been imagined by our parents.

As we have gained freedom from disease we have accumulated unforeseen challenges. Providers are faced with dispensing multiple antigens that have catchy trade names and come in various combinations made by different manufacturers, a vaccine alphabet soup that is difficult to keep straight. The business of vaccine practice has become complicated. Parents read on the Internet and hear on television that vaccines are dangerous and that vaccine policy is driven by a conspiracy of unscrupulous profiteers; this leads to vaccination hesitancy that at best prolongs the well child visit, and at worst results in refusal to vaccinate...which leads to outbreaks of disease. Translating the science of vaccinology into layman's terms has become a critical skill as patients bring more in-depth questions into the exam room and demand more sophisticated answers. Adults are not immunized as they should be. There are vaccines for persons with particular risks, and particular risks of vaccines for certain persons. Recurrent shortages, frequent changes in official recommendations, labyrinthine guidances and regulations—these things characterize today's vaccination environment.

The Vaccine Handbook has a simple purpose: to draw authoritative information about vaccines together into a simple, concise, user-friendly, practical resource that can be used in the private office or public health clinic, on the hospital wards, and in the classroom. There are already several excellent books about vaccines. The definitive textbook is *Vaccines*, edited by Stan Plotkin, Walt Orenstein, and Paul Offit (Elsevier; 2008). This book, which is encyclopedic in scope and rich in content, remains the essential reference for specialists and scientists. Two other books in particular contain authoritative recommendations: the *Red Book* (*Report of the Committee on Infectious Diseases*), published by the American Academy of Pediatrics (AAP), and the *Pink Book* (*Epidemiology and Prevention of Vaccine-Preventable Diseases*), published by the Centers for Disease Control and Prevention.

Unlike *Vaccines*, which is geared towards academicians, and unlike books in the popular press, which are geared exclusively towards parents and patients, *The Vaccine Handbook* is geared towards practicing pediatricians, family physicians, internists, obstetrician/gynecologists, nurses, nurse practitioners, physician's assistants, clinic staff, students and residents (some parents and patients might find it useful as well!). Unlike the *Red Book*, which is about infectious diseases, *The Vaccine Handbook* is only about vaccines and the diseases they prevent. It expands on the *Red Book* by including information on the fundamentals of vaccine immunology, development, licensure, policy making, the vaccine safety net and risk-benefit communication. *The Vaccine Handbook* also addresses current public concerns about vaccines, adult vaccination, travel vaccines, billing, legal obligations, and office organization and logistics. It differs from the *Pink Book* as well in the extent to which these topics are covered. Finally, *The Vaccine Handbook* is, well, purple. You can call it *The Purple Book*.

The book has continued to evolve since the first edition was published in 2004 and the second edition in 2008. In that period of time, new vaccines, and new versions of existing vaccines, have been licensed and recommended for use. New recommendations and updates to old recommendations have been issued. There has even been a new influenza pandemic, and vaccines developed and deployed in response. New concerns about vaccine safety have been raised in the public's mind, and most if not all of these concerns have been laid to rest by definitive scientific studies. All of this is captured in the new edition of *The Purple Book*. There have also been some notable improvements. First, the book is now organized into two sections. *Section A* provides all the necessary background on vaccinology, from how vaccines work to how they are tested, licensed, recommended for use, and monitored for safety and effectiveness. There are tips on implementing vaccinations in daily practice and on addressing concerns about vaccines. *Section B* contains all the details about every vaccine (the vaccine chapters are in alphabetical order) that is available in the United States, including the biology, clinical features, and epidemiology of the disease, background on the immunization program, composition of the vaccines, details on safety, efficacy, and immunogenicity, and recommendations. There is also an *Appendix*, which lists important resources for practitioners. One other major improvement—references are now footnoted in the text and listed at the end of each chapter.

The Purple Book provides enough background for the practitioner to understand the recommendations and explain them to his or her patients. It should be noted that while official recommendations are the foundation of scientific vaccine practice, they have their limitations. They take time to develop and are constrained by precedent, the need for consensus, the big public health picture, and, in some cases, politics. In addition, not all contingencies and permutations are covered. The language is sometimes definitive (*vaccine X is recommended*), sometimes not definitive (*vaccine X should be considered*), and sometimes vague (*some experts believe vaccine X should be given*). There is even disagreement among sources—the package insert, for example, and the recommendations set forth by the Advisory Committee on Immunization Practices (ACIP) of the Centers for Disease Control and Prevention. Wherever possible, this book attempts to distill the material down to practical guidance. Where official recommendations do not exist, reasonable suggestions are offered.

One goal we all share is to prevent disease and death without causing harm. Vaccines are a means to this end, and *The Purple Book* is intended to provide help along the way.

> — **Gary S. Marshall, MD**
> Professor of Pediatrics
> Chief, Division of Pediatric Infectious Diseases
> Director, Pediatric Clinical Trials Unit
> University of Louisville School of Medicine
> Louisville, Kentucky

Conventions Used in This Book

The nomenclature and abbreviations used in this book for disease agents and their respective vaccines are given in the *Appendix*. In general, these follow ACIP standards (http://www.cdc.gov/vaccines/recs/acip/downloads/vac-abbrev.pdf; accessed 02/14/09), with some modifications. For example, the conjugate proteins used in protein-polysaccharide conjugate vaccines are added to the abbreviations as a qualifier, as in "Hib-T" for "*Haemophilus influenzae* type b vaccine, tetanus toxoid conjugate" and "Hib-OMP" for "*Haemophilus influenzae* type b vaccine, (meningococcal) outer membrane protein conjugate" (these are important to differentiate because the dosing schedules for these vaccines differ). To make things a little more complicated (but hopefully more accurate), there are times when vaccines are referred to in generic fashion, in which case the qualifier is dropped (eg, "Hib" for "*Haemophilus influenzae* type b conjugate vaccine," referring to both the "T" and "OMP" conjugates). Here's another example: "LAIV" refers to live-attenuated influenza virus vaccine, in general, whereas "LAIV-seasonal" refers specifically to the trivalent seasonal live-attenuated influenza vaccine and "LAIV-2009 H1N1" refers to the monovalent vaccine used during the 2009 pandemic.

In some cases, the abbreviation for the agent (eg, "HAV" for "hepatitis A virus") is different from the vaccine (eg, "HepA," which means "hepatitis A vaccine"). In other cases, the abbreviation for the agent (eg, "HPV," which means "human papillomavirus") may be used when referring to the vaccine (eg, "HPV vaccine," which means "human papillomavirus vaccine," or "HPV4," which means "HPV vaccine, 4-valent"). For some vaccines (eg, rabies vaccine), the abbreviation was just made up ("RAB") in fashion with established abbreviations. Specific identifying characteristics, such as the cell type in which the vaccine was produced, may be indicated, as in "RAB-HDC," which means "rabies vaccine, human diploid cell."

Premixed modern combination vaccines are denoted by dashes between the components (eg, "DTaP-HepB-IPV" for Pediarix, which contains DTaP, HepB, and IPV). Modern combination vaccines that require reconstitution are denoted by a slash mark (eg, "DTaP-IPV/Hib-T," where the liquid DTaP-IPV is used to reconstitute the lyophilized Hib-T, creating a combination vaccine [Pentacel]). In general, vaccine trade names use initial capitals only, except where upper and lower case letters are interspersed in the name, as in "RotaTeq." Trademark symbols are not used. Uncommon abbreviations used in the book are defined in the text upon first use; commonly used abbreviations are used in the text without definition but are listed in the *Appendix*.

In general, "age" means that the individual has passed one mark in time but has not yet reached the next relevant mark. For example, "2 months of age" means at or beyond the 2-month birthday but not yet at the 3-month birthday. Age intervals may be indicated by a dash or the word "to"; thus, "4-6 years of age" and "4 to 6 years of age" mean "4 years of age through 6 years of age," or "from the 4th birthday until the day before the 7th birthday. As far as time intervals are concerned, "weeks" means 7 days and "months" means 28 days, unless specified as "calendar months." In that case, the interval is to the same date in the appropriate month. For example, for an infant vaccinated on January 6, an interval of 6 calendar months would be on July 6. These definitions are particularly relevant when referring to age indications for vaccines and minimum intervals (eg, **Table 5**.1). In general, if an interval is <4 months, then weeks or days are used to denote the time period; for 4 months and beyond, calendar months are used.

Many organizations provide guidance regarding immunizations. The most generally applicable, authoritative recommendations come from the ACIP, the AAP, and the American Academy of Family Physicians. The recommendations from these organizations are usually very similar, and as such, the ACIP recommendations are referenced in this book. Any differences with the recommendations of other agencies, or the respective package inserts, are highlighted.

Referencing is enough to give interested readers someplace else to go but is not intended to be exhaustive.

Disclaimers

Care has been taken to confirm the accuracy of the information presented herein and to describe generally accepted practices. However, the author, editor, and publisher are not responsible for errors or omissions or for any consequences from application of the information in this book and make no warranty, expressed or implied, with respect to the currency, completeness, or accuracy of the contents of the publication. Application of this information in a particular situation remains the professional responsibility of the practitioner.

The author, editor, and publisher have exerted every effort to ensure that drug selection and dosage set forth in this text are in accordance with current recommendations and practice at the time of publication. However, in view of ongoing research, changes in government regulations, and the constant flow of information relating to drug therapy and drug reactions, the reader is urged to check the package insert and published or posted recommendations for each drug or vaccine discussed, being aware that there may be changes in indications, dosage, or schedule, and that added warnings and precautions may have been issued.

This is particularly important when the recommended agent is a new or infrequently employed drug. Some drugs and medical devices presented in this publication may have Food and Drug Administration (FDA) clearance for limited use in restricted research settings. It is the responsibility of health care providers to ascertain the FDA status of each drug or device planned for use in their clinical practice.

Some of the material from the first edition (*The Vaccine Handbook: A Practical Guide for Clinicians*; 2004, Lippincott Williams & Wilkins; Philadelphia, PA), contributed by Drs. Penelope H. Dennehy, David P. Greenberg, Paul A. Offit, and Tina Q. Tan, is retained here with the respective authors' express permission. In addition, some of the material in this book was previously published in *The Vaccine Quarterly* (©2007-2010, Wolters Kluwer Health) and is reprinted here with permission.

Acknowledgements

The author is deeply indebted to Drs. Dennehy, Tan, Greenberg, and Offit for their contributions to the first edition. Appreciation is also extended to the many other people who contributed to this work through conversation and comment, including Dr. Litjen Tan from the American Medical Association and Drs. Yabo Beysolow and Bill Atkinson from the Centers for Disease Control and Prevention. Finally, the author would like to thank Dr. Sharon Humiston from the University of Rochester and Dr. Jim Conway from the University of Wisconsin for their superb, comprehensive review of the manuscript and many helpful suggestions.

Dedication

For Cherie, Emily, and Cullen.
And for Grandpop, who got his flu shot
even though his friend said
it would give him the flu.

1   Introduction to Vaccinology

Immunization

Immunization is the process of protecting individuals from disease by making them immune. This is most often accomplished *actively* through *vaccination*, the delivery of antigens to the host for purposes of stimulating an immune response. It can also be accomplished *passively* by the administration of antibodies. While not technically correct in all instances, the terms *vaccination* and *immunization* are often used interchangeably.

■ Active Immunization

Table 1.1 gives one approach to classifying vaccines that have been used in humans. *Live vaccines* replicate in the host and generate immune responses that mimic those induced by natural infection. They are generally *attenuated*, or weakened, in some fashion such that they cause subclinical infection with very little risk of disease. Three approaches to attenuation are represented in our current repertoire of vaccines.

- *Serial passage*—This is the classical method of attenuating viruses, dating back to the 1930s when Thieler passaged yellow fever virus in eggs 200 times in order to weaken it. For viruses, serial passage is now most often accomplished in animal or human cell cultures. The mechanisms of attenuation are not clear but probably involve the accumulation of deletions and mutations that, while adapting the virus to growth in vitro, render the virus less fit (but still capable of replicating) in vivo. The modern prototype live-attenuated virus vaccine was developed by Sabin, who passaged the poliovirus serially in monkey cells and demonstrated that oral administration of the attenuated virus protected against polio. Serial passage also was used to attenuate measles, mumps, and rubella viruses for use in vaccines. The virus used to make VAR was originally isolated from a child in Japan in the early 1970s. It was serially passaged in human embryonic lung, embryonic guinea pig, and WI-38 (human diploid) cells in order to achieve attenuation, and it is currently produced in MRC-5 (human diploid) cells. The most recent example of the use of serial passage is the human rotavirus vaccine RV1, which was derived from a strain of rotavirus that circulated in Cincinnati in the late 1980s. That virus was initially passaged 26 times in Vero (African green monkey kidney) cells in order to achieve attenuation.

TABLE 1.1 — Classification of Vaccines Currently Available in the United States

Live-Attenuated			Inactivated				
					Component		
Classical Bacterial	Classical Viral	Engineered Agent	Whole Agent	Toxoid	Purified Subunit	Engineered Subunit	Recombinant Subunit
None	MMR[a]	LAIV[b]	HepA	Diphtheria	Anthrax[c]	Hib[d]	HepB[e]
	RV1[f]	RV5[f]	IPV	Tetanus	IIV[g]	MCV[d]	HPV[h]
	Smallpox	Ty21a[i]	JE vaccine		MPSV[j]	PCV[d]	
	VAR		RAB		Pertussis (acellular)[k]		
	YF vaccine				PPSV[j]		
	ZOS				TViPSV[j]		

Listed vaccines are administered parenterally unless otherwise noted. The following vaccines never were or are no longer available in the United States: BCG (tuberculosis)—live-attenuated, classical bacterial; adenovirus—live-attenuated, classical viral, orally administered; cholera—inactivated, whole cell; cholera (CVD 103-HgR)—live-attenuated, engineered, orally administered; cholera (WC/rBS)—inactivated, whole agent plus recombinant-derived subunit, orally administered; OPV (polio)—live-attenuated, classical viral; influenza (whole virus)—inactivated, whole agent; hepatitis B (plasma-derived)—inactivated, whole agent; Lyme disease (rOspA)—inactivated, recombinant-derived subunit; Hib polysaccharide—inactivated, purified subunit; pertussis (whole cell)—inactivated, whole agent; plague—inactivated whole agent; typhoid—inactivated whole agent.

[a] Contains a mixture of classically-attenuated measles, mumps, and rubella viruses.

[b] Influenza virus engineered to attenuation, then reassorted to include hemagglutinin and neuraminidase of circulating influenza strains. In 2009, this was available as a 3-valent seasonal and a monovalent H1N1 vaccine, intranasally administered.

[c] Produced from cell-free filtrate.

[d] Protein-polysaccharide conjugates. Valency varies. For example, Hib contains only one polysaccharide derived from the capsule of *H influenzae* type b, whereas MCV contains polysaccharides derived from the capsule of 4 different *N meningitidis* serogroups. Carrier proteins also vary. For example, Hib uses either tetanus toxoid or an outer membrane protein from *N meningitidis*; MCV uses either diphtheria toxoid or CRM$_{197}$, a mutant diphtheria toxin.

[e] HBsAg expressed in yeast.

[f] RV1 contains a classically-attenuated human rotavirus strain and is monovalent. RV5 contains bovine-human reassortants and is 5-valent. Both are orally administered.

[g] Contains physically-purified hemagglutinin and neuraminidase from influenza virus. In 2009, this was available as a 3-valent seasonal and a monovalent H1N1 vaccine.

[h] Human papilloma virus L1 protein expressed in yeast (HPV4) or baculovirus (HPV2); these vaccines are 4-valent and 2-valent, respectively.

[i] Mutagenized *S typhi*, selected for attenuation, orally administered.

[j] Contains physically-purified polysaccharides. Valency varies. For example, MPSV contains polysaccharides derived from the capsule of 4 different *N meningitidis* serogroups, whereas PPSV contains polysaccharides from 23 different *S pneumoniae* serotypes.

[k] All pertussis vaccines contain physically-purified, inactivated pertussis toxin and filamentous hemagglutinin; some also contain pertactin and fimbriae.

Attenuation of bacteria dates back to the mid 1800s, when Pasteur protected animals from anthrax using a form of the bacterium that had been weakened using chemicals. In vitro passage also has been used to attenuate bacteria. For example, Bacille Calmette-Guérin (BCG), a vaccine that protects against disseminated tuberculosis, was a strain of *Mycobacterium bovis* originally isolated from a cow in 1908 and passaged over 200 times in culture (*M bovis* is related to *M tuberculosis*).

• *Heterologous host*—This method dates back to the late 1700s, when Jenner used cowpox to protect humans from smallpox. The modern smallpox vaccine, consisting of a virus called vaccinia, is not the cowpox virus per se but rather a hybrid of cowpox and variola virus (the scientific name for smallpox) that does not exist in nature. Nevertheless, Jenner established the principle that animal viruses can induce immunity to human diseases. Cowpox is not necessarily attenuated for humans—it does cause lesions, as does vaccinia (in fact, if smallpox vaccination does not result in a lesion, it is not considered to have been effective). However, other animal viruses are naturally attenuated for humans. For example, the other available rotavirus vaccine, RV5, was derived from a bovine strain of rotavirus (WC3) that can replicate in humans but does not cause disease. It also does not induce sufficient protective antibody to human strains, so it had to be engineered to express immunogenic surface proteins of human rotaviruses. This was accomplished through *reassortment*, whereby the parental strain was cocultured with natural human strains. Bovine viruses that "accidentally" packaged genes for the human G or P proteins (the dominant protective antigens) were selected and propagated. The vaccine strains, then, consist of viruses that in every way are identical to the naturally attenuated bovine virus, except for the fact that each one expresses an immunogenic human protein instead of the corresponding bovine protein.

• *Engineered attenuation*—Today, the attenuated phenotype can be engineered into vaccines. A good example of this is the oral typhoid (Ty21a) vaccine, which was derived from *Salmonella typhi* strain Ty2 after treatment with a mutagenic agent and selection for attenuation. Another example is LAIV. Here, influenza virus was serially passaged in chick embryo cells at successively lower temperatures, selecting for mutants that grow well in the cold (77°F [25°C)]). As it happens, these strains grow poorly at core body temperature. After intranasal inoculation, they replicate well in the relatively cooler nasal passages, thereby generating broad-based systemic and mucosal immune responses. Their attenuation comes in the fact that they cannot replicate in the lower airways and therefore cannot cause pneumonia or more serious influenza syndromes. Each year, a new set of live-attenuated viruses must be constructed, incorporating genes for the hemagglutinin and neuraminidase (the dominant protective antigens) for the strain anticipated in the next season. This can be accomplished through reassortment, as described earlier, or through direct transfer of the genetic material.

Other approaches to attenuation have been used. For example, the attenuated phenotype can be achieved by something as simple as using an unnatural route of inoculation. The best example of this was the adenovirus vaccine used in the military in the 1970s and 1980s. This consisted of enteric-coated tablets, one containing live (intrinsically unattenuated) adenovirus type 4, and the other, type 7. These viruses are pathogenic in the respiratory tract, but when given in the gastrointestinal tract they replicate without causing disease.

Inactivated vaccines may consist of whole, inactivated microbial agents or specific microbial components that are derived through physical, chemical, or molecular means. Inactivated *whole agent* vaccines date back to the late 1800s, when Pasteur used killed rabies virus (derived from dried rabbit spinal cords) to protect animals and, eventually, humans against rabies. The modern prototype inactivated whole-virus vaccine was developed by Salk, who grew the poliovirus in cell culture, purified it, inactivated it with formaldehyde, and demonstrated that intramuscular injection of the inactivated virus protected against polio. The hepatitis A, Japanese encephalitis, and modern rabies vaccines are made in much the same way. The modern prototype whole bacterial vaccine is whole-cell pertussis, which was made from suspensions of cultured *Bordetella pertussis* organisms that were killed and detoxified. Because it contained every antigen from the live organism, this vaccine was both effective and reactogenic.

Component vaccines include *toxoids*, which are protein toxins that are immunogenic but have been chemically modified to reduce pathogenicity. The only current toxoid vaccines are those for diphtheria, tetanus and pertussis. Other component vaccines are made from *purified subunits* of the organism. The original hepatitis B vaccine, for example, consisted of HBsAg that was purified from the blood of persistently infected individuals (these individuals overproduce HBsAg, which is released from the liver into the plasma). Of course, steps were taken to inactivate any live virus that might have also been present. In order to reduce reactogenicity of the whole cell pertussis vaccine, specific immunogenic proteins (inactivated pertussis toxin, filamentous hemagglutinin, pertactin, and fimbriae) were purified from whole organisms and formulated into acellular vaccines. For *S pneumoniae*, *H influenzae*, *N meningitidis*, and *S typhi*, it was known that the

15

capsular polysaccharide was the immunogenic part of the bacterium. Subunit vaccines were therefore developed using capsular polysaccharide that was stripped from the cell and purified.

Pure polysaccharide vaccines, however, induce only short-term immunity, do not produce immunologic memory, and are not immunogenic in young infants. *Engineered subunits* in the form of protein-polysaccharide conjugates are necessary to overcome these problems (see below). Subunits can also be produced through *recombinant DNA* technology. The prototype here is the recombinant-derived hepatitis B vaccine, in which the gene for HBsAg was inserted into yeast cells, which then produced large quantities of the protein for purification. A similar method was used to produce the HPV vaccine. In this case, the gene for the L1 protein was expressed in either yeast cells (HPV4) or insect cells using a baculovirus vector (HPV2). The nice thing about L1 is that it spontaneously aggregates into virus-like particles, which in every way look like viruses on the outside but which carry no genetic material and are, therefore, incapable of replicating.

Table 1.2 lists general characteristics of live and inactivated vaccines. These properties have very real consequences in practice, affecting storage conditions, scheduling, expected efficacy, contraindications, and the potential for adverse reactions. Some implications of these characteristics, as well as exceptions to the generalizations, are given in the footnotes, and the following section on vaccine immunology provides explanations for some of these characteristics.

■ Passive Immunization

Passive immunization is the process by which short-term protection from disease is conferred through the administration of antibodies. This process occurs naturally during the last 2 months of pregnancy, when large quantities of IgG are transferred across the placenta to the fetus, and it explains the relative protection that newborns enjoy against invasive *S pneumoniae* and *H influenzae* type b infections, among others. Passive immunization is necessary for patients with humoral immune defects who cannot synthesize their own antibody; in these cases, *polyclonal immune globulin* is used. For example, patients with agammaglobulinemia receive regular infusions of immune globulin to prevent a broad range of infections. Polyclonal immune globulin is also used to prevent certain specific infections, such as measles and hepatitis A, because the level of antibody to these agents is sufficiently high in the general population from whom the immune globulin is derived.

Passive immunization also is useful for persons at risk for particular infections; in such cases, *hyperimmune globulins*, derived from donors with high antibody levels to the pathogen, are used. One example is varicella zoster immune globulin

(VariZIG), which is used for prevention of chickenpox in exposed immunocompromised individuals. Another example is hepatitis B immune globulin (HBIG), which is used in neonates born to mothers who are chronic hepatitis B carriers and also in other susceptible individuals who are exposed to the virus. It should be understood that hyperimmune globulins also contain antibodies to pathogens besides the one they target; this is true because the individuals from whom they are derived, while selected for their high antibody levels to specific pathogens, also have antibodies to other agents. Although immune globulin products are made from blood, current donor screening and processing of the antibodies make the risk of transmission of blood-borne pathogens negligible. Antibodies can be *engineered* for prevention of specific diseases, as in the case of RSVmAB (Synagis), a monoclonal antibody that has the effector (constant) region of human IgG but the combining (antigen recognition) region of a mouse monoclonal antibody specific for the RSV F protein (which mediates fusion of the viral envelope to the host cell membrane—blocking this prevents infection). *Antitoxins*, also known as *heterologous hyperimmune sera*, are also used for passive immunization. These are produced in animals like horses and target toxins such as diphtheria, botulism, and tetanus.

Whether passive immunization occurs *intentionally*, as when IGIM is administered for prevention of hepatitis A, or *unintentionally*, as when antibodies accompany blood products transfused for other reasons (eg, IGIV for Kawasaki disease), passively acquired polyclonal antibodies can inactivate live-attenuated viral vaccines, such as MMR and VAR. RSVmAB, which is specific for RSV alone, does not inactivate live vaccines. Yellow fever vaccine (which is also live-attenuated) does not appear to be inactivated by commercially available polyclonal immune globulin products in the United States, since the amount of yellow fever antibody in the donors from whom these products are derived is low. **Table 5.2** gives the recommended intervals between receipt of antibody-containing blood products and certain live vaccines.

Basic Vaccine Immunology

Entire textbooks have been written about the immune response, and many of the details have been worked out at the molecular level. Despite the complexity, only a few basic concepts are necessary in order to understand how vaccines mediate protection against disease. These concepts shed light on the differences between various types of vaccines, the duration of protection, dosing schedules, and other aspects of vaccine practice that are delineated elsewhere in this book.

Vaccines are designed to generate pathogen-specific antibodies and T-cells by stimulating the *adaptive immune system*, which

17

TABLE 1.2 — Generalizations About Live and Inactivated Vaccines

Characteristic	Live Vaccines	Inactivated Vaccines
Immune response	Humoral and cell-mediated[b]	Mostly humoral[a]
Dosing	1 dose usually sufficient[b]	Multiple-dose primary series and booster doses usually required[c]
Adjuvant[d]	Not necessary	May be necessary[e]
Route of administration	IN, PO, or SC	IM or SC
Duration of immunity	Potentially lifelong	Booster doses may be required[f]
Person-to-person transmission	Possible[g]	Not possible
Inactivation by passively acquired antibodies	Possible[h]	Less likely[i]
Use in immunocompromised hosts	May cause disease	Cannot cause disease
Use in pregnancy[j]	Fetal infection theoretically possible[k]	Fetal damage theoretically unlikely
Storage requirements	Reflect need to maintain viability	Reflect need to maintain chemical and physical stability
Simultaneous administration at separate sites	Acceptable[l]	Acceptable
Interval between doses of the *same* vaccine given in sequence	Minimum intervals apply[m,n]	Minimum intervals apply[m]
Interval between doses of *different* vaccines given in sequence	Minimum intervals apply[n]	No minimum intervals[o]

18

a Some inactivated vaccines stimulate limited humoral responses. For example, polysaccharide vaccines (eg, MPSV4 and PPSV23) induce short-lived IgM responses and do not result in immunologic memory. Engineering can overcome these limitations, as in the conjugation of polysaccharides to protein carriers. Protein vaccines can induce memory responses that are T-helper cell dependent.

b Although 1 dose of MMR or VAR may be sufficient to induce long-lasting immunity, second doses are given before school entry to ensure that children who did not seroconvert to the first dose have another chance to do so (the second dose is therefore not considered a "booster" in the classic sense). Live oral vaccines such as RV1, RV5, and typhoid Ty21a are given in multiple-dose series.

c Some inactivated vaccines, such as PPSV23 for older adults, are given as a single dose. In this case, individuals have probably been previously primed by natural exposure to S pneumoniae. Another example is MCV4, which is routinely given as a single dose to children at 11 to 12 years of age to "cover" them during the high-risk adolescent years.

d Adjuvants are substances that enhance the immune response to vaccine antigens.

e One Hib vaccine, IIV, MCV4-D, MCV4-CRM, MPSV4, PPSV23, IPV, JE-MB, and RAB do not contain adjuvants.

f Long-term protection has been demonstrated for some inactivated vaccines, such as HepA and HepB, in the absence of booster doses.

g This phenomenon was relevant for OPV, where horizontal transmission probably contributed to immunity at the population level but also on rare occasion caused disease in contacts. Transmission of vaccinia from smallpox vaccinees represents a real risk to susceptible close contacts. Transmission of VAR, LAIV, and RV has been documented but is extremely rare. Transmission of MMR, Ty21a, and YF vaccine has not been documented.

h This phenomenon is most relevant for MMR and VAR and is the reason why these vaccines are not given in the first year of life, when passively acquired maternal antibodies can interfere with "take". Receipt of antibody-containing products does not affect the take of LAIV, RV, smallpox vaccine, Ty21a, YF vaccine, or ZOS. See **Table 5.2** for recommended intervals between antibody-containing products and certain live vaccines.

i Passively acquired maternal antibodies may interfere with the take of HepA; vaccination is therefore recommended in the second year of life.

j To avoid antigen-antibody interactions, antibody-containing products are not administered at the same site as inactivated vaccines.

k Most vaccines are classified as Pregnancy Category C (see *Chapter 6: Vaccination in Special Circumstances—Pregnancy*).

l This possibility leads to the general recommendation that live vaccines are contraindicated in pregnancy, although there are some exceptions (see *Chapter 7: Vaccination in Special Circumstances—Pregnancy*).

l The only examples of two live vaccines that cannot be given at the same time are varicella and smallpox and LAIV-seasonal and LAIV-2009 H1N1.

Continued

TABLE 1.2 — *Continued*

m Proper spacing between the doses is necessary to maximize the immune response.

n Replication of the first vaccine can interfere with replication of the second.

o The AAP suggests a minimum interval of 1 month between Tdap and MCV4-D if the vaccines are not given on the same day (the concern here is that both vaccines contain diphtheria toxoid [it is used as the carrier protein in MCV4-D]—too many doses of diphtheria toxoid in sequence can cause increased reactogenicity). However, the ACIP does not recommend a minimum interval.

recognizes and remembers specific pathogens and learns to respond to them more strongly after each exposure. What follows is a simplified version of the immune mechanisms that underpin vaccination—in essence, what you need to know to understand how vaccines work.[1,2]

■ Antibodies

Antibodies are proteins that bind to 3-dimensional patterns, or *epitopes*, that are present on *antigens* (substances on the microbe that are foreign to the host and engender immune responses). Antibodies constitute the humoral, or soluble, arm of the adaptive immune system, and are produced as several different immunoglobulin *isotypes* (IgG, IgA, IgM, IgE, IgD) that differ in function. A given antibody with a given antigenic specificity can be produced as one of several different isotypes. Antibody binding is *specific* in that each antibody molecule binds best to one particular epitope; any given antigen may have many different epitopes, and any given microbe may have hundreds of different antigens. Binding of antibodies to a virus or toxin can lead to *neutralization*, ie, the blocking of ligands or receptors that are critical for infectivity or toxicity. Binding of antibodies to a bacterium can lead to *opsonization* (coating of the organism) so that it can be pulled out of circulation by cells of the reticuloendothelial system or so that it can be killed by *complement-mediated lysis* (fixing of complement proteins on the surface, forming a *membrane attack complex* that kills the organism). Binding of antibodies to a virus-infected cell can lead to *antibody-dependent cell-mediated cytotoxicity*, whereby the infected cell is flagged for destruction by natural killer cells, monocytes, and eosinophils.

Antibodies are the only element of the adaptive immune system that can *prevent* viral infection because they can neutralize the virus before it has a chance to replicate in cells. They are also the mainstay of protection against bacterial invasion since they facilitate destruction of the inoculating organism before it has a chance to reproduce. The battle between antibodies and pathogens takes place at different sites. At mucosal surfaces, where most pathogens try to gain entry, secretory IgA and serum IgG antibodies that leak across from the vascular space are important. Live vaccines that replicate at the mucosal surface (eg, LAIV) have the advantage of inducing strong local IgA responses that can neutralize pathogens before invasion. Vaccines given intramuscularly or subcutaneously are not as good at generating secretory IgA at mucosal surfaces, although this does happen. A vaccine that induces high levels of serum IgG not only can protect against bloodstream invasion or infection in extravascular spaces, but also can block infection at mucosal sites before the organism gains a foothold.

Antibodies are produced by plasma cells, which are derived from B lymphocytes or B-cells. B-cells have immunoglobulins

21

on their surface (mostly IgM) that express one and only one antibody specificity. During ontogeny, genetic rearrangements lead to a diversity of B-cell clones, each with its own unique antibody specificity (those B-cells that emerge from this process with surface immunoglobulins that recognize self antigens are deleted). People are, therefore, walking around with millions of B-cells, each precommitted to recognizing one and only one epitope. When a given B-cell binds to its antigenic match, it becomes activated and proliferates; this is known as *clonal expansion*. The daughter cells eventually differentiate into plasma cells, the factories that secrete large amounts of antibody.

There are two basic pathways through which antibody production occurs, and the differences between them are important to understanding how vaccines work.

■ The Extrafollicular Reaction

The extrafollicular reaction, one of the pathways for antibody production, is best exemplified by the immune response to polysaccharides (**Figure 1.1**). A precommitted B-cell encounters its polysaccharide match (at the site of inoculation with a vaccine or perhaps in a lymph node to which the vaccine antigen was transported), leading to activation, proliferation, and rapid differentiation into plasma cells, which migrate to the red pulp of the spleen and intramedullary areas of lymph nodes. There the plasma

FIGURE 1.1 — Polysaccharide Antigens and the Extrafollicular Reaction

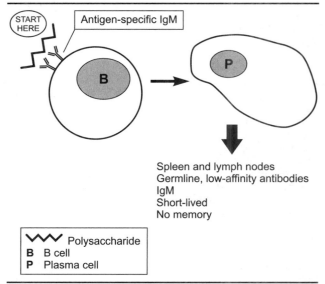

START HERE

Antigen-specific IgM

B

P

Spleen and lymph nodes
Germline, low-affinity antibodies
IgM
Short-lived
No memory

︿︿︿	Polysaccharide
B	B cell
P	Plasma cell

cells begin to produce antibodies. It is important to understand that these are *germline* antibodies, ie, antibodies transcribed from genes that were present in the B-cell to begin with. Germline antibodies have low affinity for their corresponding antigens because the genes from which they are transcribed, the sequence of amino acids, the shape of their combining site, and thus their ability to bind to the antigen was determined by a random process way back when the person was a fetus. These B-cells (and their genes) were selected during ontogeny because they recognized nonself antigens, not because they would someday bind especially tightly to those particular antigens. Furthermore, most of the antibodies produced in the extrafollicular reaction are of the same isotype that was present on the B-cell surface, namely IgM, which does not offer the functional benefits of other isotypes such as IgG. Finally, the plasma cells produced through the extrafollicular reaction ultimately die out—no more antibodies produced, no more protection, no ability to remember the encounter and respond more quickly or decisively the next time.

This is called the *extrafollicular reaction* because it takes place outside of the germinal centers of lymph nodes. Antigens that elicit this response are called *T-cell independent* because the responding B-cells differentiate without much T-cell interaction. The characteristics of T-cell independent responses—rapid production (days to weeks) of short-lived, low-affinity, predominantly IgM antibodies without induction of memory—are hallmark features of the response to pure polysaccharide antigens, such as those in the original *H influenzae* vaccine, PPSV, and MPSV. To compound the problem with polysaccharides, children <2 years of age do not mount robust T-cell independent responses, making these vaccines poor immunogens in that age group. And there's one other problem—*hyporesponsiveness*. This refers to the observation that children who initially receive pure polysaccharide vaccines seem to respond less well to future doses of polysaccharide and protein-polysaccharide vaccines, as if they have permanently "used up" some of their polysaccharide-specific B-cells. This phenomenon has been referred to as *original polysaccharide sin*.

It is important to point out that there is some crossover between the immunologic pathways. For example, some degree of T-cell help (see below) may be available to extrafollicular B-cells, such that some isotype switching occurs and some memory may be generated.

■ The Germinal Center Reaction

Underpinning the adaptive immune system is the much more primitive *innate immune system*, capable of initiating the battle against an invading microorganism in a nonspecific fashion. Cells of the innate immune system—most notably dendritic cells and monocytes—carry receptors that recognize conserved patterns among pathogens (*pathogen-specific molecular patterns*) that are not found in self tissues. Among the most important of these are *Toll-like receptors* (TLRs), each of which recognizes a different pattern. TLR3, for example, recognizes double-stranded viral RNA; TLR2 binds lipopolysaccharide, and TLR6 binds bacterial flagellins. Engagement of pattern-recognition receptors activates the cell, which then secretes *cytokines* (intercellular communication molecules) that activate and recruit other cells, setting up an inflammatory reaction. The end result might be destruction of the invader through processes such as phagocytosis. Importantly, this is a one-time occurrence—once the pathogen is destroyed, there is no memory of the encounter that might facilitate a response the next time around.

Why do vaccinologists care about innate immunity if it provides no memory? The answer lies in the fact that activation of the innate immune system can trigger an adaptive immune response. The key link is provided by *antigen-presenting cells* (APCs), the most important of which are dendritic cells (**Figure 1.2**). Immature APCs circulate through the body or reside in tissues (immature dendritic cells in the dermis are called *Langerhans cells*). When a pathogen-specific molecular pattern is encountered—in the form, for example, of an injected vaccine antigen—the APC cells begin to mature, express new receptors on their surface, and migrate through lymphatic vessels to regional lymph nodes. Some of them also engulf the antigen, degrade the proteins into small peptides, load the peptides into the groove of *major histocompatibility complex* (MHC) *class II molecules* (MHC-II), and express those molecules on their surface (MHC molecules are also referred to as *human leukocyte antigens* or HLAs).

The mature APC is now activated (secreting proinflammatory cytokines and expressing costimulatory molecules on its surface), flagged (by the surface expression of antigen-derived peptides in the context of MHC-II), and has migrated to the follicular region of the lymph node. At this stage the APC is ready to engage immature *helper T lymphocytes* (Th-cells) by interacting with the *T-cell receptor* (TCR) and the *CD4 coreceptor* (both are on the Th-cell). Each Th-cell is predetermined to recognize a particular peptide/MHC-II flag by virtue of its TCR and CD4 coreceptor (like the surface immunoglobulin of B-cells, the TCR has a unique antigenic specificity; the diversity of TCRs is generated during fetal development by a random process, much like the generation of germline antibodies, and those T-cells that emerge from this process with receptors that recognize self antigens are deleted or inactivated). Through soluble cytokines and costimulatory receptor-ligand interactions, contact with the right APC results in activation and maturation of the Th-cell into one of two antigen-specific subtypes: Th1- or Th2-cells. Th2-cells have some direct antimicrobial functions, particularly against parasites.

FIGURE 1.2 — Antigen-Presenting Cells and the Germinal Center Reaction

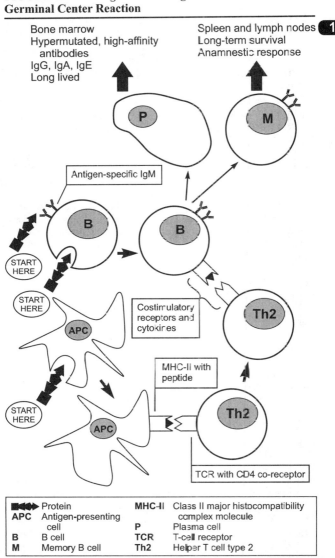

Bone marrow
Hypermutated, high-affinity
    antibodies
IgG, IgA, IgE
Long lived

Spleen and lymph nodes
Long-term survival
Anamnestic response

Antigen-specific IgM

START HERE

START HERE

Costimulatory receptors and cytokines

START HERE

MHC-II with peptide

TCR with CD4 co-receptor

		MHC-II	Class II major histocompatibility complex molecule
APC	Antigen-presenting cell	P	Plasma cell
B	B cell	TCR	T-cell receptor
M	Memory B cell	Th2	Helper T cell type 2

Protein

More importantly, though, Th2-cells seek out their unique B-cell matches in order to help them make antibody (to the antigen from which the peptide in the MHC groove was originally derived). B-cells are primed to be helped by engulfing some of the bound antigen, digesting the proteins, and presenting the peptides on their surface in the context of MHC-II, much like dendritic cells do.

Th1-cells also have direct antimicrobial functions, particularly against viruses. More importantly, though, Th1-cells seek out *cytotoxic T-cells* (Tc-cells) and macrophages, coaxing them into performing cytotoxic functions (see below). Several factors determine whether a Th-cell differentiates into a Th1 or Th2-cell during immunization; among these are the dose of antigen, route of administration, and the effect of *adjuvants* (see below). These factors, therefore, also determine whether humoral or cellular responses will predominate.

The interaction between B-cells and Th-cells takes place in the germinal centers of lymph nodes, hence the name of the reaction. The signals provided by Th2-cells, as well as the persistence of antigen shuttled there by APCs, drive B-cells to undergo massive clonal proliferation—producing millions of daughter cells capable of making the same antibodies. As they proliferate under these conditions, the B-cells undergo a process of somatic hypermutation, whereby the genes encoding the immunoglobulin combining region mutate at exceptional rates, randomly producing a spectrum of antibodies with varying affinities for the antigen. Those B-cells expressing high-affinity antibodies are selected for and clonally expanded. The end result is a set of dominant B-cell clones that produce high-affinity antibodies, ones that bind the antigen better than the germline antibodies produced in the extrafollicular reaction. The only problem is that this process takes a week or two to get rolling.

Two other things happen in the germinal center. First, signals from Th2-cells drive *isotype switching* as B-cells transform into plasma cells. The end result is large numbers of plasma cells that migrate to the bone marrow and produce high-affinity IgG (as well as other isotypes). Second, Th2-cells drive the parallel evolution of *memory B-cells*, which migrate to the spleen and lymph nodes and wait there—sometimes for decades—until they again encounter the antigen, at which time they rapidly proliferate and differentiate into plasma cells that produce antibody. This is called the *anamnestic response*. It should be mentioned that memory Th-cells are also generated, but their numbers wane with time.

The germinal center reaction has many implications for vaccination.

- *Stimulating innate immunity*—The more innate immunity is stimulated, the more robust the adaptive immune response will be. For example, intradermal vaccination, which has not yet made its way into routine practice, generally stimulates more robust responses than intramuscular injection, probably because there are more immature dendritic cells lying in wait in the dermis.[3] As another example, we know that live viral vaccines are more immunogenic than inactivated ones. One reason is that live viruses can disseminate and encounter dendritic cells at multiple sites, ultimately establishing multiple foci of germinal center reactions. Another reason is that live vaccines carry more recognizable pathogen-specific molecular patterns that are capable of activating innate immune cells.

- *Adjuvants*—Adjuvants are substances that potentiate the innate immune response by slowing the release of antigen or by enhancing delivery to, increasing uptake by, and inducing maturation of antigen-presenting cells.[4] They are necessary in some inactivated vaccines in order to engender robust immune responses. There is no predicting which antigens will need adjuvants and which ones will not. In fact, similar vaccines may differ with regard to adjuvants—for example, take the *H influenzae* type b conjugate vaccines: PedvaxHIB contains an adjuvant whereas ActHIB and Hiberix do not. For many decades, the only adjuvant used in human vaccines was alum, an amorphous mixture of aluminum salts that adsorbs antigen, promotes inflammation, and facilitates uptake by APCs. In 2009, the door to newer adjuvants was opened with the licensure of HPV2 (Cervarix), which contains AS04, an adjuvant composed of 3-*O*-desacyl-4'-monophosphoryl lipid A (MPL, a derivative of bacterial lipopolysaccharide) adsorbed to an aluminum hydroxide salt. MPL activates Toll-like receptor-4 on APCs, promoting cytokine expression, antigen presentation, and migration of APCs to lymph nodes. Adjuvants may allow for *antigen sparing*. For example, an adjuvanted vaccine against the 2009 H1N1 influenza virus was just as immunogenic as a nonadjuvanted version, even though it contained one fourth the amount of antigen (as might be expected, though, the adjuvanted vaccine produced more local and systemic symptoms, but these were transient and mild to moderate in intensity).[5] Finally, newer adjuvants may cause *epitope spreading*, a broadening of the antibody repertoire such that more epitopes on a given antigen are recognized.[6]
- *Priming and boosting*—Ultimately, the magnitude and duration of the antibody response to inactivated vaccines depends on the immunologic set point following primary immunization. In other words, the more germinal centers that are formed, the more long-lived plasma cells and memory B-cells there will be. In addition to optimizing antigen dose and using adjuvants, *primary immunization* is enhanced by multiple doses of the vaccine given in succession, classically separated by 1 or 2 months (as in the 2-, 4-, and 6-month schedule for primary DTaP immunization). These doses are given too soon

to exploit memory responses, but they do drive the process of affinity maturation in the germinal centers. Following priming, vaccine schedules take advantage of anamnestic responses, which boost the level of high-quality antibody (**Figure 1.3**). The need to wait until the germinal center reaction is complete explains the longer interval between the primary series of a vaccine and the booster doses (as in the 15- to 18-month dose of DTaP). The response to booster doses of vaccine mimics what happens when the natural pathogen is encountered.

- *Specificity*—Hypermutated, high-affinity antibodies specifically target single epitopes. For this reason, most inactivated vaccines are very specific in the protection they afford. For

FIGURE 1.3 — Time Course of Antibody Responses

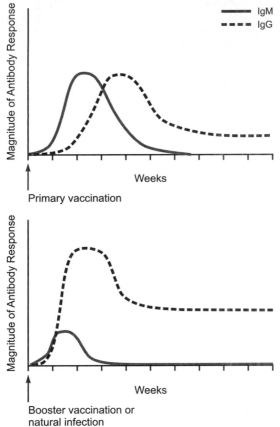

example, IPV contains formalin-inactivated, disrupted viral particles from three different serotypes of poliovirus because the antigens from any given serotype do not induce antibodies that will neutralize the other serotypes. Germinal center reactions by and large generate *homotypic* responses, ones directed against the antigen used as the vaccine. *Heterotypic*, or *cross-protective*, responses occur only if there is sufficient similarity between the antigens of different strains, or if there is a common antigen between them. Tc-cells offer much more potential for cross-strain protection (see below).

• *Persistence of antibody*—The germinal center reaction peaks in several weeks, after which it is terminated. The mechanisms by which serum antibodies persist for long periods of time—something so critical to maintaining protection—are not yet worked out. Some models suggest that there is more or less constitutive differentiation of memory B-cells into plasma cells, stimulated by persistent antigen, reinfection, or exposure to cross-reactive antigens. Other models propose there is nonspecific, or so-called "bystander," activation of memory B-cells, although recent data suggest this mechanism is less important. These models have important implications for vaccine programs. For example, early studies of VAR showed persistent if not *rising* titers of antibody over time. But these studies were done at a time when the wild-type virus was still circulating; therefore, immunized individuals might have experienced repeated subclinical reinfections with natural virus, coaxing memory B-cells to differentiate into plasma cells and boosting antibody production. As transmission of natural varicella decreased, some studies began to show waning immunity over time (this observation made it less likely that antibody persisted because of boosting from periodic reactivation of latent vaccine virus). Although technically intended to immunize those who failed to seroconvert after the first dose (so-called *primary vaccine failures*), the second dose of VAR that is now recommended also serves to boost immunity in those individuals whose antibody levels have fallen low enough to allow *take*, or replication of the vaccine virus.

Other models suggest that plasma cells derived from the germinal center reaction can live for a very long time. Either way, for some vaccines, it is necessary to periodically conjure up the anamnestic response through booster vaccination.[8] One thing is clear—to prevent infections with a short incubation period (*N meningitidis* is a good example), one must have a sufficient amount of circulating antibody at the time of encounter with the pathogen. Anamnestic responses, while brisk, are not fast enough to be of much help when dealing with rapidly replicating bacteria. They may be sufficient, however, for pathogens with longer incubation periods. Thus, for example, although antibodies to HBV, and along with them protection from *infection*, may wane with time, protection against *disease* does not wane—there is plenty of time for memory responses to kick in before the virus can do damage.

• *Making better immunogens*—As mentioned above, polysaccharides are poor immunogens. Vaccinologists have learned, however, to harness the power of the germinal center reaction to enhance their immunogenicity (**Figure 1.4**). The polysaccharides are chemically attached to protein carriers—among the variety of carriers used are an outer-membrane protein from *N meningitidis* (Hib-OMP [PedvaxHIB]), a mutant diphtheria toxin called CRM_{197} (PCV7-CRM [Prevnar], MCV4-CRM [Menveo]), tetanus toxoid (Hib-T [ActHIB, Hiberix]), and diphtheria toxoid (MCV4-D [Menactra]). B-cells that are precommitted to producing anti-*polysaccharide* antibody are stimulated by their encounter with the antigen. They also engulf the bound antigen, digest it, and present peptides from the *protein* portion of the vaccine on their surface in the context of MHC-II (polysaccharides cannot be presented in this context). So what you have is a B-cell committed to making anti-*polysaccharide* antibodies that is displaying a *peptide* flag on its surface. All it takes now is for APCs to display the same peptides and stimulate Th2-cells, which then find their B-cell matches and help them make antibody through the germinal center reaction. In essence, the Th2-cells "think" they are helping B-cells make antibodies to the protein antigen from which the peptides are derived, but in fact the flagged B-cells make *polysaccharide* antibody. By converting a *T-cell independent* response to a *T-cell dependent* one, the shortcomings of polysaccharides as antigens are overcome. **Table 1**.3 summarizes the advantages of protein-polysaccharide conjugate vaccines.

■ **Cytotoxic T Cells**

Tc-cells are the main effectors of the adaptive cellular immune response. Like Th-cells, they express the TCR on their surface, which has a unique antigenic specificity encoded in the germline. Unlike Th-cells, which express CD4, Tc-cells express the CD8 coreceptor, which directs engagement with *MHC class I molecules* (MHC-I). Like MHC-II, MHC-I loads pathogen-derived peptides into its groove and presents those peptides on the cell surface. However, instead of coming from the digestion of exogenous proteins that were engulfed by the cell, the peptides loaded into MHC-I are actually made inside the cell—by infecting viruses or other intracellular pathogens.

MHC-I is expressed on APCs as well as on all nucleated host cells. Naïve Tc-cells, predetermined to recognize a particular

FIGURE 1.4 — Response to Protein-Polysaccharide Conjugate Vaccines

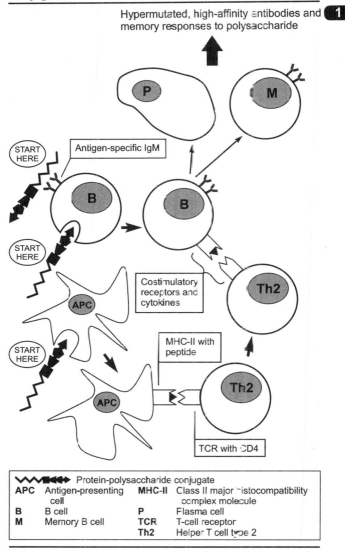

Hypermutated, high-affinity antibodies and memory responses to polysaccharide

START HERE

Antigen-specific IgM

START HERE

START HERE

Costimulatory receptors and cytokines

MHC-II with peptide

TCR with CD4

〜〜〜〜◄◄◄►	Protein-polysaccharide conjugate	
APC	Antigen-presenting cell	**MHC-II** Class II major histocompatibility complex molecule
B	B cell	**P** Plasma cell
M	Memory B cell	**TCR** T-cell receptor
		Th2 Helper T cell type 2

31

TABLE 1.3 — Advantages of Protein-Polysaccharide Conjugate Vaccines

Property	Type of Vaccine	
	Polysaccharide	Protein-Polysaccharide Conjugate
B-cell response	T-cell independent	T-cell dependent
Pathway	Extrafollicular	Germinal center
Antibody generation in young infants	No	Yes
Induction of immune memory	No	Yes
Anamnestic or booster responses	No	Yes
Long-term protection	No	Yes
Reduced carriage of the organism at mucosal surfaces	No	Yes[a]
Herd immunity	No	Yes[b]

[a] Robust serum IgG levels allow for leakage onto mucosal surfaces, where colonizing bacteria are killed.
[b] Fewer colonized people means less transmission of the pathogen from person to person, indirectly protecting people who are not immune.

peptide/MHC-I flag, engage infected APCs that express those particular peptides in the context of MHC-I (**Figure 1.5**). While this leads to activation of the Tc-cell, the Tc-cell does not become a killer until it receives additional signals—those coming in the form of cytokines from Th1-cells, which in turn have been activated by engagement of APCs expressing pathogen-derived peptides in the context of MHC-II (Th1-cells have other functions as well, such as activation of macrophages). The respective, critical role of the two different types of Th-cells is obvious—Th2-cells help B-cells produce high-quality antibodies and memory cells, and Th1-cells help Tc-cells become killers (and memory cells as well).

FIGURE 1.5 — Cytotoxic T-Cell Response

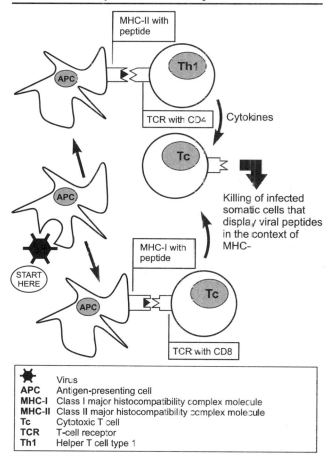

✸	Virus
APC	Antigen-presenting cell
MHC-I	Class I major histocompatibility complex molecule
MHC-II	Class II major histocompatibility complex molecule
Tc	Cytotoxic T cell
TCR	T-cell receptor
Th1	Helper T cell type 1

What does a Tc-cell kill? Remember that Tc-cells recognize peptides in the context of MHC-I, and all cells express MHC-I. Therefore, Tc-cells find and destroy infected cells that express pathogen-derived peptides on their surface in the context of MHC-I. How does a Tc-cell kill? One mechanism is through the release of *cytotoxins* that create holes in the cell membrane. In addition, Tc-cells can induce *apoptosis*, or programmed cell death, through the release of certain enzymes and through cell-surface receptor-ligand interactions.

It is important to point out that there is some crossover between the immune mechanisms delineated above. For example, some exogenous peptides can be presented to a limited extent in the context of MHC-I; therefore, some inactivated vaccines can induce Tc responses.

The unique characteristics of Tc-cells and their generation have several implications for vaccination:

- *Viruses versus bacteria*—Tc-cells are much more important in controlling viral infections than in controlling bacterial infections. The reason is simple—most bacteria are fully capable of replicating independently outside of cells, and therefore do not generate APCs or somatic cells flagged with peptide/MHC-I ("somatic cells" refers to all cells in the body except gametes, or sex cells). Viruses, on the other hand, are obligate intracellular pathogens—they can only replicate by usurping the host cell machinery for protein synthesis. Therefore, infected APCs and somatic cells are routinely flagged with peptide/MHC-I—unless the virus has evolved a mechanism to cloak the infected cell in anonymity by preventing the surface expression of peptide/MHC-I (cytomegalovirus and adenovirus, for example, evade the immune response in this fashion).

  Vaccines against bacterial pathogens are designed to maximize high-quality antibody production (some part of this involves the generation of large pools of Th2-cells). The ideal vaccine for a viral infection would maximize high-quality antibody production as well as lead to the generation of Tc-cells.

- *Preventing versus limiting infection*—Tc-cells operate *after* infection has taken place; they limit but do not prevent infection. Unlike antibody, a Tc-cell cannot kill a free virion that lands on a mucosal surface or enters the bloodstream. It must first wait until a cell is infected and expressing viral peptides. If a vaccinated person is exposed to a virus, the first line of defense is the antibody that resides at the site of inoculation or in the immediate local environment. That antibody could neutralize the virus, thus preventing *infection*. If it does not, and the virus gains entry into cells and begins to replicate, memory Tc-cells are called into action to destroy those cells, thus preventing *disease*. Antibody may also play a role in

34

the destruction of infected cells through antibody-dependent cell-mediated cytotoxicity.

Differences between VAR and ZOS, which contains the same live-attenuated virus as VAR but at a higher dose, are instructive. First, the main goal of ZOS is to expand the pool of memory Tc-cells. By definition, people who get herpes zoster (shingles) are already infected with VZV (herpes zoster is the reactivation of endogenous, natural VZV that has been latent in the person since he or she had chickenpox). Early in the process of reactivation, infected cells begin to express viral peptides on their surface, and the idea is to have Tc-cells ready to pounce on those cells before the disease can manifest. Second, in order for the vaccine itself to stimulate Tc-cells, it must first infect host cells so that its peptides can be expressed in the context of MHC-I. The reason ZOS has so much more virus in it (14 times the amount) than VAR is precisely the fact that it must avoid neutralization by any naturally occurring antibody in order to gain entry into host cells.

- *Live versus inactivated vaccines*—Because they replicate within cells, live viral vaccines are much better at inducing Tc-cells than are inactivated vaccines. This is in addition to other factors that have already been mentioned, such as their enhanced ability to stimulate innate immune responses and their ability to amplify and disseminate antigens.
- *Cross-protection*—B-cells recognize epitopes that are conformational in nature, in essence 3-dimensional structures that are represented on antigens on the pathogen surface. A good example of such an antigen is the hemagglutinin (H) molecule of influenza virus, a glycoprotein that protrudes from the viral envelope and mediates attachment to cells. IIV is very good at eliciting antibodies to H that can block infectivity—but those antibodies are specific to the strain of influenza virus that was used to make the vaccine. If antigenic drift occurs during a given season—that is, if the H of the prevailing virus has a slightly different sequence and conformation—the vaccine will not be as effective.

Tc-cells, on the other hand, recognize peptides that are derived from any protein made by the pathogen, some of which are more conserved between strains than are surface molecules. Just like IIV, LAIV elicits strain-specific antibodies directed at H. However, it can also induce Tc-cells that recognize peptides derived from the nucleocapsid of the virus. The advantage here is that nucleocapsid proteins are well conserved from one strain to another. Thus LAIV can induce Tc-cell responses capable of limiting infection due to strains whose H has drifted from the vaccine strain.

■ Correlates of Protection

Ideally, vaccines are shown to be effective in randomized, blinded, placebo-controlled trials, where one group of subjects gets the vaccine, another gets the placebo, and the measured outcome is *efficacy*, or ability to prevent the disease (or infection). This works if the disease is prevalent, such that the number of subjects needed in a clinical trial is within reach. For diseases that are relatively rare, demonstrating efficacy may not be feasible.[9] In such situations, *immunogenicity*, or the ability to generate an immune response, is relied upon as a predictor of efficacy. Such predictors may be *correlates* of immunity, that is responses that are closely related to protection, or *surrogates* of immunity, qualifiable immune responses that, while not in themselves protective, nevertheless can substitute for the true correlate.[10] As will be seen, however, the connection between immunogenicity and efficacy is not that straightforward.

Correlates of protection against a disease are useful for other reasons as well. For example, it may not be possible to study vaccine efficacy in every population that will ultimately be targeted for immunization. How can we be sure that a vaccine demonstrated to be effective in one age group will be effective in another, or, for that matter, in persons of different ethnic groups, those with underlying medical conditions, or those living in different geographic areas? If we knew which immunologic tests predicted protection, we could be reassured that if the immunologic criteria were met, protection would likely ensue. Immune correlates or surrogates also drive preclinical development, in the sense that scientists choose antigens, delivery systems, and dosing schedules that maximize immune responses thought to be important in protecting people from disease. Correlates also are critical to quality assurance—each new production lot of vaccine cannot be studied for efficacy, but it *can* be studied for immunogenicity and, in particular, for its ability to generate responses that are relevant in some way to protection. Likewise, there are many vaccination scenarios that must be studied in practice. For example, a new vaccine might be effective in clinical trials, but in real life it needs to be given concomitantly with other vaccines. It would be very difficult to study efficacy under every permutation of concomitant use; instead, investigators rely on correlates to determine if concomitant use is likely or unlikely to compromise protection. For new combination vaccines, noninferiority (with respect to a relevant immune response) to concomitant administration of the separate vaccines must be demonstrated (see *Chapter 2: Vaccine Infrastructure in the United States—Vaccine Development and Licensure*).

Table 1.4 shows some generally accepted quantitative correlates of protection after vaccination. For some diseases, there are generally accepted, albeit imperfect, correlates of protection. For example, studies in the prevaccine era showed that children who had naturally occurring anticapsular polysaccharide (polyribosylribitol phosphate [PRP]) antibody levels ≥0.15 mcg/mL were protected from invasive *H influenzae* disease; those with levels <0.15 mcg/mL were not. Studies utilizing the pure (unconjugated) PRP vaccine showed that antibody levels ≥1.0 mcg/mL immediately following vaccination correlated with protection against disease. So, which is the correlate of protection, 0.15 mcg/mL or 1.0 mcg/mL? Some have referred to 0.15 mcg/mL as the "short-term" correlate of protection, meaning that this is the level of circulating anti-PRP antibody you need at any given time to kill *H influenzae* that happens to gain entry into the bloodstream; 1.0 mcg/mL is referred to as the "long-term" correlate of protection, meaning that this is the amount of antibody you need after vaccination with a pure polysaccharide vaccine to be protected for a long time. The question is, what antibody levels are necessary immediately after vaccination with a *conjugate* vaccine to achieve long-term protection? One cannot directly infer this from studies of polysaccharide vaccine, because conjugate vaccines induce higher quality antibodies.

The situation becomes even more complex. Protection may be mediated before the organism enters the bloodstream, at the site of mucosal colonization. Little is known, however, about mucosal correlates of protection. How much secretory IgA or extravascular IgG is enough to prevent colonization? What role does prevention of colonization play in prevention of disease? How about the role of inoculum size (assuming there is a correlate of protection necessarily assumes there is an average inoculum)?

Another example of the problem with interpreting correlates of protection comes from observations made with HepB. Studies suggest that circulating levels of HBsAb ≥10 mIU/mL at the time of exposure to HBV perfectly predict protection from infection. In this sense, then, HBsAb ≥10 mIU/mL is a correlate of protection. However, studies also show that antibody wanes with time—often to levels <10 mIU/mL—even though protection does not. Therefore, there must be another (unmeasured) correlate of long-term protection.

One also needs to ask how antibodies are being measured. Clearly, quantitation of high-avidity antibodies that kill or opsonize *H influenzae* would correlate more closely with protection than measurement of antibodies that bind to PRP in an enzyme-linked immunosorbent assay. Similarly, we are much more interested in the levels of serum bactericidal antibodies to *N meningitidis*, a functional immune response endpoint, than we are in quantitating antibody binding to the capsular polysaccharide.

TABLE 1.4 — Generally Accepted Correlates of Protection After Vaccination

Disease	Test	Correlate of Protection
Diphtheria	Toxin neutralization	0.01-0.1 IU/mL
Hepatitis A	Enzyme-linked immunosorbent assay	10 mIU/mL
Hepatitis B	Enzyme-linked immunosorbent assay	10 mIU/mL
H influenzae (polysaccharide vaccine)	Enzyme-linked immunosorbent assay	1 mcg/mL
H influenzae (conjugate vaccine)	Enzyme-linked immunosorbent assay	0.15 mcg/mL
Influenza	Hemagglutination inhibition	1:40 dilution
Japanese encephalitis	Plaque reduction neutralization	1:10 dilution
Lyme	Enzyme-linked immunosorbent assay	1100 EIA U/mL
Measles	Microneutralization	120 mIU/mL
N meningitidis (serogroup C)	Serum bactericidal assay using human complement	1:4 dilution
Polio	Serum neutralization	1:4-1:8 dilution
Rabies	Serum neutralization	0.5 IU/mL
Rubella	Immunoprecipitation	10-15 mIU/mL
S pneumoniae	Enzyme-linked immunosorbent assay	0.20-0.35 mcg/mL (for children)
	Opsonophagocytosis	1:8 dilution
Tetanus	Toxin neutralization	0.1 IU/mL
Varicella	Serum neutralization	1:64 dilution
	Glycoprotein enzyme-linked immunosorbent assay	5 IU/mL

Adapted from Plotkin SA. *Pediatr Infect Dis J.* 2001;20:63-75.

Quantitation of antibodies that neutralize viruses in vitro might be more relevant than measurement of antibodies that bind to viral proteins—unless one knows exactly which proteins are involved in generating neutralizing antibody. Even then, there is no guarantee that a protein-binding assay will measure antibodies that bind to the neutralizing epitopes, and that binding to those epitopes actually correlates with neutralization in a functional assay. For some infections (eg, tetanus), antibodies to the *organism itself* are not relevant, but antibodies to *toxins produced by the organism* are. The situation becomes even more complex when one considers that for some diseases, protection may be mediated as much by Th- and Tc-cells as by antibody. In as much as Th-cells help B-cells make antibodies, antibody levels may be an indirect measure of cellular immunity.

Fortunately, vaccine development does not depend on establishing immunologic correlates of protection. For example, there is no consensus on correlates of protection against rotavirus (candidates include mucosal IgA and T-cells), even though highly effective vaccines have been developed. Likewise, debate continues about the correlates of protection against pertussis. Most agree that antibody to pertussis toxin is necessary; some say it is sufficient, but some say immunity is incrementally enhanced by antibodies to filamentous hemagglutinin, pertactin, and fimbrial antigens. No one really agrees on the actual levels of antibody that are necessary. Yet pertussis vaccines in various iterations have been in use since the 1940s—licensed based on demonstrated efficacy against disease in clinical trials.

Interestingly, the newest pertussis vaccine, Tdap, was licensed without proof of efficacy—and despite the fact that there are no agreed-upon correlates of protection. For both available products, the basis for licensure was the demonstration of levels of antibodies to pertussis antigens that were similar to the levels found in infants who had received DTaP, a vaccine already proved to be effective against disease. Similarly, MCV4-D was licensed because the levels of antibody following vaccination were equivalent to those achieved after immunization with MPSV4, which was also known to be protective. MCV4-CRM, in turn, was licensed after demonstration of noninferiority with MCV4-D.

■ Herd Immunity

Vaccines protect people in two ways. First, they stimulate adaptive immunity in vaccinated individuals. The level of protection depends on the quality, magnitude, and duration of the individual's response. Since no vaccine is 100% effective, even vaccinated individuals can become infected—*if* they are exposed. Exposure, in turn, depends on transmission of the pathogen from person-to-person (an exception is tetanus, which is acquired from the environment, not other people). What if transmission were interrupted because there were enough immune individuals in the population? Then everyone—susceptible vaccinated and unvaccinated individuals alike—would be indirectly protected.

The term *herd immunity* was coined in 1923 by Topley and Wilson in drawing a distinction between (but acknowledging the relatedness of) the immunity of individuals and protection of the community in which the individuals live. It refers to the fact that susceptible members of "the herd" are protected by the presence and proximity of immune members who prevent propagation of the infection.[11] For every disease that is transmitted from person to person, there is a *herd immunity threshold*—a critical proportion of the population that must be immune in order for transmission to be squelched. Although simple in concept, the herd-immunity threshold depends on a complex interplay of many factors, including contagiousness of the pathogen, mode of transmission (eg, fecal-oral vs respiratory droplet), how people interact with each other, and whether the disease is endemic or comes in epidemic waves. Ideally, one would want to know what proportion of a population needs to be vaccinated in order to protect the entire population. This will depend on the above factors, as well as on the efficacy of the vaccine and the reality that neither vaccination nor exposure is evenly distributed within a population. For example, there may be pockets of susceptible individuals (eg, undervaccinated inner-city residents) or foci of close contact (eg, college dormitories).

In addition, the microbial ecology of the pathogen must be taken into account. For measles virus, there is no carrier state and there is no reservoir per se. Thus a vaccine that prevents individual infection will prevent transmission and amplify the protective effect on individuals through herd immunity. For *H influenzae*, in contrast, there *is* a reservoir—the nasopharynx of young children. A vaccine that prevents invasive infection but not nasopharyngeal colonization arguably would not result in herd immunity, since transmission could still occur from vaccinated children who remain colonized. Fortunately, protein-polysaccharide conjugate vaccines are very effective at reducing colonization. In the case of Hib, herd immunity effects are dramatic. A Danish study, for example, estimated that by 3.5 years of age, the protection afforded unvaccinated children through herd immunity was about the same as the direct protection afforded through vaccination, approximately 94%.[12]

Figures 1.6 and **1.7** give modern-day examples of herd immunity in action. In the early 1990s, the incidence of hepatitis A in Butte County was six times higher than in California as a whole. Beginning in 1995, children 2 through 17 years of age were routinely immunized with HepA. Within 5 years, the incidence of hepatitis A had fallen dramatically among children, as one might have expected (**Figure 1.6**). However, the incidence also had

FIGURE 1.6 — Average Annual Age-Specific Incidence of Hepatitis A in Butte County, California

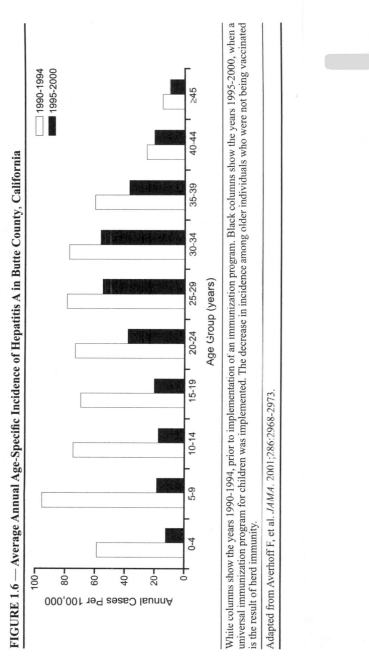

White columns show the years 1990-1994, prior to implementation of an universal immunization program for children was implemented. The decrease in incidence among older individuals who were not being vaccinated is the result of herd immunity.

Adapted from Averhoff F, et al. *JAMA*. 2001;286:2968-2973.

FIGURE 1.7 — Mean Annual Incidence of Pneumococcal Meningitis Due to PCV7 Serotypes (4, 6B, 9V, 14, 18C, 19F, and 23F) at United States Surveillance Sites

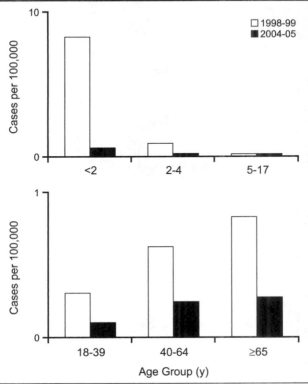

Routine use of PCV7 at 2, 4, 6, and 12-15 months of age was introduced in 2000. The dramatic reduction in incidence among children *(top panel)* was due to both direct and herd effects. The reduction seen in adults *(bottom panel)* was due to herd effects alone, since they were not being immunized with PCV7 (note the difference in scale between the two panels).

Adapted from Hsu HE, et al. *N Engl J Med.* 2009;360:244-256.

fallen in all other age groups—groups that were not targeted for immunization. Preventing hepatitis A in children was enough to prevent transmission to, and infection among, adults. Economic models suggest that herd immunity effects more than double the cost savings from universal HepA immunization of young children.[13]

Similarly, **Figure 1.7** illustrates the impact that routine childhood PCV7 immunization has had on *S pneumoniae* meningitis in unimmunized older individuals. In this case, herd immunity was mediated by decreases in nasopharyngeal colonization among vaccinated children.[14] However, there is a cautionary tale to tell here. Vaccination only affects colonization with vaccine serotypes. When these serotypes disappear from the nasopharynx, other serotypes take over, something called *serotype replacement*. Some of those serotypes—19A, for example, in the case of *S pneumoniae*—are themselves capable of causing invasive disease. In fact, invasive disease due to nonvaccine serotypes has *increased* in the PCV7 era, although the overall rate of invasive disease (all serotypes included) has dramatically declined. The challenge is to stay one step ahead of the organism by developing vaccines that include the emerging serotypes, which, in the case of PCV7, has been accomplished with the licensure of PCV13. Interestingly, *H influenzae* serotype replacement has not occurred in the Hib vaccine era, despite similar effects of Hib on nasopharyngeal colonization with that organism.[15]

Dramatic herd effects have also been seen in the United Kingdom[16] and Canada[17] with the introduction of serogroup C meningococcal conjugate vaccines.

■ Genetics of Vaccine Responses and Adverse Events

Immune responses depend on the interplay of various cells that engage each other through MHC molecules loaded with peptides derived from the pathogen (or vaccine). The genes encoding MHC molecules demonstrate a large degree of diversity, such that one person's MHC molecules might be better able to present a given peptide than another person's. Thus, for example, individuals with a particular HLA allele called DQB1*0303 appear to be less competent at producing mumps antibody after 2 doses of vaccine than those who possess other alleles.[18] Other HLA alleles, however, such as DRB1*0301, DRB1*0801, DRB1*1201, and DRB1*1302, are associated with lower lymphoproliferative responses. Polymorphisms in cytokine and cytokine receptor genes may also predict immune responses. Importantly, these polymorphisms are not something you would necessarily know about ahead of time, since they (probably) do not result in a particular disease phenotype. However, the information could someday be used to predict which individuals are at risk for suboptimal vaccine responses.

Likewise, genetic analyses might someday be used to predict which individuals might have adverse reactions to vaccines. One study, for example, showed that specific haplotypes in the IL-1 gene complex on chromosome 2 and the *IL18* complex on chromosome 11 were associated with fever after smallpox vaccination.[19] The application of genetic analyses to the prediction of immune responses and adverse events has been termed *vaccinomics*.[20]

43

■ **Goals of Immunization Programs**

Some historians believe that smallpox has killed more people since civilization began than all other infectious diseases combined. Although global eradication through vaccination was conceived by Jenner as early as 1801, it did not become a real possibility until 1967, when the following factors converged: 1) the World Health Assembly resolved to eradicate the disease and increased funding was secured; 2) large amounts of stable, lyophilized vaccine became available and reference testing centers were established; 3) a highly effective bifurcated needle was adopted for administration; and 4) the strategy of ring vaccination was developed, wherein active cases were hunted down and their contacts vaccinated. As a result, the last natural case of smallpox on the planet occurred in 1977 (the last case in the United States was in 1949), and on December 9, 1979, the WHO certified that smallpox had been eradicated. It was remarked that smallpox eradication was one of the few things that needed to be done only once in the history of the world.

Vaccination programs progress from *control* of disease to *elimination* of disease and infection to *eradication*, defined as a permanent reduction to zero of the worldwide incidence of infection as the result of deliberate efforts.[21] Because there is no reservoir of variola virus in nature and there is no human carrier state, the elimination of smallpox was felt to be definitive. In the United States, routine vaccination of civilians ceased in 1972, health care personnel in 1976, and military personnel in 1990. Until 2001, the only persons in the United States who continued to be vaccinated were laboratory and animal care workers with potential exposures to orthopox viruses and health care personnel conducting clinical trials with recombinant vaccinia virus vaccines. Between 1984 and 2001, no country routinely immunized civilians.

The terrorist attacks of September 11, 2001, raised the concern that the end game for smallpox should not have been eradication but rather *extinction*, where the specific agent no longer exists in nature or the laboratory. After eradication, worldwide stocks of variola virus were consolidated at the CDC and the Institute of Virus Preparations in Moscow (now the Russian State Centre for Research on Virology and Biotechnology, Koltsovo, Novosibirsk Region, Russian Federation). It is now known that the Soviet Union had an active program to weaponize variola virus, and with the political unrest and economic hardship that ensued in Russia during the 1990s, it remained possible that the virus and the technology to deliver it may have fallen into the hands of terrorists or rogue nations. Even a single case of smallpox anywhere in the world would strongly imply an intentional release and would be considered an international medical and strategic emergency.

The destruction of remaining lots of variola virus was debated in the 1990s, but on December 20, 2001, the WHO recommended against this—the virus was spared execution in order to facilitate continued research into molecular diagnosis, genetic analysis, serologic assays, animal models, antiviral drugs, and vaccines.

Many diseases have been *controlled* through vaccination. Beyond smallpox, three diseases—polio, measles, and rubella—have been *eliminated* from the United States, meaning that indigenous cases no longer occur. Because infection can still be imported from outside the country, as was demonstrated by the measles outbreaks in Arizona, California, Wisconsin, and elsewhere in 2008, elimination should be viewed as a step along the way to the ultimate goal of global eradication. Worldwide efforts to eliminate and ultimately eradicate hepatitis B, measles, rubella, and polio are under way. One could argue, though, that in the post-9/11 era, the ultimate goal should be *extinction*. Even that, however, may not be enough—the genome of polio virus is known, and live virus could theoretically be reconstructed from the raw genetic materials.

What does it take to eliminate or eradicate a vaccine-preventable disease? First, it takes favorable disease characteristics, including a readily recognizable clinical syndrome, easy diagnosis, few subclinical infections, a short period of contagion, absence of persistence and nonhuman reservoirs, little strain variability, and lifelong immunity after natural infection. Then it takes a safe, effective, stable, easily stored and transported, cheap vaccine. Then it takes political will and the collaboration of governments, organizations, and many individuals. Finally, eradication takes money—while it requires intensive effort and expense over a short period of time, eradication can be viewed as very cost-effective when you consider that once achieved, vaccination may no longer be necessary.

■ Public Health Impact of Vaccines

It is difficult to summarize the tremendous impact that vaccines have had on our general wellbeing. Vaccination ranks among the top ten great achievements in public health during the 20th century and is partially responsible for the dramatic increase in life expectancy that was seen during that period of time.[22] **Table 1.5** shows the impact on specific diseases by comparing the peak number of cases and deaths in the prevaccine era to data from 2004 to 2006. The decline in cases for almost all of these diseases has been nothing short of spectacular, although a few things are worth pointing out. Pertussis, for example, declined to historic lows in the 1970s but has resurged since then. Some part of this is more awareness, active surveillance, and better diagnostic tools, such that more cases are being detected. Part of it is also the fact that immunity induced by childhood vaccination wanes,

TABLE 1.5 — Annual Morbidity and Mortality From Vaccine-Preventable Diseases

Disease	Historical Peak		2004-2006[a]	
	Cases	Deaths	Cases	Deaths
Vaccine Programs Initiated Before 1980				
Diphtheria	30,508	3065	0	0
Measles	763,094	552	55	0
Mumps	212,932	50	6584	0
Pertussis	265,269	7518	15,632	27
Poliomyelitis (acute)	42,033	2720	0	0
Poliomyelitis (paralytic)	21,269	3145	0	0
Rubella	488,796	24	11	0
Congenital rubella syndrome	20,000	2160	1	0
Smallpox	110,672	2510	0	0
Tetanus	601	511	41	4
Vaccine Programs Initated After 1980				
Hepatitis A	254,518	298	15,298	18
Hepatitis B	74,361	267	13,169	47
Invasive:				
H influenzae type b	>20,000	>1000	<50	<5
S pneumoniae	64,400	7300	41,550	4850
Varicella	5,358,595	138	612,768	19

[a] For programs initiated before 1980, reported cases in 2006 and deaths in 2004 are given; for programs initiated after 1980, estimates for cases and deaths in 2006 are given.

Adapted from Roush SW, Murphy TV; Vaccine-Preventable Disease Table Working Group. *JAMA*. 2007;298:2155-2163.

and that until recently there have been no vaccines available to boost immunity in adolescents and adults. **Table 1.5** also reflects the abrupt resurgence of mumps that occurred in the Midwest in 2006, which was probably due to a virus imported from Europe. That outbreak, which disproportionately affected young adults, was driven by waning vaccine-induced immunity and the close-contact living situation of college students.

New strategies have been adopted for diseases that have stubbornly persisted. For example, HepA targeted at high-risk individuals and communities could only bring us so far; the adoption of a universal childhood immunization program in 2006 should bring the number of cases down much further. Similarly, the one-dose VAR program initiated in 1995 was very success-ful, but because of breakthrough disease in vaccinees (primary vaccine failure) could only bring us so far; the adoption of a routine 2-dose childhood schedule and catch-up immunization for everyone else should close the deal. In the case of invasive *S pneumoniae* disease, the recent licensure of PCV13 should take care of many of the serotypes that emerged after 2000, when PCV7 was licensed; it is possible that more serotypes will need to be added in the future.

Studies have shown that the *clinically preventable burden*, which is the proportion of disease aborted by a preventive service in usual practice, is higher for the routine childhood immunization schedule than for virtually every other routine public health inter-vention.[23] Vaccines also make economic sense—a study of the 2001 US birth cohort showed that for every $1 spent on routine childhood immunizations (which at the time did not include RV, HepA, PCV, influenza vaccine, MCV, or HPV), $5 was saved in direct costs and an additional $11 was saved in societal costs.[24]

REFERENCES

1. Huang AYC, et al. In: Stiehm ER, et al, eds. *Immunologic Disorders in Infants & Children*. 5th ed. St Louis, MO: Elsevier; 2004.

2. Siegrist CA. In: Plotkin SA, et al, eds. *Vaccines*. 5th ed. St Louis, MO: Elsevier; 2008.

3. Arnou R, et al. *Vaccine*. 2009;27:7304-7312.

4. Garcon N, et al. *Sci Amer*. 2009;301:72-79.

5. Roman F, et al. *Vaccine*. 2010;28:1740-1745.

6. Khurana S, et al. *Sci Transl Med*. 2010:2:1-7.

7. Amanna IJ, et al. *N Engl J Med*. 2007;357:1903-1915.

8. Pichichero ME. *Pediatrics*. 2009;124:1633-1641.

9. Qin L, et al. *J Infect Dis*. 2007;196:1304-1312.

10. Plotkin SA. *Pediatr Infect Dis J*. 2001;20:63-75.

11. Fine PE. *Epidemiol Rev*. 1993;15:265-302.

12. Hviid A, et al. *Vaccine*. 2004;22:378-382.

13. Armstrong GL, et al. *Pediatrics*. 2007;119:e22-e29.

14. Millar EV, et al. *Clin Infect Dis*. 2008;47:989-996.

15. Ladhani S, et al. *Lancet Infect Dis*. 2008;8;275-276.

16. Ramsay ME, et al. *BMJ*. 2003;326:365-366.

17. Kinlin LM, et al. *Vaccine*. 2009;27:1735-1740.

18. Ovsyannikova IG, et al. *Pediatrics*. 2008;121:e1091-e1099.

19. Stanley SL, et al. *J Infect Dis*. 2007;196:212-219.

20. Poland GA. *Clin Pharmacol Ther*. 2007;82:623-626.

21. Hinman A. *Annu Rev Pub Health*. 1999;20:211-229.

22. CDC. *MMWR*. 1999;48:243-248.

23. Coffield AB, et al. A*m J Prev Med*. 2001;21:1-9.

24. Zhou F, et al. *Arch Pediatr Adolesc Med*. 2005;159:1136-1144.

Vaccine Infrastructure in the United States

Vaccine Development and Licensure

A tremendous amount of effort is involved in developing vaccines. The biology of the infectious agent and pathogenesis of the disease must be elucidated. Correlates of immunity, and the laboratory tools to measure them, must be developed. Animal models of vaccine efficacy need to be investigated. Issues such as immunopotentiation, formulation, and delivery need to be worked out, and consistent test lots must be produced. These steps in preclinical development may take place in academia, industry, governmental research institutions, or collaborations between these groups. **Figure 2.1** illustrates the process of vaccine development and licensure in the United States.

Once candidate vaccines are ready for testing in humans, the process is rigorously overseen by the Food and Drug Administration (FDA). In general, the financial risk of clinical development is borne by industry. The risk is substantial—for example, the estimated, inflation-adjusted, capitalized, total research and development costs for RotaTeq (RV5) were as high as $644 million[1]—and there was no guarantee that the investment would pay off. It is important to understand that no vaccines reach the public without industry, since pharmaceutical companies—not academic medical centers or governmental agencies—manufacture and distribute the final products.

The FDA group that sets the standards for vaccine development is the Center for Biologics Evaluation and Research (CBER). The World Health Organization (WHO) provides guidance for products that are used internationally. Laboratory testing for vaccine purity and consistency is required before and after licensure. An intensive search is performed for contaminating viral, bacterial, and fungal agents, potency tests are applied, and biochemical identity is assured. Manufacturers are required to conform to Good Manufacturing Practices (GMPs), a vast collection of rules and guidances that cover everything from raw-materials quality assurance to record keeping, cleanliness standards, personnel qualifications, inhouse testing, process controls, warehousing, and distribution. They must also adhere to Good Laboratory Practices (GLPs), an analogous set of guidances for the laboratory that involves everything from assay reproducibility to interpretation. Several large lots of vaccine (each containing tens of thousands of doses) with identical potencies and demonstrated safety must be produced in a manner that is consistent and reliable. In addi-

FIGURE 2.1 — Schematic of the Process of Vaccine Development and Licensure in the United States

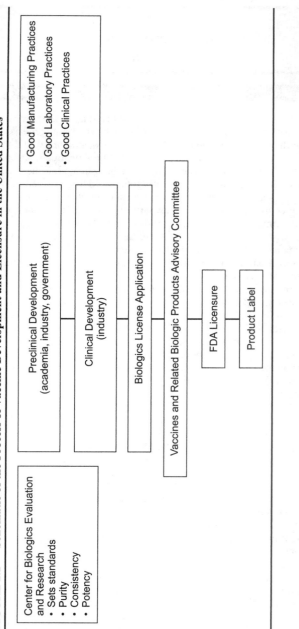

Center for Biologics Evaluation and Research
• Sets standards
• Purity
• Consistency
• Potency

Preclinical Development (academia, industry, government)

Clinical Development (industry)

Biologics License Application

Vaccines and Related Biologic Products Advisory Committee

FDA Licensure

Product Label

• Good Manufacturing Practices
• Good Laboratory Practices
• Good Clinical Practices

tion, manufacturers are required to provide information regarding appropriate storage and handling. Fulfilling the requirements of CBER may take 5 and 10 years.

After a candidate vaccine is approved as an investigational new drug for use in clinical trials, studies for safety, immunogenicity, and efficacy are performed. Good Clinical Practices (GCPs) set the standard for the conduct of clinical trials. Some trials are conducted by the National Institutes of Health (NIH) through Vaccine and Treatment Evaluation Units; as of February 2010, there were eight such funded units, most of them at academic medical centers. Other studies, generally involving more mature candidate vaccines, are conducted at academic medical centers or private offices by pharmaceutical companies (or clinical research organizations contracted by these companies) using local principal investigators who are overseen by institutional review boards or human studies committees. Strict federal guidelines apply regarding the protection of human subjects and the management of potential conflicts of interest.

Prelicensure trials proceed in three phases, followed by a postmarketing phase (**Figure 2.2**):

- *Phase 1*—These trials usually involve <100 volunteers and are intended to provide basic information on safety and tolerability. Because of their small size, they can detect only extremely common adverse events. Subjects are often not drawn from the intended vaccine target population. For

FIGURE 2.2 — Sequential Stages in the Testing of Vaccines in Humans

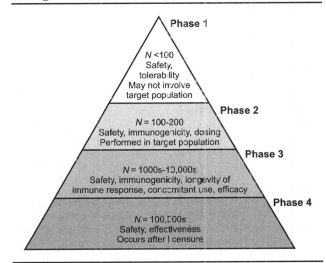

Phase 1
$N < 100$
Safety, tolerability
May not involve target population

Phase 2
$N = 100\text{-}200$
Safety, immunogenicity, dosing
Performed in target population

Phase 3
$N = 1000\text{s-}10,000\text{s}$
Safety, immunogenicity, longevity of immune response, concomitant use, efficacy

Phase 4
$N = 100,000\text{s}$
Safety, effectiveness
Occurs after licensure

example, pediatric vaccine candidates might undergo initial testing in adults until basic safety is assured.

• *Phase 2*—These trials enroll hundreds of subjects and provide information about the vaccine's immunogenicity, dose, and common side effects. Studies are performed in the proposed target group and may also provide some information on efficacy.

• *Phase 3*—These studies enroll thousands to tens of thousands of subjects, using sample sizes large enough to ensure that questions about safety and efficacy will be answered (they are often referred to as pivotal studies). Subjects are carefully followed for adverse events in the immediate postvaccination period, usually as long as 42 days out. Longer periods of observation allow for assessment of protection from disease and persistence of immune responses. Large trials also evaluate the consistency of responses and look at concomitant use with other vaccines. This phase of development includes the transfer of manufacturing to full-scale facilities, which must operate under GMPs and are subject to rigorous inspections (the plant itself must be licensed).

Phase 3 trials of new vaccines, that is, vaccines for diseases that previously were not vaccine-preventable, include placebo recipients; therefore, efficacy against disease can be determined and adverse events related to the vaccine can be pinpointed. Phase 3 trials of new versions of existing vaccines generally pit the new vaccine against the existing one. Here, prevention of disease may not be a feasible end point, since the disease itself may be unusual. The end point, therefore, may be immunogenicity, the inference being that if the new vaccine is as immunogenic as the existing one (which is known to be protective), it should provide equal protection; these are often called *immunogenicity bridging* studies. *Noninferiority* is statistically defined for each study and is usually agreed upon before the trial is conducted.

Pressure to make sure that vaccines are as safe as possible before licensure has driven the size of Phase 3 trials upward—the studies that went into the licensure of RV5 and RV1, for example, each involved >70,000 children, more than any other prelicensure studies since the Salk vaccine trials of the early 1950s. As illustrated in **Table 2.1**, huge numbers of subjects are needed to detect adverse events that have a low background rate in the general population and a rare association with a vaccine. For example, assuming that a given event occurs in 1 out of 100,000 people in the general population, a clinical trial would need to enroll 1,238,000 subjects in order to detect a 2-fold higher rate of the event in vaccinees. Such trials are obviously not feasible, necessitating postmarketing safety surveillance mechanisms (see below).

TABLE 2.1 — Number of Subjects Needed to Test for Increased Relative Risk of an Adverse Event Relative to Background Rates

Background rate in general population	Rate in vaccinated population		
	2-fold higher	10-fold higher	100-fold higher
1 in 10,000	141,000	5,500	500
1 in 100,000	1,238,000	53,500	2,500
1 in 1,000,000	12,951,500	532,500	23,500

Adapted from Evans D, et al. *J Infect Dis.* 2009;200:321-328. Assumes a 5% risk of comitting a Type I error and 90% power to detect a difference.

- *Phase 4*—Prelicensure trials cannot detect very rare side effects, adverse events with delayed onset, or potential reactions in culturally or ethnically diverse populations. Formal postmarketing studies, which may involve large cohorts of vaccinated children followed prospectively, are designed to detect such rare events. Guidance for postmarketing activities is provided by Good Pharmacovigilence Practices (GPPs), which are analogous to GCPs. These studies are supplemented by the surveillance systems described below. Postmarketing studies also may look at *effectiveness*, or how a vaccine performs in real life, outside the context of a controlled clinical trial.

After Phase 1 through 3 studies are completed, the manufacturer submits a Biologics License Application (BLA) to the FDA. The BLA contains all of the data necessary to determine if a license should be granted. It is important to point out that the file is not submitted blindly—rather, its content is determined in a dynamic process of evaluation and negotiation between the FDA and the manufacturer. Around the time of the BLA submission, the manufacturing facilities are inspected and all aspects of vaccine production are evaluated. Once the BLA is accepted, the formal evaluation process begins—a process that generally takes a year or two, depending on whether supplemental information or additional studies are requested by the FDA. In 1992, the Prescription Drug User Fee Act (PDUFA) went into effect, authorizing the FDA to collect fees from manufacturers submitting a file. The continued reauthorization of PDUFA has allowed FDA to expand its staff and shorten the time to approval—the current goal is to act on 90% of standard new BLAs within 10 months.

Eventually, the manufacturer may be invited to present the entire case for licensure to the Vaccines and Related Biological Products Advisory Committee (VRBPAC), especially if the vaccine is the first in a class or if there are questions about safety or efficacy. VRBPAC consists of 12 core voting members appointed by the FDA Commissioner. Although most members have recognized expertise in fields related to vaccinology, one member who is identified with consumer interests may be appointed. In addition, a nonvoting representative of the pharmaceutical industry may be invited; this ensures that all interested parties have input into vaccine licensure decisions. VRBPAC makes recommendations to the FDA Commissioner regarding whether to license the product, what the indications should be, and whether any additional data are needed.

In general, the FDA Commissioner follows the VRBPAC recommendations, and licensure is usually granted within a few months. The FDA also approves a package insert (PI), synonymously referred to as the product information or label.

The PI contains official indications, statements about efficacy, contraindications, warnings, precautions, and adverse events. When people refer to labeled indications, they are referring to the specifics contained in the PI.

There are several things to bear in mind regarding the PI:

- The labeled indications are based on the data in the BLA. So, for example, if the studies on file only included persons in a certain age group, the label will specify approved use only in that age group. That will not change, even if new studies are published, unless the manufacturer submits a supplemental BLA that is subsequently approved.

- Official recommendations are sometimes at odds with the PI. For example, Comvax (HepB-Hib-OMP) is labeled for use only in infants of HBsAg-negative mothers, but use in infants of HBsAg-positive mothers is considered acceptable by the Advisory Committee on Immunization Practices (ACIP). Thus there is a difference between the labeled *indications*—which are derived strictly from the PI, and therefore from the FDA—and the *recommendations*, which are derived from authoritative professional bodies (see below). One question to consider is which of the two—the PI or the recommendations—sets the authoritative reference standard in malpractice litigation. Most people would agree that the *recommendations* supersede the *PI* in this respect because they are based on a more comprehensive dataset and they represent the opinion of medical peers.

- The PI does not provide guidance for all situations. For example, the Boostrix (Tdap) PI (January 2009) states that there are no immunogenicity or safety data for the concomitant administration of Boostrix with other vaccines (although data are provided for concomitant use of Fluarix). The next sentence reads, "When Boostrix is administered concomitantly with other injectable vaccines, they should be given with separate syringes and at different injection sites." While this would seem self-evident, one is still left to wonder if other vaccines—MCV4 and HPV vaccine in particular—can be given at the same time. Fortunately, ACIP recommendations usually answer these questions; in this case, concomitant administration of Tdap, MCV4, and HPV vaccine is recommended.

- Taking a conservative approach, the PI often mentions adverse events that have been reported but not proved to be caused by the vaccine. Thus, for example, the RotaTeq (RV5) PI mentions Kawasaki disease as an adverse event that has been reported postmarketing. While this is true at face value, the number of cases reported does not exceed what one would expect as background, and data from postmarketing studies do not support a causal relationship (see *Chapter 7: Addressing*

Concerns About Vaccines—Do Vaccines Trigger Kawasaki Disease [KD]?). Nevertheless, the mere fact that Kawasaki disease was added to the PI has led to unnecessary concern on the part of parents and providers.

• The PI determines how a vaccine can be advertised and marketed. Company field representatives must restrict their claims about the product to the information contained in the PI. Likewise, promotional programs must remain within the label, and it must be specified during continuing medical education programs when off-label uses of a product are mentioned.

With the above caveats, the PI does contain valuable information. The provider should be familiar with its contents, including the specifics regarding proper storage and handling.

Policy and Recommendations

Figure 2.3 gives an overview of the various agencies and committees involved in making and executing vaccine policy in the United States. The Centers for Disease Control and Prevention (CDC) includes the National Center for Immunization and Respiratory Diseases (NCIRD, formerly known as the National Immunization Program), an interdisciplinary program that merges vaccine-preventable disease science and research with immunization program activities. NCIRD provides leadership in the planning, coordination, and conduct of immunization activities throughout the country. It assists health departments in implementing immunization programs, supports establishment of vaccine supply contracts for state and local programs through the Vaccines For Children (VFC) Program, assists in the development of information-management systems, administers research and operational programs, provides clinician educational programs, and supports surveillance for vaccine-preventable diseases.

The ACIP is the principal body that makes recommendations for vaccine use. It provides advice and guidance to the Secretary of Health and Human Services, the Assistant Secretary, and the Director of the CDC regarding the most appropriate application of vaccines and related agents to control communicable diseases in the civilian population. ACIP recommendations also provide an evidence base for providers and programs regarding how vaccines should be used. There are 15 voting members who are appointed by the Secretary; persons who are knowledgeable about consumer perspectives and/or social and community aspects of immunization programs are included, as are infectious diseases specialists. In addition, there are eight *ex officio* members representing a variety of other governmental agencies involved in vaccine policy, distribution, and financing, as well as 26 nonvoting liaison mem-

FIGURE 2.3 — Governmental Agencies and Advisory Committees Involved in Vaccine Development, Policy, and Implementation

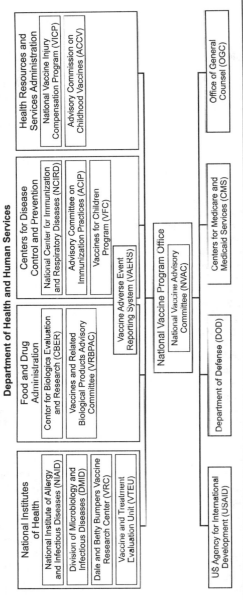

Department of Health and Human Services

National Institutes of Health
- National Institute of Allergy and Infectious Diseases (NIAID)
- Division of Microbiology and Infectious Diseases (DMID)
- Dale and Betty Bumpers Vaccine Research Center (VRC)
- Vaccine and Treatment Evaluation Unit (VTEU)

Food and Drug Administration
- Center for Biologics Evaluation and Research (CBER)
- Vaccines and Related Biological Products Advisory Committee (VRBPAC)

Vaccine Adverse Event Reporting System (VAERS)

Centers for Disease Control and Prevention
- National Center for Immunization and Respiratory Diseases (NCIRD)
- Advisory Committee on Immunization Practices (ACIP)
- Vaccines for Children Program (VFC)

Health Resources and Services Administration
- National Vaccine Injury Compensation Program (VICP)
- Advisory Commission on Childhood Vaccines (ACCV)

National Vaccine Program Office
- National Vaccine Advisory Committee (NVAC)

US Agency for International Development (USAID)

Department of Defense (DOD)

Centers for Medicare and Medicaid Services (CMS)

Office of General Counsel (OGC)

bers from professional organizations. Members with financial conflicts of interest concerning particular vaccines cannot vote on recommendations that pertain to those products. This includes members who receive research funding from the manufacturer.

The committee meets three times each year. In making its recommendations, the ACIP considers a product's labeled indications and dosing schedule, disease burden, safety data, feasibility, and input from other stakeholder groups. In 2008, a standardized approach to the presentation of health economics studies was adopted.[2] Oftentimes, data that are not included in the product BLA are considered, which explains why the recommendations may differ from the label. The process usually involves the formation of working groups on specific topics; these groups are chaired by ACIP members but often include outside experts. For some issues, such as vaccination during pregnancy and breastfeeding, specific guiding principles have been adopted.[3]

There are four permanent working groups:

- *Childhood/Adolescent Immunization Schedules*—This group recommends changes to the routine childhood and adolescent schedules, which are published every January. Since 1995, the ACIP schedule has been harmonized in its characteristic graphic layout with the recommendations of the American Academy of Pediatrics (AAP) and the American Academy of Family Physicians (AAFP).
- *Adult Immunization Schedule*—This group recommends changes to the routine adult schedule, which are also updated every year.
- *Influenza Vaccine*—This group makes recommendations regarding influenza immunization for the upcoming influenza season, which are usually published in late spring or summer.
- *General Recommendations*—Every 3 to 5 years, the ACIP publishes a document entitled *General Recommendations on Immunization*, commonly referred to as the "General Recs," which provides background and technical guidance regarding vaccination.[4] Specific topics include timing and spacing of doses, contraindications and precautions, administration technique, storage and handling, special situations, record keeping, and adverse-event reporting, among others. These topics are elaborated upon elsewhere in this book (see *Chapter 5: General Recommendations*).

Recommendations pertaining to newly licensed vaccines, programmatic issues, changes in previous recommendations, and informational items ("Notice to Readers") are published periodically in the *Morbidity and Mortality Weekly Report (MMWR)* and on the CDC Web site, which also posts provisional recommendations, oftentimes many months before the full recommendations are published in the *MMWR*. A comprehensive summary of ACIP recommendations is released every 1 to 2 years in a book entitled *Epidemiology and Prevention of Vaccine-Preventable Diseases*, commonly known as the "Pink Book."[5]

ACIP recommendations usually come in three varieties. First, there are recommendations for *routine immunization*, whereby every person in the specified age group should be vaccinated (eg, all children should receive Hib at 2, 4, 6, and 12 to 15 months of age). Second, there are recommendations for *catch-up immunization*, which apply to defined cohorts and time periods (eg, a second dose of VAR should be given to all persons who previously received one dose). Third, there are *risk-based immunization* recommendations, which apply to persons with specific risk factors for the disease or complications (eg, PPSV23 should be given to persons 19 to 64 years of age who smoke). Occasionally, there are *anti-recommendations* (for lack of a better term), which provide the rationale why a vaccine should not be routinely administered to certain age groups (eg, MCV4-D should not be routinely given to healthy children 2 through 10 years of age, even though it is licensed in that age group). Finally, there are *permissive statements*, which allow for use of a vaccine but do not make a recommendation (eg, HPV4 may be used in boys for prevention of genital warts).

The AAP Committee on Infectious Diseases also develops policy recommendations on the use of vaccines. While these are developed independently, every attempt is made to achieve congruity with the ACIP recommendations. From time to time, however, there are subtle but important differences. AAP recommendations on vaccination are included the *Report of the Committee on Infectious Diseases*, a comprehensive summary of infectious diseases that is published every 3 years and is commonly called the "Red Book."[5] The AAP also partners with the CDC in the Childhood Immunization Support Program, with goals to promote quality improvement and best immunization practices, improve delivery, and enable effective communication.

The ACIP has one other important function: it determines which vaccines should be added to the VFC program (see below). In order for a vaccine to be covered under the VFC program, a specific resolution must be passed. Resolutions may be passed even when the ACIP position on a given vaccine is permissive.

The National Vaccine Program Office (NVPO) was created in 1986 to coordinate the activities of all federal agencies in developing and implementing the National Vaccine Plan. In so doing, the NVPO strives to improve collaboration with the commercial vaccine industry, global organizations, consumer groups, and academic institutions. The Plan was created in 1994 and an updated plan was drafted in 2008.[7] Since then, input from the public and other stakeholders has been sought, and in December 2009 recommendations from the Institute of Medicine were released.[8]

The Plan has five main goals:
- Develop new and improved vaccines
- Enhance the safety of vaccines and vaccination practices
- Support informed vaccine decision-making by the public, providers, and policy-makers
- Ensure a stable supply of recommended vaccines, and achieve better use of existing vaccines to prevent disease, disability, and death in the United States.
- Increase global prevention of death and disease through safe and effective vaccination

The National Vaccine Advisory Committee (NVAC) makes recommendations to the NVPO regarding the supply of safe and effective vaccines, research priorities, areas of cooperation, and ways to achieve optimal prevention of infectious diseases through vaccine development while minimizing adverse reactions. The 17 members include physicians, researchers, and people involved in manufacturing and public health, and representatives from parent organizations.

Monitoring Delivery

Once vaccines are licensed and recommended for use, delivery to the appropriate people needs to be monitored. *Coverage* refers to the proportion of eligible persons who receive a recommended vaccine. *Timeliness* assesses whether vaccinated persons receive the recommended doses of a vaccine within the recommended age range, measured as the proportion of individuals who receive the vaccine on time or as the cumulative number of days a given vaccine or vaccine series is delayed. Both coverage and timeliness are important measures of the quality of immunization care. Through effective monitoring, racial and ethnic disparities can be discovered, underserved groups can be identified, the effectiveness of intervention programs can be assessed, uptake of new vaccines and the effect of shortages can be tracked, and correlates of quality can be determined.[9]

■ National Immunization Survey (NIS)

Conducted annually since 1994, the NIS is a random digit dialing telephone survey of households in the United States. Historically focused on vaccine coverage among children 19 to 35 months of age, it was expanded in 2006 to include adolescents 13 to 17 years of age (NIS-Teen) and again in 2007 to include adults (NIS-Adult). Respondents provide information about vaccinations as well as sociodemographic information. For those who give permission, validating data are obtained from the providers. The survey includes all 50 states and selected urban and county areas. **Figure 2.4** shows the results of the NIS over the past decade.

FIGURE 2.4 — Immunization Coverage Rates Among Young Children

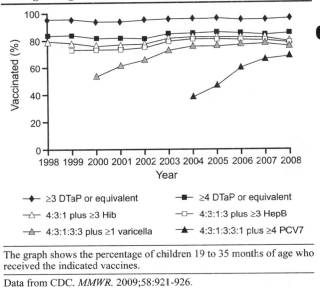

The graph shows the percentage of children 19 to 35 months of age who received the indicated vaccines.

Data from CDC. *MMWR.* 2009;58:921-926.

The 2008 report included data from 18,430 provider-reported vaccination records.[10] Coverage rates for most routinely recommended vaccine series remained ≥90%, with only ≥4 DTaP lagging behind at 84.6%. Coverage for the series of ≥4 DTaP, ≥3 IPV, ≥1 MMR, ≥3 Hib, ≥3 HepB, and ≥1 VAR (4:3:1:3:3:1) was 76.1%, essentially unchanged from 77.4% the year before. State-to-state variability was evident, with 4:3:1:3:3:1 coverage ranging from 59.2% in Montana to 82.3% in Massachusetts. As might be expected, coverage was lower among children living below the poverty level, but little variability was seen based on ethnicity or race when controlling for poverty. Coverage for 4:3:1:3:3:1:4 (4:3:1:3:3:1 plus ≥4 doses of PCV7) was 68.4%, up from 66.5% (coverage for ≥4 PCV7 alone was 80.1%, up from 75.3%). However, coverage for ≥3 Hib declined from 92.6% to 90.9%, possibly a result of the Hib shortage.

2008 marked the beginning of routine reporting of coverage for the birth dose of HepB (55.3%) and for ≥2 HepA (40.4%) under the most current recommendations. The proportion of children receiving no vaccinations remained stable at 0.6%, which is reassuring in light of continuing public challenges to the necessity and safety of vaccinations (see *Chapter 7: Addressing Concerns About Vaccines*).

Good news also derived from the 2008 NIS-Teen.[11] Coverage for ≥1 MCV4 went from 32.4% to 41.8%; ≥1 Tdap from 30.4% to 40.8%; and ≥1 HPV vaccine from 25.1% to 37.2%. The proportion of teenagers with ≥2 doses of VAR went from 18.8% to 34.1%. Finally, for the first time, the *Healthy People 2010* target of 90% coverage was reached for MMR and HepB among adolescents.

NIS data have been instrumental in uncovering poor timeliness as an issue in vaccine delivery, one that is masked by good coverage rates. A study using 2003 NIS data and involving 14,810 children showed that during the first 2 years of life, children spent a median of 172 days underimmunized; 37% of underimmunized children had cumulative delays of >6 months.[12] Eighteen percent of children who were considered fully covered by 24 months of age were actually undervaccinated for >6 months. In some states, <5% of children had received the 4:3:1:3:3 (4 DTaP, 3 IPV, 1 MMR, 3 Hib, 3 HepB) series exactly as recommended. Poor timeliness could leave children vulnerable to disease.

NIS data rely on provider-reported vaccination histories, which may be incomplete. In addition, coverage estimates for state and local areas may be imprecise because of small sample size.

■ National Health Interview Survey (NHIS)

This survey covering a broad range of health issues has been conducted by the CDC's National Center for Health Statistics since 1957. The current sample size target is 35,000 households containing about 87,500 persons. The NHIS is an important source of information about adult vaccine coverage.

■ Behavioral Risk Factor Surveillance System (BRFSS)

This state-level, random digit dialing telephone survey of noninstitutionalized civilians 18 years of age and older has been conducted by the CDC since 1984. More than 350,000 adults are surveyed every year, making the BRFSS the largest ongoing health survey in the world. The data obtained are very useful for issues such as influenza and pneumococcal vaccine coverage (**Figure 2.5**). The BRFSS showed that influenza vaccine coverage during the 2008-2009 season for persons 18 to 49 years of age with high-risk conditions was only 32.1%.[13] Coverage was 42.3% for adults 50 to 64 years of age and 67.2% for those ≥ 65 years of age. These rates represented no gains over previous years.

■ School Surveys

Retrospective school entry surveys are the most common form of state and local level surveillance. Coverage data are collected from the health records of randomly selected schools, and an assessment is made of vaccine coverage. Audits are performed to validate school entry data. The data necessarily lag several years behind current performance because children are 5 or 6 when

FIGURE 2.5 — Immunization Coverage Rates Among US Adults

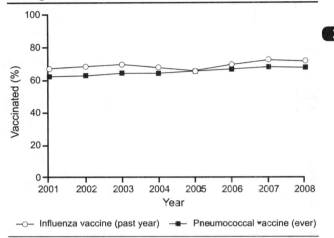

The graph shows the percentage of adults ≥65 years of age who received an influenza vaccine in the past year and the percentage who ever received pneumococcal vaccination.

Data from Prevalence and trends data. National Center for Chronic Disease Prevention and Health Promotion Web site. http://apps.nccd .cdc.gov/BRFSS/page.asp?yr=2008&state=UB&cat=IM#IM. Accessed January 20, 2010.

they enter school. In addition, no information on the timing of immunizations is obtained. A recent study looked at coverage rates for kindergarten students during the 2006-2007 school year.[14] Approximately 75% of states had reached the *Healthy People 2010* objective of ≥95% coverage for all vaccines among kindergarten attendees (this goal is higher than the general goal of 90% because settings such as kindergarten represent a higher risk of spread of vaccine-preventable disease). These data highlighted the success of school mandates in ensuring that children are fully immunized.

■ Special Area and Population Surveys

These studies involve small geographic units such as counties or census tracts or specific populations in a local area, such as Medicaid participants. Largely supported by federal grants, special surveys can target needy groups and ensure accountability within the public and private health care sectors. The National Nursing Home Survey, which is conducted on an episodic basis, is an example of a targeted survey.

■ Healthcare Effectiveness Data and Information Set (HEDIS)

The National Committee for Quality Assurance, an independent nonprofit organization, monitors the performance of managed health care plans through HEDIS, a set of standardized measures. Immunization rates on preschoolers, children, adolescents, and adults are captured through administrative claims, encounter data, and chart review.

Monitoring Effectiveness

Vaccine-preventable disease activity must be monitored in order to assess the effectiveness of immunization programs. A variety of mechanisms are in place to accomplish this at the population level. Efforts are coordinated by the CDC's Epidemiology Program Office and the NCIRD, in collaboration with groups such as the Council of State and Territorial Epidemiologists. Over 60 diseases are now reportable through the National Notifiable Disease Surveillance System (NNDSS).[15] Disease reporting by the states is voluntary, and reporting of diseases within states is mandated through legislation or regulation; for these reasons, the list of notifiable diseases varies from state to state. Reporting to the CDC occurs weekly through the National Electronic Telecommunications System for Surveillance; the CDC analyzes the data and launches investigations when appropriate. Active surveillance systems are in place for certain diseases such as measles, mumps, rubella, congenital rubella syndrome, diphtheria, tetanus, pertussis, poliomyelitis, and varicella. Laboratory-based surveillance programs, such as that for influenza, supplement these programs. Additional surveillance for invasive bacterial infections, such as those due to *S pneumoniae*, *H influenzae*, and *N meningitidis*, is done through the Active Bacterial Core surveillance (ABCs), which is part of the CDC's Emerging Infections Program Network.[16] This system stores demographic information on cases and collects bacterial isolates for further laboratory testing.

The New Vaccine Surveillance Network (NVSN) was established in 1999 in order to evaluate the impact of new vaccines and new recommendations.[17] The network currently consists of three sentinel sites at academic medical centers: the University of Rochester in Rochester, NY, Vanderbilt University in Nashville, TN, and the Cincinnati Children's Hospital Medical Center in Cincinnati, OH. These sites conduct inpatient and outpatient surveillance for vaccine-preventable diseases, including seasonal surveillance for acute respiratory illness and acute gastroenteritis. Special targeted studies look at vaccine effectiveness.

Other systems can contribute to our understanding of changes after immunization programs are implemented. For example, the impact of rotavirus vaccine has been monitored using the National

Respiratory and Enteric Surveillance System (NREVSS), a passive laboratory system that provides data on rotavirus testing. A similar program, the National Rotavirus Strain Surveillance System (NRSSS), looks at the geographic occurrence of rotavirus genotypes over time.

The Vaccine Safety Net

No medical intervention is 100% safe. For therapeutic interventions—antibiotics, for example—there is an inherent tolerance for risk, because without therapy, the infection will intensify. Preventive interventions such as vaccines, in contrast, are usually given to people who are perfectly healthy; as a consequence, the tolerance for adverse events is much lower. Moreover, everyone gets vaccines but only selected people get medicines. Therefore, the consequences of even rare adverse events are significant at the population level. It has been said that when a medicine is given, *disease is treated*, but when vaccines are given, *nothing happens*. The truth is, of course, that disease prevention through vaccination is an action, just as is treating pneumonia with antibiotics. The difference is that with antibiotics, it is about what you see happen (*the pneumonia improves*), whereas with vaccines, it is about what you do not see happen (*disease does not occur*).

Major components of the vaccine safety net in the United States are listed in **Table 2.2**. Monitoring for safety begins as soon as a

TABLE 2.2 — The Vaccine Safety Net in the United States

- FDA Center for Biologics Evaluation and Research (CBER)
- Good Manufacturing Practices (GMPs)
- Good Laboratory Practices (GLPs)
- Good Clinical Practices (GCPs)
- Phase 1, 2, and 3 prelicensure trials
- Review and licensure by the FDA
- Review and recommendation by authoritative bodies such as the Advisory Committee on Immunization Practices (ACIP), the American Academy of Pediatrics (AAP), and the American Association of Family Physicians (AAFP)
- Phase 4 (postlicensure) studies
- Good Pharmacovigilence Practices (GPPs)
- Vaccine Adverse Event Reporting System (VAERS)
- Vaccine Safety Datalink (VSD)
- Clinical Immunization Safety Assessment (CISA) Network
- Brighton Collaboration
- Ad-hoc groups such as the Task Force on Safer Childhood Vaccines and the Immunization Safety Review Committee (ISRC) of the Institute of Medicine (IOM)
- Enhanced efforts such as those employed during the 2009 H1N1 influenza vaccination program

candidate vaccine is proposed for testing. Prelicensure evaluation is described earlier in this chapter. Aspects of postlicensure safety monitoring are described below.

■ Vaccine Adverse Event Reporting System (VAERS)

VAERS is a postmarketing surveillance system created by the National Childhood Vaccine Injury Act of 1986 and coadministered by the FDA and the CDC. Anyone can submit a report about any event that they feel is related to vaccination, and reporting of certain events is mandated by law (see *Chapter 3: Standards, Principles, and Regulations—National Childhood Vaccine Injury Act*). Information from VAERS reports is entered into a database, and selected serious events and deaths are compiled and analyzed. Between 1991 and 2001, a total of 128,717 reports were received, representing approximately 11.4 reports per 100,000 net doses distributed.[18] The most common adverse events reported were fever (25.8%), injection site hypersensitivity (15.8%), rash (11.0%), injection site edema (10.8%), and vasodilatation (10.8%). Approximately 14% of reports described serious adverse events. Most reports were from vaccine manufacturers (36.2%), health departments (27.6%), and providers (20.0%). The proportion reported by providers increased from 11.4% in 1991 to 35.3% in 2001. Overall, only 4.2% of reports were filed by parents or patients.

A significant limitation of VAERS is that it only receives information regarding vaccinated persons in whom an adverse event occurs. Because it does not receive information about the number of vaccine doses administered or the occurrence of adverse events in unvaccinated persons, causal relationships between vaccines and particular adverse events cannot be established.[19] In addition, underreporting, poor data quality, incomplete reports, differences between public and private sector reporting rates, lack of consistent diagnostic criteria for disease, and simultaneous administration of multiple vaccines limit the information that can be derived from VAERS. Moreover, significant reporting biases exist. For example, increased reporting is seen immediately after licensure and when particular vaccines are "in the news." As another example, many of the reports of autism following administration of thimerosal-containing vaccines have been filed by attorneys. For all of the above reasons, VAERS is vital for hypothesis *generation*, but not useful for hypothesis *testing*.

Despite these limitations, VAERS is the only surveillance system that covers the entire US population, and it includes the largest number of case reports temporally associated with vaccination. It serves to generate the signal that triggers further investigation, and can provide early warning of potential problems, including new, rare, or unusual adverse events. A good example of the utility of VAERS data was in prompting investigation of the relationship between the rhesus rotavirus vaccine and intussusception. Unfortunately, VAERS data have also been misunderstood by the media and misused by antivaccine activists, who have made the erroneous supposition that temporal association means causation (see *Chapter 7: Addressing Concerns About Vaccines*).

■ Vaccine Safety Datalink (VSD)

The VSD is an active surveillance system created by the CDC in 1990 and operated by the CDC's Immunization Safety Office.[20] Information regarding vaccination, medical outcomes, birth history, and census is collected through large, linked, computerized databases from eight health maintenance organizations in Seattle, WA, Portland, OR, Oakland, CA, and Los Angeles, CA, Denver, CO, Minneapolis, MN, Marshfield, WI, and Boston, MA. Approximately 6 million people of all ages are studied through this process, amounting to 2% of the entire US population. Given these numbers, relatively rare adverse events can be detected. Strengths of the VSD include improved reporting, reduced recall bias, and the ability to study unvaccinated control subjects. For these reasons, the VSD is an excellent way to test hypotheses and determine if the relationship between a vaccine and an adverse event is causal or coincidental. A recent priority has been to develop mechanisms for rapid-cycle analysis to reduce the lag time between the occurrence of adverse events and assessment of risk factors. This methodology will be particularly useful for monitoring the safety of newly licensed vaccines.

■ Clinical Immunization Safety Assessment (CISA) Network

Before the creation of the first CISA centers in 2001, there was no coordinated effort to evaluate and treat vaccine adverse events in individual patients. The CISA network is a partnership between academic medical institutions and the CDC that systematically evaluates patients who experience adverse events after immunization. Major goals include studying the pathophysiologic basis of adverse events, understanding risk factors (including host genetics), and providing evidence-based guidelines for vaccination, revaccination, and evaluation of adverse events following vaccination. CISA centers as of 2010 are located at Johns Hopkins University (Baltimore, MD), Northern California Kaiser Permanente (San Francisco, CA), Vanderbilt University (Nashville, TN), Boston University Medical Center (Boston, MA), Stanford University (Palo Alto, CA), and Columbia University Medical Center (New York, NY).

■ Brighton Collaboration

The Brighton Collaboration, launched in 2000, is an international organization that aims to facilitate the development, evaluation, and dissemination of high-quality information about the safety of vaccines.[21] Participants are volunteers from patient care, public health, pharmaceutical, regulatory, scientific, and professional organizations. The primary objective is to develop standardized definitions of adverse events following immunization, which should enhance comparability of data. In addition, Brighton aims to establish guidelines for collection, analysis, and presentation of safety data.

■ Special Surveillance Efforts

The 2009 H1N1 influenza immunization campaign, during which tens of millions of individuals were vaccinated in a short period of time, called for unprecedented safety surveillance efforts, especially in light of the association between the 1976 swine flu vaccine and Guillain-Barré syndrome (see *Chapter 7: Addressing Concerns About Vaccines—Do Vaccines Cause Guillain-Barré Syndrome [GBS]?*). Some of the measures employed included the following:

- Enhanced VAERS reporting, facilitated by report cards given to vaccinees and collaboration with the American Academy of Neurology
- Near-real time rapid-cycle analysis by the VSD
- Surveillance through the Vaccine Analytic Unit, a collaboration between the CDC, FDA, and Department of Defense, covering 1.5 million active US military personnel
- GBS case finding through the Emerging Infections Program, a collaboration between the CDC and 10 state health departments

As of January 2010, over 120 million doses of 2009 H1N1 vaccine had been distributed; 8294 VAERS reports had been received, the vast majority of which were not serious (eg, sore arms).[22] Six-percent of the reports were serious events, including 40 deaths; this is similar to what is seen with seasonal vaccine. Preliminary analysis showed no unique pattern of events, and there was no evidence that the deaths were caused by the vaccine. Fifty-six cases of GBS were reported, which is less than the expected 80 to 160 background cases that should occur each week.

■ Ad-Hoc Committees and Task Forces

From time to time, ad-hoc committees and task forces are constituted to address particular issues. The National Childhood Vaccine Injury Act of 1986, for example, mandated the establishment of the Task Force on Safer Childhood Vaccines, comprising representatives of several PHS agencies. The charge was to make recommendations promoting the development of safer vaccines and assuring improvement in licensing, manufacturing, processing, testing, labeling, warning, use instructions, distribution, storage, administration, field surveillance, adverse reaction reporting, recall of reactogenic lots, and research. The task force report, released in 1998, emphasized the need to assess and address public concerns about the risks and benefits of vaccines, conduct research on the biological basis for vaccine reactions, foster partnership between stakeholders, enhance the ability to detect adverse events, and improve coordination of effort between agencies.[23]

Another good example of an ad-hoc committee is the Immunization Safety Review Committee (ISRC), convened in 2001 by the Institute of Medicine (IOM), a private, nonprofit, nongovernmental organization of distinguished scholars. The ISRC consisted of 15 members with expertise in pediatrics, internal medicine, infectious diseases, immunology, epidemiology and biostatistics, public health, nursing, ethics, and risk communication, among other disciplines. Committee members were subject to strict selection criteria in order to avoid real or perceived conflicts of interest. The committee was charged with reviewing nine different vaccine safety hypotheses. Each review assessed scientific plausibility based on epidemiologic and clinical evidence of causality and experimental evidence for biologic mechanisms, as well as the significance of the issue in a broader societal context. Before release, the committee's reports were reviewed and critiqued by an independent panel of experts overseen by the National Research Council's Report Review Committee. **Table 2**.3 summarizes the findings of the ISRC.

In April 2009, the IOM convened a new committee to review the epidemiological, clinical, and biological evidence regarding adverse events associated with HPV vaccine, VAR, HepB, and influenza vaccine. A consensus report will be issued at the conclusion of the project.

■ The Safety Net in Action

The release of rhesus-human reassortant rotavirus vaccine-tetravalent (RRV-TV; RotaShield) in the United States and its rapid withdrawal illustrate how well the safety net works. The vaccine was licensed based on demonstrated safety and efficacy in clinical trials wherein nearly 11,000 children received the vaccine in its final formulation. With universal use, the vaccine was expected to prevent 55,000 hospitalizations and 25 deaths each year. Before licensure, an ACIP Working Group, the NIH, and the AAP considered the possibility of an association between the vaccine and intussusception but rejected a causal relationship based on statistical analyses of the few cases that did occur. Nevertheless, the package insert listed intussusception as a possible adverse reaction and postlicensure surveillance was mandated. The vaccine was licensed in August 1998. By July 1999 there were 15 reports of intussusception in the VAERS database, and several population-based investigations suggested a causal relationship. The CDC recommended suspension of vaccination, and by October 1999 the product was withdrawn from the market.[24]

TABLE 2.3 — Immunization Safety Review Committee Findings

Report Date	Topic	Findings
April 2001	*Measles-Mumps-Rubella Vaccine and Autism*	Reject causal relationship at the population level Cannot exclude possibility that MMR contributes to autism in a small number of children
October 2001	*Thimerosal-Containing Vaccines and Neurodevelopmental Disorders*	Hypothesis is biologically plausible Evidence is inadequate to accept or reject a causal relationship
February 2002	*Multiple Immunizations and Immune Dysfunction*	Reject causal relationship for increased risk of heterologous infections and type 1 diabetes Evidence is inadequate to accept or reject a causal relationship for allergic diseases Evidence for proposed mechanisms of allergy and autoimmunity is weak or theoretical
May 2002	*Hepatitis B Vaccine and Demyelinating Neurological Disorders*	Reject causal relationship for incident multiple sclerosis and multiple sclerosis relapse Evidence is inadequate to accept or reject a causal relationship for other demyelinating diseases Evidence for proposed mechanisms is weak
October 2002	*SV40 Contamination of Polio Vaccine and Cancer*	Evidence is inadequate to accept or reject a causal relationship for cancer Evidence is moderate that SV40 exposure could lead to human cancer

Date	Report	Findings
March 2003	Vaccinations and Sudden Unexpected Death in Infancy	Reject causal relationship for DTwP and for multiple simultaneous vaccinations Evidence is inadequate to accept or reject a causal relationship for DTaP, Hib, HepB, OPV, and IPV Evidence for proposed mechanisms is theoretical
October 2003	Influenza Vaccines and Neurological Complications	Accept causal relationship between 1976 swine influenza vaccine and Guillain-Barré syndrome Evidence is inadequate to accept or reject a causal relationship for other influenza vaccines Reject causal relationship for relapse of multiple sclerosis Evidence is inadequate to accept or reject a causal relationship for incident multiple sclerosis, optic neuritis, and other demyelinating disorders Evidence for proposed mechanisms is weak or theoretical
May 2004	Vaccines and Autism	Reject causal relationship between MMR and thimerosal-containing vaccines and autism Evidence for proposed mechanisms is theoretical

Adapted from Immunization Safety Review. Institute of Medicine of the National Academies Web site. http://www.iom.edu/Activities/PublicHealth/ImmunizationSafety.aspx. Accessed January 20, 2010.

It is estimated that intussusception attributable to RRV-TV occurred once for every 10,000 children vaccinated, although some argue that the risk was actually much less. In any event, the risk was so small that it could not have been detected in the pre-licensure trials, given the number of children enrolled. However, the vaccine safety net performed remarkably well, such that in a very short period of time the potential danger signal was detected, studies were conducted, and use of the vaccine was suspended. As a result of this experience, new-generation rotavirus vaccines were tested in tens of thousands of children before licensure in order to detect even a weak association with intussusception. Even these massive trials, however, could not detect extremely small associations, and rigorous postmarketing studies are being conducted. Ultimately, the decision to use any new vaccine will necessarily need to balance the known risks, however small, with the known complications of disease, and society will need to answer the question as to where the threshold for risk tolerance should be set.

Financing

Table 2.4 illustrates a simple truth: for any given individual in the United States, the total cost for all routinely recommended vaccines has skyrocketed, driven by the increased number of vaccines that are recommended for universal use and the increased cost of newer vaccines. Layered on top of the purchase price for vaccines are the costs associated with administration, from personnel time, storage, and equipment to wastage and insurance.

The system for financing immunization in the United States rests on a unique partnership between the public and private sectors—more than half of the purchase cost is borne by public

TABLE 2.4 — Cost of Vaccines (US$) in the Routine Childhood Schedule

Sector	1987	2003	2009 Boys	Girls
Public	34	437	1086	1403
Private	116	705	1602	1918

The total cost of all recommended vaccines from birth to 18 years of age (including influenza for 2009) is given. Public and private sector costs are from Hinman AR, et al. *Clin Infect Dis.* 2004;38:1440-1446, and CDC Vaccine Price List. Centers for Disease Control and Prevention Web site. http://www.cdc.gov/vaccines/programs/vfc/cdc-vac-price-list .htm. Accessed January 20, 2010. The least expensive vaccination strategies and products were used in the calculations. The difference between boys and girls in 2009 is due to the HPV vaccine, which is only routinely recommended for girls.

entities, but most of the vaccinating is done in private settings. As seen in **Figure 2.6**, only 47% of the purchase cost of routine childhood vaccines is borne by the private sector; most of this is reimbursed through private insurance, but some comes directly out-of-pocket. Many states have laws requiring insurers to cover childhood immunizations, at least to some degree. Some mandate coverage in accord with the recommended childhood immunization schedule, while others make reference to appropriate pediatric vaccines. Some states prohibit deductibles and coinsurance, and while self-insured employers may be exempt from such regulation, federal statutes prohibit employers providing vaccine coverage as of May 1, 1993 from reducing that coverage. Insurance plans vary in terms of which vaccines they cover for both children and adults and to what extent they reimburse for vaccine administration. In general, managed care plans are more likely than indemnity plans to cover vaccines and to promote their use. Delays in covering new vaccines are common—some insurers wait until official recommendations are published before they will provide reimbursement.

FIGURE 2.6 — Childhood Vaccine Doses According to Funding Source, 2007

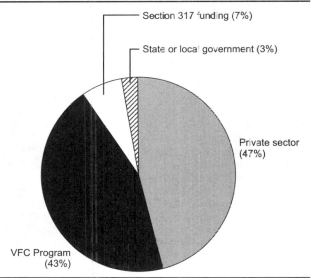

Includes vaccines for children 0 to 6 years of age, excluding influenza vaccine.

Data from Shen AK, et al. *Pediatrics*. 2009;124:S540-S547.

■ Children

Public sector funds for vaccination include the following sources:

- *The Vaccines for Children (VFC) Program*—Created in 1993 by the Omnibus Budget Reconciliation Act, VFC is a federal program that guarantees immunization services for children 18 years of age and younger who are 1) Medicaid-eligible; 2) uninsured; 3) underinsured and receiving immunizations at federally-qualified health centers (FQHCs) or rural health clinics (RHCs); or 4) American Indian or Alaska Native.

  Through this program, vaccines are purchased by the CDC at reduced rates and provided to participating private practices and public clinics free of charge. Providers are prohibited from charging the patient for the vaccine itself. Whereas they *can* charge patients administration fees, within limits established by the Centers for Medicare and Medicaid Services, they cannot *deny* vaccination if the patients cannot pay the fee (claims for these fees can still be submitted to Medicaid for those children who are enrolled). There are no regulations regarding charges for the office visit itself or nonvaccination services.

  Any private provider who sees eligible children can participate in the program; this has resulted in a shift toward private sector delivery of vaccines, establishing an anchor point for the medical home for many children. Covered vaccines are determined by ACIP resolutions; such resolutions may pertain to routinely recommended or permissively recommended vaccines, with some differences on the resulting actions (see **Table 2.5**). Even when a VFC resolution is passed, significant delays in securing a federal contract may occur. During such delays, state Medicaid programs are bound to cover ACIP-recommended vaccines. Common questions about the VFC program are addressed in **Table 2.6**.

  It is important to remember that VFC is an *entitlement program*, which means that Congress is obliged to appropriate the funds necessary to purchase the covered vaccines, no matter how much they cost. At the same time, there are an increasing number of children who are falling out of the system, namely those who qualify for VFC because their private insurance does not cover all routinely recommended vaccines (the *underinsured*) but who must receive their VFC vaccines at FQHCs or RHCs. The simple fact is that many of these children do not make it to these sites, and the fall-back position—namely, to receive the uncovered vaccines at the local health department—is less of an option as the other public funding sources listed below become more inadequate.

  There is no VFC-equivalent program for adults.

TABLE 2.5 — Actions Required Under VFC Resolutions

Action	ACIP Recommendation	
	Affirmative	Permissive
Provider *expected to* offer the vaccine proactively to VFC-eligible children	Yes	No
Provider *may* offer the vaccine proactively to VFC-eligible children	Yes	Yes
Provider *expected to* vaccinate VFC-eligible children on request	Yes	Yes, if the provider stocks the vaccine; if not, the child should be referred
Immunization programs *expected to* promote the recommendation	Yes	No
Uptake is taken as a measure of provider or program performance	Yes	No

Adapted from Rodewald LE. ACIP Meeting, October 21, 2009, Centers for Disease Control and Prevention Web site. http://www.cdc.gov/vaccines/recs/acip/slides-oct09.htm#hpv. Accessed November 28, 2009.

TABLE 2.6 — Common Questions About the VFC Program

Question	Answer
Are providers required to post a sign stating that eligible children will not be denied vaccine?	No.
Can a provider refuse to administer VFC vaccine to an eligible child?	Private VFC providers, unless otherwise required by state law, do not have to vaccinate walk-ins who are not established patients. For established patients, vaccination cannot be denied because of inability to pay the administration fee.
How does a medical or health savings account affect eligibility?	Patients with such accounts must also be insured. If their insurance does not cover vaccines, they can receive VFC vaccine at FQHCs or RHCs.
Is an uninsured child eligible if his parents plan to insure him in the near future?	Yes. Eligibility is determined on the day of vaccination. Eligibility screening must take place at every vaccination visit.
Are all children from birth through 18 years of age who are enrolled in Medicaid automatically eligible?	Yes.
What about children who have Medicaid as a secondary insurance?	Yes, they are also eligible.
If a child starts a vaccine series at 18 years of age, can the series be completed with VFC vaccine if he turns 19?	No.
Are American Indian/Alaska Native children still eligible for VFC vaccine even if they have insurance?	Yes.

If a child's insurance covers a percentage of the cost of vaccination, can he receive VFC vaccine? No.

Can all children at a school-based clinic receive VFC vaccine? No. They must still be screened for eligibility (this can be incorporated into the consent process).

If a child has exceeded his insurance coverage for provider visits in a given year, is he considered underinsured for VFC purposes? Yes.

Adapted from VCF: frequently asked questions. Centers for Disease Control and Prevention Web site. http://www.cdc.gov/Vaccines/programs/vfc/projects/faqs-doc.htm. Accessed February 26, 2010.

- *Section 317 Funds*—States, territories, protectorates, and several designated cities may purchase vaccines through block grants under Section 317 of the Public Health Service Act. The majority of these funds are used for childhood immunization, but adolescent and adult programs may be supported as well. Section 317 funds may also be used to support infrastructure and programmatic activities such as quality assurance, immunization information systems (IISs), disease surveillance, and school- or community-based delivery services. The main intent of the 317 program is to provide vaccines to people who fall outside of the VFC program. The problem is that this program—in contrast to VFC—represents *discretionary federal spending*. The amount allocated by Congress, therefore, varies from year to year, and as the costs of vaccination have increased, so has the financing gap.[25]
- *State and Local Funds*—States may appropriate funds to support both childhood and adult immunizations, but in general the contribution of this source to the whole funding picture is small (**Figure 2.6**). The State Children's Health Insurance Program (SCHIP), enacted in 1997, is a federal block grant program targeted to low-income children who are not eligible for Medicaid and are otherwise uninsured. States can use SCHIP funds to expand Medicaid or to create separate, freestanding children's insurance programs.

As of 2006, 18 states and territories had some type of universal purchase policy. Under these plans, federal, state, and local monies are used to purchase recommended childhood vaccines at the CDC-negotiated price. The vaccines are then distributed to providers free of charge for administration to children, regardless of insurance status. Providers may still charge administration fees but reimbursement varies. Supporters argue that universal purchase removes financial barriers to immunization, improves coverage rates, reinforces the concept of the medical home, increases immunization rates, improves efficiency, reduces overhead at the provider level, and facilitates participation in IISs. Detractors argue that public funds should not be used to pay for vaccines that insurers would otherwise cover. In addition, concerns have been raised about potential restrictions on product choice and provider autonomy, as well as loss of financial incentives for manufacturers to bring new vaccines to market. Importantly, no states have adopted new universal purchase policies since the 1990s, and many states have weakened existing ones.

■ Adults

Most private insurance plans cover vaccination of adults.[26] Medicare, an entirely federal insurance program for adults 65 years of age and older, covers influenza vaccine, PPSV23, and HepB (for persons of any age with end-stage renal disease or other high-risk conditions) under Part B (medical insurance). Other vaccines may be covered under Part D (prescription drug coverage), depending on the plan, but there may be requirements for prior authorization to determine medical necessity. Moreover, Part D involves pharmacies, not physicians. So options include writing a prescription and having a pharmacist administer the vaccine, or purchasing and administering the vaccine and billing the patient directly so that Medicare can be petitioned for reimbursement. In general, Medicare reimbursement includes the cost of administration.

The vast majority of Section 317 funds are used to purchase vaccines for children, not adults. Medicaid is a source of vaccine funding for adults, but coverage and reimbursement rates vary widely from state to state. States also may use their own funds to purchase vaccines for adults, but only a minority of states do so. Finally, some vaccine manufacturers have assistance programs for qualifying patients.

■ The Future of Vaccine Financing

The current system for funding vaccine services has achieved high levels of childhood immunization, but new challenges exist, including the increased number of recommended vaccines, high prices, disparities in coverage, low levels of adult immunization, the growing burden of vaccine practice on clinicians, shortages, and the increased costs of bringing new products to market. With these factors in mind, the CDC asked the IOM to study vaccine financing. In a 2003 report, the Committee on the Evaluation of Vaccine Purchase Financing in the United States recommended replacement of existing government vaccine purchasing programs with a new vaccine insurance mandate, subsidy, and voucher plan.[27] In 2005, the NVAC issued a response to the IOM report.[28] While agreeing on many points—including the need for action in ensuring easy access to vaccines, stabilizing the market so that it remains attractive to manufacturers, and the need for additional funding—NVAC suggested incremental improvements in the current system rather than replacing it with something else. In 2006, NVAC established a Vaccine Financing Working Group to obtain stakeholder input and formulate an approach to financing childhood and adolescent vaccinations.[29] The final recommendations, released in 2008, are summarized in **Table 2.7**.

Supply

The last decade has seen unique and unprecedented shortages in the supply of many routinely used vaccines.[30] The impact of these shortages has included frequent and sometimes confusing changes in the recommended immunization schedule, temporary revision of state school entry requirements, parental frustration,

TABLE 2.7 — NVAC Recommendations on Financing Childhood and Adolescent Vaccinations

Public-sector vaccine purchasing for the underinsured—Expand VFC program to include VFC-eligible, underinsured patients receiving immunizations at public health department clinics; these patients must now receive VFC vaccines at federally qualified health centers and rural health clinics

Vaccine administration reimbursement for VFC-eligible patients—Expand VFC program to cover the costs of vaccine administration; provider costs for vaccination services are summarized in **Table 4.8**

Vaccine administration reimbursement for VFC-eligible patients enrolled in Medicaid
- Publish actual Medicaid vaccine administration reimbursement rates by state each year (CDC and CMS)
- Update the maximum allowable Medicaid administration reimbursement amounts for each state, to include all appropriate nonvaccine-related costs (CMS)
- Increase federal matching rate for vaccine administration reimbursement to levels comparable with other public health services

Vaccine delivery in the medical home
- Review RVU coding to ensure that nonvaccine costs are accurately reflected, including potential costs and cost savings through use of combination vaccines (AMA Relative Value Scale Update Committee)
- Reduce financial burden for initial and ongoing vaccine inventories, particularly for new vaccines, using mechanisms like extended payment periods (manufacturers and distributors)
- Provide technical assistance regarding efficient business practices, including contracting, billing, and identifying best practices (professional medical organizations)
- Participate in buying pools to obtain volume-ordering discounts (providers)

Underinsurance rates and financial barriers
- Develop and support employer health education efforts that communicate the value of good preventive care (CDC, professional medical organizations, and other stakeholders)
- Develop flexible contract language to permit coverage and reimbursement for new or altered recommendations as well as price changes (insurers and health care purchasers)
- Provide first-dollar coverage (ie, no deductibles or copayments) for vaccines (insurers)

Continued

TABLE 2.7 — *Continued*

Underinsurance rates and financial barriers *(continued)*
- Base reimbursement policies on methodologically sound cost studies of efficient practices that include all costs associated with vaccination (insurers and health care purchasers)

Federal agencies and offices
- Report annually the size and scope of the Section 317 program and appropriate funds at the level specified in that report (CDC and Congress)
- Collect and publish data on the costs associated with vaccination according to the NVAC standards, including information about reimbursement, provider type, geographic region, and insurance status; use this information in determining state Medicaid reimbursement rates (CDC and CMS)
- Calculate the marginal increase in insurance premiums if plans were to cover all routinely recommended vaccines (NVPO)
- Convene a panel to consider whether tax credits could be used to reduce or eliminate underinsurance (NVAC)
- Decrease the time from the creation of recommendations to their publication (CDC)
- Expand Section 317 funding to support additional local, state, and national public health infrastructure (Congress)
- Continue federal funding for cost-benefit studies

State agencies and offices
- Encourage provider participation in the VFC program (state, local and federal governments and professional medical organizations)
- Develop mechanisms for billing insured patients served in the public sector, and reinvest reimbursements in immunization programs (states and localities, with CDC support)

Complementary venues
- Cover all costs associated with compliance with school immunization requirements
- Promote shared public-private approaches to fund school-based and other complementary-venue efforts

Parentheses indicate the primary target of the recommendations.

Adapted from National Vaccine Advisory Committee. *Pediatrics.* 2009; 124:S558-S562.

and a burden placed on providers to track interrupted schedules and recall patients when vaccine supplies returned to sufficiency. To date, there is no evidence that shortages have caused disease outbreaks.

Shortages result from a convergence of factors, including the following[31]:

- *Fewer manufacturers*—Vaccines are low-profit products compared with other pharmaceuticals. The costs of development have skyrocketed, the time line from preclinical testing to market may be longer than a decade, and the risks are substantial—a licensed vaccine may or may not be recommended for use in large numbers of people. Moreover, the risk of failure persists for some time after marketing—the low tolerance for adverse events leaves manufacturers vulnerable to market failure after millions of doses have been distributed. In the late 1960s, there were >20 major vaccine manufacturers licensed in the United States; today, there are only six—GlaxoSmithKline, AstraZeneca (which acquired MedImmune in 2007), Merck, Novartis, Sanofi Pasteur, and Pfizer (which acquired Wyeth in 2009). Some of this decrease was due to mergers but some resulted from companies simply getting out of the business. With so few manufacturers, disruptions at one company can have a major effect on supply. For single-source products like PCV and VAR, the effect is magnified.

- *Business decisions*—Some companies have chosen to pull products from the market rather than invest in costly changes in manufacturing processes or facilities. Such changes might be mandated in order to adhere to GMPs; others might be prompted by new recommendations. An example of the latter was the 1999 recommendation to remove thimerosal from childhood vaccines (see *Chapter 7: Addressing Concerns About Vaccines—Did the Thimerosal Used as a Preservative in Vaccines Cause Autism?*), which led some companies to pull out rather than retool their manufacturing and packaging processes (ie, to make single-dose vials or prefilled syringes) and demonstrate equivalency of the reformulated products in clinical trials.

- *Production problems*—Production problems may have a biologic basis. For example, the influenza A(H3N2) strain used for the 2000-2001 vaccine grew slowly in culture, delaying vaccine production. Similarly, a low yield of vaccine strain VZV in culture led to shortages of MMRV. Production problems can also result from routine physical plant maintenance activities.

- *Underestimated demand*—The recommendation in April 2000 to decrease the age for routine influenza vaccination from 65 to 50 years compounded production problems by increasing demand. Similarly, greater-than-expected demand for PCV7 and MCV4-D after each of these vaccines was licensed contributed to shortages.

Recent vaccine shortages are summarized in **Figure 2.7**. When deferral of doses is recommended because of shortages, providers should keep lists of patients who will need to be recalled once supplies improve.

The CDC has maintained stockpiles of vaccines since 1983. These might be more accurately termed *storage and rotation contracts* or *dynamic strategic inventories*—some portion of vaccine production lots enters the stockpile, and older vaccine with at least 12 months of shelf life left is released onto the market. Between 1983 and 2002, only single-source vaccines were stockpiled. Since 2002, the goal has been to stockpile 6 months' worth of each routine childhood vaccine (except for influenza vaccine, which changes in composition from year to year). The stockpile has been accessed on at least 8 occasions because of supply issues.

In 2003, the NVAC suggested the following short-term measures to improve vaccine supply[32]:
- Increase funding for vaccine stockpiles that would include all routinely administered vaccines
- Increase support for CBER in order to enhance review of the scientific evidence supporting the safety, efficacy, and quality of vaccines
- Highlight the function of NVPO and NVAC in identifying vaccine priorities
- Maintain and strengthen the National Vaccine Injury Compensation Program, which removes liability concerns as a barrier to manufacturers; include coverage for injuries due to preservatives, additives, and excipients, not just the vaccine antigens
- Require manufacturers to warn HHS of intent to withdraw a product from the market
- Improve availability of accurate supply information for opinion leaders and consumers
- Enhance the valuation of vaccines through educational campaigns

84

FIGURE 2.7 — Recent Vaccine Shortages in the United States

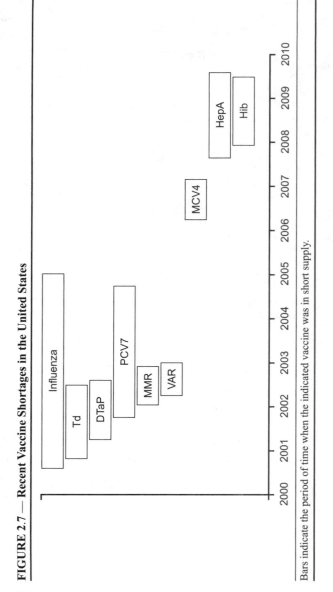

Bars indicate the period of time when the indicated vaccine was in short supply.

1. Light DW, et al. *Vaccine*. 2009;27:6627-6633.

2. Lieu T, Meltzer MI, Messonnier ML. Guidance for health economics studies presented to the Advisory Committee on Immunization Practices (ACIP). Centers for Disease Control and Prevention Web site. http://www.cdc.gov/vaccines/recs/acip/downloads/economics -studies-guidance.pdf. Accessed March 16, 2010.

3. Advisory Committee on Immunization Practices Workgroup on the Use of Vaccines During Pregnancy and Breastfeeding. http://www .cdc.gov/vaccines/recs/acip/downloads/preg-principles05-01-08.pdf. Accessed February 27, 1010.

4. Kroger AT, et al. *MMWR*. 2006;55(RR-15):1-48.

5. Centers for Disease Control and Prevention. *Epidemiology and Prevention of Vaccine-Preventable Diseases*. 11th ed. Atkinson W, et al, eds. Washington, DC: Public Health Foundation, 2009.

6. Pickering LK, Baker CJ, Kimberlin DW, Long SS, eds. *Red Book: 2009 Report of the Committee on Infectious Diseases*. 28th ed. Elk Grove Village, IL: American Academy of Pediatrics; 2009.

7. Draft Strategic National Vaccine Plan. National Vaccine Program Office Web site. http://www.hhs.gov/nvpo/vacc_plan/2008plan /draftvaccineplan.pdf. Accessed February 26, 2010.

8. Priorities for the National Vaccine Plan. Institute of Medicine Web site. http://www.iom.edu/Reports/2009/Priorities-for-the-National -Vaccine-Plan.aspx. Accessed February 26, 2010.

9. Immunization Coverage in the U.S. Centers for Disease Control and Prevention Web site. http://www.cdc.gov/vaccines/stats-surv /imz-coverage.htm#nis. Accessed January 20, 2010.

10. Molinari NA, et al. M*MMWR*. 2009;58:921-926.

11. Stokley S, et al. *MMWR*. 2009;58:927-1001.

12. Luman ET, et al. *JAMA*. 2005;293:1204-1211.

13. Euler GL, et al. *MMWR*. 2009;58:1091-1095.

14. Stanwyck C, et al. *MMWR*. 2007;56:819-821.

15. Roush SW, McIntyre L, Baldy LM, eds. *Manual for the Surveillance of Vaccine-Preventable Diseases*. 4th ed, 2008. http://www.cdc .gov/vaccines/pubs/surv-manual/default.htm#compressed. Accessed January 21, 2010.

16. Active bacterial core surveillance. Centers for Disease Control and Prevention Web site. http://www.cdc.gov/abcs. Accessed January 20, 2010.

17. New vaccine surveillance network. Centers for Disease Control and Prevention Web site. http://www.cdc.gov/vaccines/stats-surv/nvsn /default.htm. Accessed January 20, 2010.

18. Zhou W, et al. *MMWR*. 2003;52(SS-1):1-24.

19. Varricchio F, et al. *Pediatr Infect Dis J*. 2004;23:287-294.

20. Chen RT, et al. *Pediatrics*. 1997;99:765-773.

21. Bonhoeffer J, et al. *Vaccine*. 2002;21:298-302.

22. Summary of 2009 monovalent H1N1 influenza vaccine data—Vaccine Adverse Event Reporting System. Centers for Disease Control and Prevention Web site. http://vaers.hhs.gov/resources/2010H1N1Summary_Jan22.pdf. Accessed February 27, 2010.

23. National Institute of Allergy and Infectious Diseases; National Institutes of Health. Task Force on Safer Childhood Vaccines: Final Report and Recommendations (1998). http://permanent.access.gpo.gov/lps22576/safevacc.pdf. Accessed January 21, 2010.

24. Peter G, et al. *Pediatrics*. 2002;110:e67.

25. Lee GM, et al. *JAMA*. 2007;298:638-643.

26. Orenstein WA, et al. *Clin Pharmacol Ther*. 2007;82:764-768.

27. Committee on the Evaluation of Vaccine Purchase Financing in the United States, Board on Health Care Services, Institute of Medicine of the National Academes. Financing Vaccines in the 21st Century: Assuring Access and Availability. http://www.nap.edu/catalog.php?record_id=10782. Accessed January 21, 2010.

28. Hinman AR, et al. *Am J Prev Med*. 2005;29:71-75.

29. National Vaccine Advisory Committee. *Pediatrics*. 2009;124:S558-S562.

30. Hinman AR, et al. *Annu Rev Public Health*. 2006;27:235-259.

31. Klein JO, et al. *Pediatrics*. 2006;117:2269-2275.

32. Santoli JM, et al. *JAMA*. 2003;290:3122-3128.

3

Standards, Principles, and Regulations

Healthy People 2010: Objectives for Improving Health, issued January 25, 2000, was a comprehensive set of health objectives for the first decade of the new century issued by the US Department of Health and Human Services (HHS). An extension of the 1979 Surgeon General's Report entitled *Healthy People* and *Healthy People 2000: National Health Promotion and Disease Prevention Objectives*, the updated *Healthy People 2010* identified the most significant preventable threats to health and focused public and private efforts to address those threats. The agenda was developed over several years by scientists, federal and state agencies, and national professional organizations, with input from the public.

Healthy People 2010 aimed to increase quality and years of healthy life and to eliminate health disparities. Twenty-eight focus areas were identified, one of which was *Immunization and Infectious Diseases*, wherein the following aspects of vaccines were emphasized:

- Vaccines can prevent disease and death from infectious diseases, but they do not necessarily eliminate the causative organisms; by extension, decreased vaccine coverage can lead to reemergence of disease.
- Vaccines protect individuals, and vaccinated individuals protect society through herd immunity.
- Vaccines provide significant cost-benefits.

Tremendous progress in reducing indigenous cases of vaccine-preventable diseases was noted, successes mediated by outreach to underserved populations, expansion of school entry requirements, public financing of childhood vaccinations, and the widespread use of novel, highly effective vaccines. However, the report highlighted the persistence of underserved groups and the fact that most vaccine-preventable diseases in the United States occur in adults, who are much less likely to be appropriately immunized.

The *Healthy People 2010* report set general objectives for prevention of disease through universal and targeted vaccination; in addition, the goal for coverage with universally recommended vaccines was set at 90%. Objectives for *Healthy People 2020* are expected in early 2010.

Standards for both pediatric and adult immunization practices have been developed. Rather than setting a mark for the minimum standard of care, they represent the most desirable practices that pediatric health care professionals should strive to achieve. Providers also should be aware that extensive evidence-based guidelines on immunization, such as those from the Infectious Diseases Society of America (IDSA), have been published.[1]

■ Pediatric Standards

In 1992, a working group convened by the National Vaccine Advisory Committee (NVAC) developed a set of standards for pediatric immunization practices, largely in response to the measles resurgence in the late 1980s. These standards were revised and updated in 2003 and have been endorsed by most professional organizations that deal with pediatric immunization.[2]

Key elements of each standard are listed below. The means to implement many of these standards are elaborated upon elsewhere in this book.

- *Standard 1—Vaccination services are readily available.* Routinely recommended vaccines should always be part of primary care. Vaccination status should be assessed at all points of contact with the health care system, including sub-specialty practices, schools, and specialty clinics. If vaccines cannot be offered at these sites, patients should be referred elsewhere. Primary care providers should be notified about vaccines given outside the medical home.

- *Standard 2—Vaccinations are coordinated with other health care services and provided in a medical home when possible.* Vaccinations should be coordinated with routine well-child visits or other visits. Patients who receive vaccines outside the medical home should be encouraged to receive subsequent vaccines from their primary care provider. Those who do not have a primary care provider should receive assistance in finding one.

- *Standard 3—Barriers to vaccination are identified and minimized.* Vaccine visits should be scheduled promptly and, if necessary, independently of visits for other well-child services. Long waiting periods in the office should be avoided and culturally and age-appropriate educational materials should be available. A physical examination is not required for immunization—observation and screening are sufficient. Providers should ask parents and patients how they could make vaccinations more accessible.

- *Standard 4—Patient costs are minimized.* Money should not be a barrier to vaccination. Free vaccines are available through public programs like the Vaccines for Children

(VFC) Program, Public Health Service Section 317 grants to states, and state and local programs. Providers utilizing these resources should make it clear that even though the patient may be charged for administration of the vaccines, they will not be denied vaccination because of inability to pay. Health and insurance plans should cover all routinely recommended vaccines and reimbursement to providers should be enough to cover all expenses associated with delivering vaccines in practice.

- *Standard 5—Health care professionals review the vaccination and health status of patients at every encounter to determine which vaccines are indicated.* Any and all health care visits are an opportunity to review vaccination status and minimize missed opportunities. This might include, for example, emergency room visits, hospitalizations, and appointments with specialists. Undervaccination should be documented in the patient's chart. Providers who do not give vaccines should refer patients to a primary care provider who does.
- *Standard 6—Health care professionals assess for and follow only medically accepted contraindications.* There are very few true contraindications to vaccination. Decisions to withhold vaccination should be supported by published guidelines and should be documented in the medical record.
- *Standard 7—Parents/guardians and patients are educated about the benefits and risks of vaccination in a culturally appropriate manner and in easy-to-understand language.* Sufficient time should be allowed to discuss the benefits of vaccines, the diseases they prevent, and the known risks. The schedule should be reviewed and the importance of bringing the hand-held vaccination record should be emphasized. Parents should be told how to report adverse events. Vaccine Information Statements (VISs) should be provided and supplemented by oral or visual explanations when appropriate, and the parent's questions and concerns should be addressed. Reporting of adverse events should be encouraged.
- *Standard 8—Health care professionals follow appropriate procedures for vaccine storage and handling.* This is critical to maintaining potency and effectiveness.
- *Standard 9—Up-to-date, written vaccination protocols are accessible at all locations where vaccines are administered.* Protocols should detail vaccine storage and handling; the recommended schedule; contraindications; administration technique; treatment and reporting of adverse events; risk-benefit communication; and record maintenance and accessibility.
- *Standard 10—People who administer vaccines and staff who manage or support vaccine administration are knowledgeable and receive ongoing education.* Vaccine recommendations change frequently, and all personnel involved

in the process of vaccine delivery should remain abreast of these changes. Many resources are available for this purpose, including free e-mail listservs and distance-based training opportunities through the CDC.

- *Standard 11—Health care professionals simultaneously administer as many indicated vaccine doses as possible.* There are essentially no routine vaccines that cannot be administered at the same time at separate sites. When vaccines are not given simultaneously, arrangements should be made for the patient's earliest return to receive the needed vaccines. Although not specifically mentioned in the standard, combination vaccines allow delivery of multiple antigens with fewer shots and are generally preferred to separately administered components.

- *Standard 12—Vaccination records for patients are accurate, complete, and easily accessible.* This standard goes beyond the record keeping mandated by law. It calls for a permanent record that the parents carry with them and verification of vaccines received from other providers. All vaccinations should be reported to state or local immunization information systems (IISs or registries). Vaccine refusal also should be documented.

- *Standard 13—Health care professionals report adverse events after vaccination promptly and accurately to the Vaccine Adverse Events Reporting System (VAERS) and are aware of a separate program, the National Vaccine Injury Compensation Program (VICP).* These programs are described below. The law requires reporting of certain events, and reporting of all significant events is encouraged, even if causality is not established. Health care professionals should be aware that parents and patients could report adverse events to VAERS on their own.

- *Standard 14—All personnel who have contact with patients are appropriately vaccinated.* Offices and clinics should have policies to review and maintain the vaccination status of their staff.

- *Standard 15—Systems are used to remind parents/ guardians, patients, and health care professionals when vaccinations are due and to recall those who are overdue.* Computerized or manual tracking, recall, and reminder systems should be in place.

- *Standard 16—Office- or clinic-based patient record reviews and vaccination coverage assessments are performed annually.* A simple random survey of patient records can yield information about coverage rates, missed opportunities, and record quality; in general, physicians will find that they overestimate the proportion of their patients who are appropriately immunized. Systematic assessments should be conducted.

Feedback and incentives are important elements of quality improvement.

- *Standard 17—Health care professionals practice community-based approaches*. Providers should be responsive to the needs of their patients, but it should be recognized that high coverage rates protect the entire community. Partnering with other service providers, such as the US Department of Agriculture's Special Supplemental Nutrition Program for Women, Infants, and Children (WIC), advocacy groups, schools, and service organizations should be encouraged.

In 1996, the ACIP, AAP, AAFP, and AMA called for routine health care visits for all children at 11 to 12 years of age. Before 2005, vaccinations during adolescence consisted for the most part of catch-up, with the exception of the Td booster. Since then, new vaccines (MCV, Tdap, and HPV vaccine) have been recommended for adolescents, and since 2006, the National Immunization Survey has reported coverage rates for adolescents. In 2007, the routine schedule for the first time included a stand-alone chart for older children and adolescents. While there are as yet no adolescent standards per se, it is worth emphasizing that optimally immunizing adolescents represents a special set of challenges for providers, not the least of which is the fact that adolescents make infrequent visits for preventive health services.

■ **Adult Standards**

The National Coalition for Adult Immunization first offered standards for adult immunization practices in 1990. In 2003, an NVAC working group revised these standards to reflect changes in the health care system and new information regarding adult vaccine coverage.[3] Many of the standards, given in **Table 3.1**, parallel the pediatric standards.

Annual mortality from vaccine-preventable diseases among adults reaches into the tens of thousands; hospitalizations reach into the hundreds of thousands and societal costs into the billions of dollars. Yet historically, adult and adolescent immunization rates have lagged behind childhood rates.[4] In June 2007, the IDSA published a set of principles—billed as a "call to action"—designed to rectify this situation.[5] Some of the principles reiterate the adult practice standards; others extend into the area of policy. In November 2008, the IDSA and the American College of Physicians released a joint statement encouraging subspecialty physicians to take a more active role in keeping adults up-to-date.[6]

National Childhood Vaccine Injury Act

In response to growing public concern about vaccine safety and the effects that liability issues were having on the pharmaceuti-

TABLE 3.1 — Standards for Adult Immunization Practices

Standard 1—Adult vaccination services are readily available

Standard 2—Barriers are identified and minimized

Standard 3— "Out-of-pocket" costs are minimized

Standard 4—Health care professionals routinely review the immunization status of patients

Standard 5—Health care professionals assess for valid contraindications

Standard 6—Patients are educated about risks and benefits in easy-to-understand language

Standard 7—Written protocols are available at all locations where vaccines are administered

Standard 8—Persons who administer vaccines are properly trained

Standard 9—Health care professionals recommend simultaneous administration of indicated vaccine doses

Standard 10—Immunization records are accurate and easily accessible

Standard 11—All personnel who have contact with patients are appropriately immunized

Standard 12—Systems are developed and used to remind patients and health care professionals when vaccinations are due and to recall patients who are overdue

Standard 13—Standing orders are employed

Standard 14—Regular assessments of coverage levels are conducted in providers' practices

Standard 15—Patient-oriented and community-based approaches are used to reach target populations

Adapted from Poland GA, et al; National Vaccine Advisory Committee, Ad Hoc Working Group for the Development of Standards for Adult Immunization Practices. *Am J Prev Med.* 2003;25:144-150.

cal industry (threatening vaccine supply), Congress passed the National Childhood Vaccine Injury Act of 1986 (NCVIA). The NCVIA established two important programs that providers need to be familiar with, the VICP and VAERS. In addition, the NCVIA required providers to give adult vaccine recipients or the parents or guardians of minors receiving vaccines a VIS for each vaccine received.

■ **National Vaccine Injury Compensation Program (VICP)**

The VICP, which went into effect on October 1, 1988, is a no-fault alternative to the tort system for resolving claims that result from adverse reactions to mandated childhood vaccines.[7] It is administered jointly by the Health Resources and Services

Administration of HHS, the US Court of Federal Claims (the Court), and the Department of Justice (DOJ), and is funded by an excise tax levied on every dose of vaccine that is purchased.

Anyone who feels they were injured by a covered vaccine must first pursue a remedy through the VICP. In order to receive compensation, petitioners must show that any one of the following occurred: 1) they incurred an injury found in the Vaccine Injury Table (VIT)[8]; 2) the vaccine caused the injury; or 3) the vaccine significantly aggravated a pre-existing condition. The VIT, which lists specific injuries or conditions and the time frames in which they must have occurred, serves as a basis for presumption of causation (the listed events are similar to those in the Reportable Events Table [RET]; see below and **Table 3.2**). Individuals can file claims for injuries not listed in the VIT, but *proof of causation* must be given. In recent years, the standard for proof seems to have shifted from a *preponderance of the evidence* to *biologic plausibility*.

In order for a claim to be filed, the injury must have lasted for at least 6 months following vaccination, resulted in hospitalization and surgery, or resulted in death. In order to be paid, the petitioners must prove that a) they received a vaccine listed on the VIT, and b) the first signs of injury occurred within the specified time frame, or the vaccine caused the injury or caused an existing illness to get worse (it must also be determined that the injury or death did not have another cause). When a claim is filed, HHS reviews the medical aspects and makes recommendations to a DOJ lawyer representing the Secretary of Health and Human Services, who reviews the legal aspects of the case. The HHS and DOJ reviews are then forwarded to the Court, wherein a Special Master (a lawyer appointed by the Court) decides if the claim will be paid and how much money will be offered. If the medical case is straightforward—for example, an individual develops chronic arthritis (not otherwise explained) within 7 to 42 days after receiving a rubella-containing vaccine—HHS may concede the case in its review, acknowledging that the injury fits the VIT definition (this is often referred to as a *Table injury*). In this instance, the Special Masters will usually pay the claim. If it is not a Table injury and HHS contests the claim, hearings may be held. The decision of the Special Masters can be appealed by either party (HHS or the petitioner) to a judge of the Court, then to the US Court of Appeals for the Federal Circuit, and ultimately to the US Supreme Court.

Vaccines recommended by the ACIP for routine use in children are automatically covered under the VICP. Advice regarding the VICP and recommended changes to the VIT comes from the Advisory Commission on Childhood Vaccines, which consists of 9 members (3 health care professionals, 3 members of the general public, and 3 attorneys) who meet at least quarterly. Nonvoting, ex-officio members include the Director of the National Institutes

TABLE 3.2 — Reportable Events Table (Effective November 10, 2008)

Note: For all vaccines, events listed in the package insert as contraindications to additional doses are considered reportable events, even if they are not listed here. Reporting of any clinically significant or unexpected event for any vaccine is encouraged. Manufacturers are required to report all adverse events made known to them for any vaccine.

Vaccine	Event[a]	Interval From Vaccination When Event Occurs
Tetanus (in any combination)	Anaphylaxis or anaphylactic shock	7 days
	Brachial neuritis	28 days
Pertussis (in any combination)	Anaphylaxis or anaphylactic shock	7 days
	Encephalopathy or encephalitis	7 days
MMR (in any combination)	Anaphylaxis or anaphylactic shock	7 days
	Encephalopathy or encephalitis	15 days
Rubella (in any combination)	Chronic arthritis	42 days
Measles (in any combination)	Thrombocytopenic purpura	30 days
	Vaccine-strain measles virus infection in an immunodeficient recipient	6 months
OPV	Paralytic polio	Immunocompetent: 30 days
		Immunocompromised: 6 months
	Vaccine-strain poliovirus infection	Immunocompetent: 30 days
		Immunocompromised: 6 months
IPV	Anaphylaxis or anaphylactic shock	7 days

HepB	Anaphylaxis or anaphylactic shock	7 days
Hib	No specific event listed[b]	
VAR	No specific event listed[b]	
RV	No specific event listed[b]	
PCV	No specific event listed[b]	
HepA	No specific event listed[b]	
Influenza	No specific event listed[b]	
Meningococcal	No specific event listed[b]	
HPV	No specific event listed[b]	

[a] See reference below for event definitions. Any acute complications or sequelae of these events, including death, are also reportable, with no applicable interval from the date of vaccination.

[b] Where no specific event is listed, the general mandate to report any event listed in the package insert as a contraindication to additional doses still applies.

Adapted from Guidance on reportable events. Vaccine Adverse Event Reporting System Web site. http://vaers.hhs.gov/professionals/index. Accessed January 21, 2010.

of Health, the Assistant Secretary for Health, the Director of the CDC, and the Commissioner of the FDA, or their designees.

Important points about the VICP include:

- Covered vaccines as of January 2010 are listed in a footnote in **Table 3.3**.
- Injuries caused by the 2009 H1N1 influenza vaccine are covered under the Countermeasures Injury Compensation Program.[9]
- Claims can be filed by individuals, parents, legal guardians, trustees, legal representatives of the estate of deceased persons, non-US citizens, and, under certain conditions, individuals vaccinated outside of the United States.
- Adults are covered under the program if they receive one of the covered vaccines.
- After adjudication, petitioners are free to reject the decision of the Court and pursue civil litigation.
- Compensation is available for past and future nonreimbursable medical, custodial, and rehabilitation costs and lost earnings. There are no limits on compensation for attorney's fees; petitioners representing themselves can only recover legal costs, not fees. Compensation for pain and suffering, and compensation to the estate in the case of death, is capped at $250,000.

Many people had not heard of the vaccine court or the VICP until 2009 and 2010, when landmark decisions regarding vaccines and autism were handed down—see *Chapter 7: Addressing Concerns About Vaccines—Did the Thimerosal Used as a Preservative in Vaccines Cause Autism?*

■ **Vaccine Adverse Event Reporting System (VAERS)**

VAERS, in operation since 1990, is a passive surveillance program that collects and analyzes postmarketing information about adverse vaccine events.[10] Any event following vaccination can be reported, with no restriction on the interval between vaccination and the onset of illness and no requirement for medical care having been rendered. Anyone can submit a report, including health care professionals, pharmaceutical companies, parents, and patients. However, health care providers are *required* to report events that are listed by the manufacturer as a contraindication to subsequent doses as well as events listed in the RET (**Table 3.2**). Reports can be submitted directly on the Internet or forms can be downloaded and mailed in. VAERS data are available to the public for analysis, although caveats regarding interpretation are offered (see *Chapter 2: Vaccine Infrastructure in the United States—Vaccine Adverse Event Reporting System*).

■ **Vaccine Information Statements (VISs)**

A VIS is a concise (1-page, 2-sided) description of the risks and benefits of a given vaccine written for lay people and published by the CDC. **Table 3.3** summarizes use of the VIS, as well as other federal obligations that are binding on vaccine providers. Keep in mind that there may be state laws that supplement these national requirements.

Occupational Safety and Health Administration (OSHA)

Because most vaccines are injected percutaneously, vaccine providers and their employees are at risk for needlestick injuries. As such, all facilities where vaccinations are given, including doctor's offices, public health clinics, and hospitals, fall under OSHA regulations designed to minimize occupational exposure to bloodborne pathogens. Some states may have OSHA plans that exceed the federal requirements discussed below, but those plans cannot be less stringent.

In 1991, under authority of the Occupational Safety and Health Act of 1970, OSHA promulgated the Bloodborne Pathogens Standard, which mandated that employers establish and implement an exposure-control plan for their employees. This plan had to include work-practice controls, procedures for handling exposures, personal protective clothing and equipment, training, medical surveillance, HepB vaccination, signs, and labels. In addition, engineering controls designed to isolate or remove hazards, such as sharps-disposal containers, self-sheathing needles, and plastic capillary tubes, were mandated. In 2000, recognizing that occupational exposure to blood-borne pathogens was a continuing concern and that newer preventive technologies were available, Congress passed the Needlestick Safety and Prevention Act, which directed OSHA to revise the blood-borne pathogens standard. This act called for more detail in the requirements for engineered devices, added new elements to the exposure-control plan, including documentation of employee input, and required the creation of a sharps-injury log. The revised standard went into effect on April 18, 2001.[11]

The basic elements of the Bloodborne Pathogens Standard, as revised, are listed below. With respect to vaccinations, the most important element is the use of engineered sharps protections on needles and the proper disposal of sharps. However, most physicians' offices perform other procedures, such as phlebotomy, wound cleansing, and suturing, necessitating attention to many other areas of the standard.

• *Exposure-control plan*—A *written* plan needs to be in place that details all of the elements listed below. In addition, the

TABLE 3.3 — Federal Requirements Regarding Vaccination

Requirement	Details
Give a VIS	Give a current, *take-home* copy of the relevant VIS before *each* dose of *each* vaccine[a]
	Children: give to the parent or legal representative[b]
	Adults: give to the patient or legal representative[c]
	Use the VIS published by the CDC[d]
	Mandatory for vaccines covered under the National Vaccine Injury Compensation Program (VICP)[e]
	Mandatory for any vaccines purchased under a federal (CDC) contract[f]
	Encouraged for all other vaccines
	Provide VIS for each component of a combination vaccine if there is no VIS for the combination
	Use translations if necessary[g]
Document in the permanent medical record or office log	Name of the VIS, edition date, and date it was given to the recipient[h]
	Name, office address and title of the individual who administered the vaccine
	Date of administration
	Manufacturer
	Lot number
Report to VAERS	Any event listed by the manufacturer as a contraindication to subsequent doses of the vaccine
	Any event listed in the Reportable Events Table (**Table 3.2**) that occurs within the specified time period after vaccination

[a] VISs may be read *before* the immunization visit, but patients must still be given a copy *at* the immunization visit (they may choose not to take the VIS with them, but it must still be offffered). The take-home copy can be an electronic version downloaded to a mobile device. The VIS should

be supplemented as needed with oral discussions, videotapes, other printed material, and whatever else is needed for the parent or patient to gain understanding. The information on the VIS must still be conveyed to the vaccinee even if he or she is blind, deaf, or cannot read.

[b] If immunizations are to be given when the parent is not present, for example during a school-based program, the following options can be exercised: *Consent prior to administration of each dose of a series.* The VIS is mailed to the family or sent home with the student prior to each dose. A consent form is signed and returned before vaccination, and the form is placed in the medical record.
Single signature for series. Some states permit the parents to sign a single consent form for the entire vaccine series. They first receive a copy of the VIS and sign a statement acknowledging receipt of the VIS and authorizing the complete series. A VIS is still sent home prior to each dose in the series.

[c] For incompetent adults living in long term care facilities, all relevant VISs may be provided at the time of admission or at the time of consent if later than admission.

[d] Available from Vaccine Information Statements. Centers for Disease Control and Prevention Web site. http://www.cdc.gov/vaccines/pubs/vis/default.htm. January 21, 2010. Providers may not alter a VIS or make their own version of a VIS, but they can add the practice's name, address, and phone number. In January 2008, a multiple-vaccines-VIS was released that covers all of the vaccines in the first 6 months of life. Providers do not need to withhold a vaccine if a VIS for it does not yet exist. In this situation, the package insert or a homemade information sheet can be used until the official VIS is available. At that point, the VIS should be used.

[e] The basis for this is the National Childhood Vaccine Injury Act. As of January 2010, the following vaccines are included: DT, DTaP, HepA, HepB, Hib, HPV, IIV, IPV, LAIV, MCV, MMR, MPSV, PCV, RV, Td, Tdap, TT, VAR, and any component or combination of these. DTwP and OPV are covered but are no longer used in the United States.

[f] The basis for this is a "duty to warn" clause in CDC's vaccine contracts.

[g] The California and Minnesota state immunization programs have translated the VISs into 30 different languages. These are considered *de facto* equivalents of the English versions and are available from the Immunization Action Coalition Web site (Vaccine information statements. Immunization Action Coalition Web site. http://www.immunize.org. Accessed January 21, 2010).

[h] The patient's signature is *not* required and the VIS should not be construed as informed consent, which may be required in certain states.

Adapted from Mandatory instructions for use of the vaccine information statements. Centers for Disease Control and Prevention Web site. http://www.cdc.gov/vaccines/pubs/vis/default.htm#download. Accessed January 21, 2010.

procedures and job classifications where exposure to blood might occur should be delineated. An annual review and update must be conducted that takes into account innovations in medical procedures and new technological developments that reduce the risk of exposure.

- *Sharps-injury log*—Employers must maintain a log of percutaneous injuries from contaminated sharps. It must include, at a minimum, the type and brand of device, department or work area where the incident occurred, and an explanation of how the incident occurred (including, for example, the procedure being performed and the body part affected). In addition, it must protect the confidentiality of the injured employee. The log should serve as a tool to identify high-risk areas and evaluate devices.

- *Engineered sharps protections*—Devices with built-in safety features or mechanisms that effectively reduce the risk of exposure must be used for procedures that will have contact with blood. Such features should be an integral part of the device, allow the worker's hands to remain behind the needle at all times, remain in effect after the procedure and during disposal, and should be as simple as possible. Examples pertinent to immunizations include syringes with sheaths that slide forward by a single-handed operation to cover the attached needle after use, as well as retractable needles. Documentation must be provided in the exposure-control plan that appropriate, commercially available, engineered devices are evaluated each year, and justification must be provided for selecting a particular device (*not* selecting an engineered device is *not* an option). In addition, it must be documented that nonmanagerial, front-line employees with direct patient care responsibilities had input into the selection (this can take the form of meeting minutes or written evaluations filled out by employees). Selected devices must not jeopardize patient or employee safety or be medically inadvisable. Since sheaths and the like are considered temporary measures, even sharps with engineered protections must be disposed of in an approved container.

- *Universal precautions*—All blood and body fluids must be treated as if infectious for hepatitis B, hepatitis C, and HIV, even if they are from low-risk individuals. Facilities for hand-washing and personal protective equipment (eg, gloves, gowns, masks, mouthpieces, and resuscitation bags) must be available at no cost to employees. Employers must launder lab ~~~~~ and scrubs, if used as protective equipment, at no cost; laundering is not permitted. Gloves (hypoallergenic if ary) must be available and hand washing is required e. However, use of gloves is *not* required when administering intramuscular or subcutaneous injections as long as bleeding is not anticipated.

- *Procedures*—Detailed protocols must be given for all procedures with risk, including decontamination of equipment, handling of sharps-disposal containers and other regulated waste, broken glassware, and laundry. Routine cleaning of work sites should be described.
- *Sharps handling*—A protocol for handling of sharps needs to be in the exposure-control plan. Recapping contaminated needles is prohibited but this should not be an issue since needles will have engineered controls. If recapping is necessary for uncontaminated needles, such as those used to draw vaccine from a vial into a syringe, the cap should be scooped up from a flat surface using the hand that is holding the syringe and needle. Disposal containers should be closable, puncture resistant, leak proof, labeled appropriately, and located where procedures are performed. The protocol should specify how the containers are handled once they are filled.
- *Warning labels*—Orange or orange-red biohazard labels must be affixed to containers of regulated waste and refrigerators and freezers containing blood or infectious materials (labeled bags may also be used).
- *HepB vaccination*—Vaccination should be available at no cost to all employees with potential blood contact. The employee's health insurance cannot be used to pay this expense unless the employer routinely pays the entire premium. Employees must sign a declination form if they choose to opt out.
- *Postexposure evaluation*—Specific procedures should be outlined for the handling of exposures. Baseline and follow-up laboratory tests should be done after consent is obtained and must be provided free of charge. Provisions for confidential medical follow-up must be made. Postexposure HIV prophylaxis should be offered if indicated in accord with current guidelines. The source individual's blood should be tested for blood-borne pathogens after consent is obtained; if consent is not given, this needs to be documented. Medical records on employees must be kept for the duration of employment plus 30 years.
- *Training*—Training that includes background information and the exposure-control plan must be provided upon assignment and annually thereafter. Documentation of training sessions, including the dates, content, trainer, and attendees must be maintained.

Many vaccines are now available from manufacturers in prefilled syringes and needles with engineered protections. More information on implementing the Bloodborne Pathogens Standard can be obtained from the International Healthcare Worker Safety Center at the University of Virginia.[12]

School Mandates and State Legislation

There are no federal laws specifying which vaccines civilians must receive. There are, however, state laws specifying which vaccines must be received before attendance at day care, pre-school, school, or college is allowed. These requirements have been instrumental in the eradication or near-eradication of many diseases.[13] The courts have repeatedly upheld the legal basis for these statutes, which include the societal mandate to protect nonenfranchised persons (children who do not [yet] have a vote) and the rights of others to be protected from harm (transmission of disease from unimmunized individuals). The case for mandates that prevent the spread of highly contagious diseases (such as measles) in schools is relatively straightforward. The situation becomes complicated when considering infections such as HPV, which is arguably not spread in schools and which can largely be prevented by avoidance of high-risk behaviors. In fact, some have argued that characteristics like these disqualify a vaccine from consideration for school mandates.[14] Others argue that there are moral grounds for compulsory HPV vaccination, including the principles of beneficence, nonmaleficence, autonomy and justice.[15] In 2008, NVAC offered guidance for states considering adolescent vaccination mandates.[16]

There are few laws that apply to adults other than college students, those entering military service, and immigrants. However, some states, employers, or institutions might require certain vaccines or proof of immunity for selected individuals. Examples include influenza vaccine, MMR, Tdap, and HepB for health care personnel, influenza and pneumococcal vaccines for residents and employees of long-term care facilities, vaccines for laboratory workers who work with specific pathogens, and RAB for animal handlers. There is a clear moral and ethical justification for mandatory influenza immunization of health care personnel,[17] and professional societies such as the IDSA and the Association for Professionals in Infection Control and Epidemiology have called upon health care institutions to adopt mandates. The legal basis for these mandates has been questioned, something that was brought to the forefront during the H1N1 influenza pandemic in 2009. Detractors cite deprivation of liberty without due process; guarantees against illegal search and seizure; violation of the establishment clause of the First Amendment; and freedom of contract between employee and employer.[18] Proponents—including, by and large, the courts—cite precedents that uphold the state's authority to restrict privileges and personal economic, even religious, freedoms in the interest of preserving the public welfare.

In interpreting the validity of a child's immunization history, the CDC recommends a 4-day grace period for specific minimum age and interval requirements. For example, a child who receives MMR 3 days before his first birthday is considered effectively immunized; one who receives MMR a week before his first birthday is not. Some local school districts may not accept the 4-day grace period, so the best advice is to give vaccines at the recommended ages. Practitioners may have to balance the issues surrounding giving a vaccine before the exact specified age with the risk that the patient may not return to be vaccinated at the appropriate time.

All states allow either temporary or permanent exemption from school immunization requirements for medical reasons. As of 2009, some form of religious exemption was granted by 48 states (Mississippi and West Virginia were the exceptions), and 20 granted some form of philosophical exemption. In a 1997 policy statement (reaffirmed in 2009), the AAP emphasized the need for sensitivity and flexibility in dealing with parents' religious beliefs.[19] It was acknowledged that constitutional guarantees of freedom of religion do not permit children to be harmed through religious practices, and while the AAP called for the repeal of religious exemption laws, it also argued against the stringent application of medical-neglect laws when parents refuse the recommended childhood immunizations. Philosophical exemptions are more problematic because the level of proof can be minimal (it may be minimal for religious exemptions as well), amounting simply to parents being "opposed to immunization." In some cases, parents request philosophical exemptions as a matter of convenience when their children's immunizations are not up-to-date. Physicians, public health providers, and school officials should not grant philosophical exemptions in such circumstances, and in general should work toward the repeal of philosophical exemption laws. Importantly, the risk of some vaccine-preventable diseases has been shown to increase with the availability of philosophical exemptions and the ease with which these are granted. For parents considering exemption, physicians should emphasize that disease rates among exemptors are higher than among vaccinated persons; in addition, large numbers of exemptors in a community put everyone at risk, including vaccinated children. *Chapter 7: Addressing Concerns About Vaccines* has a more in-depth discussion of vaccine refusal and its attendant public health consequences.

Contact your state health department (see *Appendix*) for the most up-to-date information about local mandates.

REFERENCES

1. Pickering LK, et al. *Clin Infect Dis.* 2009;49:817-840.

2. National Vaccine Advisory Committee. *Pediatrics.* 2003;112:958-963.

3. Poland GA, et al. *Am J Prev Med.* 2003;25:144-150.

4. Hinman AR, et al. *Clin Infect Dis.* 2007;44:1532-1535.

5. Infectious Diseases Society of America. *Clin Infect Dis.* 2007;44: e104-e108.

6. ACP-IDSA Joint Statement of Medical Societies Regarding Adult Vaccination by Physicians. Infectious Diseases Society of American Web site. http://www.idsociety.org/adultimmunization.htm. Accessed February 28, 2010.

7. National Vaccine Injury Compensation Program (VICP). Health Resources and Services Administration Web site. http://www.hrsa .gov/vaccinecompensation. Accessed January 22, 2010.

8. Vaccine injury table. Health Resources and Services Administration Web site. http://www.hrsa.gov/vaccinecompensation/table.htm. Accessed January 22, 2010.

9. Countermeasures Injury Compensation Program. Health Resources and Services Administration Web site. http://www.hrsa.gov/coun termeasurescomp/. Accessed January 21, 2010.

10. US Department of Health and Human Services. Vaccine Adverse Event Reporting System. http://vaers.hhs.gov. Accessed January 22, 2010.

11. Bloodborne pathogens and needlestick prevention. Occupational Safety & Health Administration Web site. http://www.osha.gov /SLTC/bloodbornepathogens/index.html. Accessed January 22, 2010.

12. International Healthcare Worker Safety Center. University of Virginia Health System Web site. http://www.healthsystem.virginia.edu /internet/epinet/home.cfm. Accessed February 28, 2010.

13. Hinman AR, et al. *J Law Med Ethics.* 2002;30:122-127.

14. Opel DJ, et al. *Pediatrics.* 2008;122:e504-e510.

15. Balog JE. *Am J Pub Health.* 2009;99:616-622.

16. National Vaccine Advisory Committee. *Am J Prev Med.* 2008;35: 145-151.

17. Van Delden JJM, et al. *Vaccine.* 2008;26:5562-5566.

18. Stewart AM. *N Engl J Med.* 2009;361:2015-2017.

19. American Academy of Pediatrics Committee on Bioethics. *Pediatrics.* 1997;99:279-281.

4

Vaccine Practice

Mishandling of vaccines can reduce potency and leave vaccinated people susceptible to disease. The recommendations for handling and storage of each vaccine are given in *Section B*. Here are some general rules[1]:

- Designate one person (and a backup) to be in charge of inventory, handling, and storage.
- Maintain an inventory log, including product name, manufacturer, lot number, doses received, date received, condition on arrival, and expiration date.
- Inspect products on delivery, including the integrity of containers and cold chain monitoring devices.
- Store vaccines immediately under appropriate conditions.
- If there are questions about a vaccine's condition at delivery, store the vaccine under the recommended conditions and contact the manufacturer's quality-control office or the state immunization program.
- Discard mishandled and expired vaccines (vaccines can be used until the last day of the month indicated on the expiration date).
- Dispose of all vaccine materials using medical waste disposal procedures, including sharps/biohazard containers (materials coming in contact with live vaccines carry the risk of contagion).
- Consider as invalid any doses that were inadvertently given with mishandled or expired vaccine.
- Do not open more than one multidose vial at a time.
- Be aware that for some multidose vials, there is a limited recommended shelf life after the vial is first entered.
- Do not prefill syringes with vaccines that are supplied in vials.
- Discourage "brown bagging," where patients pick up their vaccines at a pharmacy and bring them to the provider for administration (this practice has become popular for ZOS).

Here are some general rules regarding refrigerators and freezers:

- A freezer used for vaccines should not be a compartment within a refrigerator (as in a "dormitory" unit). It should be a separate sealed unit and should have a separate external door, although completely separate refrigerator and freezer units are preferred. As of January 2010, the CDC no longer allowed VFC or other federally supplied vaccines to be stored permanently in dormitory-style refrigerators; these can be used, however, for the day's supply of *refrigerated* vaccines, after which the vaccines must be returned to their permanent refrigerator.

- Do not store food in the vaccine refrigerator or freezer (frequent opening of the door can cause temperature fluctuations).
- Do not store vaccines on shelves on the refrigerator door.
- Vaccines that need to be refrigerated but protected from freezing should be stored in the middle of the refrigerator, away from the freezer portion of the unit.
- Use clearly labeled, color-coded trays for each product and include separate compartments for unopened and opened vials (record the date of opening or reconstitution directly on the label).
- Rotate stock (place newly received vaccines behind current supplies).
- Post a sign that specifies which vaccines are stored in the refrigerator and which are stored in the freezer.
- Keep a thermometer in the refrigerator and one in the freezer and record the temperatures on a log when the office opens in the morning and when it closes in the evening. Alternatively, a recording thermometer can be used. *Appropriate ranges are 35°F to 46°F (2°C to 8°C) for the refrigerator and ≤5°F (-15°C) for the freezer.*
- Keep large jugs of water in the refrigerator and ice packs in the freezer to help maintain a steady temperature. This also helps maintain the temperature in the event of a power outage.
- Place a "DO NOT UNPLUG" sign near the outlet for the refrigerator and freezer units. Mark other points along the circuit (eg, fuses, circuit breakers) in a similar fashion.
- Do not use an outlet with a ground fault circuit interrupter (ie, one with test and reset buttons) or one connected to a wall switch.
- Use plug guards to prevent accidental dislodging.
- If possible, use an outlet connected to an auxiliary power source.
- **Table 4.1** gives some suggestions for managing the vaccine inventory in the event of a power failure or weather emergency.

Here are some tips on maintaining the cold chain while transporting vaccines to off-site clinics:

- FDA regulations require that multidose vials be used only by the provider's office where they were first opened (partially used vials may be moved to other sites operated by the same provider as long as the cold chain is maintained).
- The following may be used to transport vaccines at 35°F to 46°F (2°C to 8°C): original shipping containers; hard-sided plastic insulated containers; Styrofoam coolers with walls

TABLE 4.1 — Storage and Handling During Emergencies

Power Outages
- Do not open refrigerators and freezers until power is restored
- Record temperature after power is restored and note duration of outage (do not open to monitor temperature during outage)
- Transfer to alternative storage with reliable power source if possible, maintaining cold chain and monitoring temperature
- Contact state or local public health authorities or the vaccine manufacturer if there is *any* question about the potential potency of exposed vaccine
- Label exposed vaccine and keep it separated from new stock
- Remember that live vaccines are the most susceptible to inactivation by warming

Weather Emergencies
- Suspend vaccination and implement emergency procedures in advance of the event
- Identify alternative storage facilities with backup power
- Ensure availability of staff to package and transport vaccine
- Maintain appropriate packing materials
- Ensure availability of transportation
- Include the following in standard operating procedures:
  - Emergency phone numbers for power company, equipment repair, alarm monitoring companies, backup storage facility, dry ice vendor, generator repair company, National Weather Service, and vaccine manufacturers
  - Working agreements with hospitals, health departments, or other facilities to serve as emergency vaccine storage facilities
  - Procedures for entering facilities and storage areas during emergency or after hours, including location of emergency equipment and packing materials, as well as phone numbers for responsible persons
  - Procedures for packaging (including inventory documentation and cold-chain monitoring) and transporting vaccines (including preferred and alternative routes)
  - Priority list for vaccine rescue, aiming to minimize dollar loss but ensure ability to deliver the routine schedule in the short term

Adapted from Impact of power outage on vaccine storage. Centers for Disease Control and Prevention Web site. http://www.cdc.gov/vaccines/recs/storage/poweroutage.htm, and Emergency procedures for protecting vaccine inventories. Centers for Disease Control and Prevention Web site. http://www.cdc.gov/vaccines/recs/storage/vacc-weather-emerg.htm. Accessed January 27, 2010.

that are at least 2" thick (do not use the thin-walled coolers typically found in grocery stores).

- Use refrigerated or frozen gel packs, not loose or bagged ice (use enough of these to maintain the proper temperature and validate a stable temperature before using the cooler for vaccines).
- Keep the vaccines in their original boxes.
- Place bubble wrap, crumpled brown packing paper, or Styrofoam peanuts around the vaccines to prevent direct contact with the refrigerated or frozen gel packs; include a thermometer next to the vaccines.
- Varicella-containing vaccines should be transported on dry ice in order to stay frozen. If dry ice is not available, VAR and MMRV may be transported at 35°F to 46°F (2°C to 8°C) using the methods described above but must be used within 72 hours and should not be refrozen. ZOS must be transported on dry ice.
- Diluents should travel with their corresponding vaccines at all times. They can stay at room temperature. If packed inside coolers, they should be refrigerated ahead of time and should not come in direct contact with the refrigerated or frozen gel packs. The diluents for MMR, MMRV, VAR, and ZOS should not be transported in dry ice containers.

Improving Delivery

A large evidence base exists on strategies to improve immunization delivery.[2,3] Many of the following strategies for improving immunization rates are emphasized in *Chapter 3: Standards, Principles, and Regulations—Standards for Pediatric Immunization Practices* and *Standards for Adult Immunization Practices*.

■ Reminder, Recall, and Tracking Systems

Reminders are messages that immunizations are due. They may be directed at parents in the form of telephone calls (by humans or computers) or mailings (simple postcards or letters), or they may be directed at physicians, nurses, or other staff members in the form of chart or electronic medical record flags saying "vaccines are due." Recall messages are notices to parents that vaccinations are overdue. Tracking systems, which can be manual or computerized, allow each child's immunization status to be followed precisely.

Studies have consistently shown improvements in immunization rates for both children and adults if tracking and messaging systems are used, in both public and private settings.[4,5] The AAP has offered the following guidelines (among others):

- Goals should include documenting immunization status, increasing immunization rates, decreasing costs of immunization, and facilitating immunization opportunities.
- There should be accurate documentation of each child's immunization status.
- Confidentiality should be preserved.
- Immunization information should be available at all times to ensure that all opportunities to immunize are used.
- Information on coverage rates should not be used to sanction health care personnel.
- Data input and access should be easy.
- Incomplete immunization status should not be used to deny any child access to care or eligibility for insurance benefits.
- Collaboration between public and private initiatives should include the ability to link databases.

Reminder and recall systems are particularly difficult to implement in practices with high patient turnover or in populations that change residence frequently. Keep in mind that in some areas, bilingual reminders may be necessary.

■ Missed Opportunities

Providers should utilize all clinical encounters to assess immunization status and administer vaccines for which the child is eligible, as long as true contraindications do not exist. The idea is to prevent contacts with the health care system from becoming *missed opportunities* for vaccination.[6,7] Common reasons why opportunities are missed are listed below:

- Failure of providers to consider acute care visits as a time to catch up on immunizations
- Inability to accurately determine immunization status
- Adherence to erroneous contraindications (**Table 5.4**)
- Failure to give all needed vaccines simultaneously

Additional barriers may exist in emergency departments and other acute care facilities, including time constraints, insurance reimbursement, and the perception that by giving routine immunizations, the patient's relationship with his primary care provider will be disrupted. Immunization Information Systems (IISs) and standing orders can help prevent missed opportunities.

■ Expanding Access

After-hours or weekend clinics may help boost coverage rates by making it more convenient for parents to bring their children in or for adults to stop by after work. In addition, access to vaccination once a patient enters the office can be facilitated through the use of "vaccination express lanes" and drop-in clinics. Alternative venues for adolescents, from schools to—dare we say it, the mall—should be explored. Also, with proper vaccine storage and handling, there is no reason why home visits could not be used to vaccinate those persons who are receiving home health services for other reasons.

The "cocoon strategy" deserves special mention here. The idea is to surround infants in a sea of immune contacts, in essence erecting a barrier to disease transmission. This concept is most germane to preventing pertussis, since older individuals are the source of infection for infants, and influenza, since immunization does not begin until 6 months of age. However, cocooning requires thinking outside the box regarding adult immunization. Thus, for example, women may receive Tdap postpartum in the hospital through a standing order (see below) protocol. This was successfully implemented at a hospital in Houston that serves an uninsured, high-risk population, where Tdap uptake under the program was 96% among women without medical contraindications.[8] Between January 2008 and February 2010, 10,000 mothers and immediate family members were immunized.[9] Parents of infants who are hospitalized could be immunized when they visit; this takes the concept one step further, since those parents, unlike postpartum women, are not themselves patients. Nevertheless, the strategy has been successfully employed for both influenza[10] and pertussis[11] immunizations. One added value to this approach is that immunization rates among health care personnel tend to increase!

The pediatric office is also fair game as a venue for adult immunization.[12] However, in all of these settings, accurate information about the parent's medical and immunization history will need to be obtained, and a permanent record of the immunization will need to be provided. In addition, providers are likely to have questions about covering costs, billing, reimbursement, scope of practice, and liability.

■ **Standing Orders**
Standing orders enable nonphysician personnel, such as nurses and pharmacists, to prescribe or deliver vaccinations by protocol without direct physician involvement at the time of the encounter. This is one of the most consistently effective interventions for increasing adult immunization rates, and recent studies even show that the entire process can be computerized—that is, patients can be screened for eligibility electronically and the orders can be generated automatically, without investment of personnel time. Employing standing orders in nursing homes, hospitals, clinics, physicians' offices, and other institutional settings can increase coverage rates. In fact, standing orders for adult pneumococcal and influenza vaccination are recommended.[13] Standing orders are also applicable to pediatric patients. In fact, it is recommended that all birthing hospitals have standing orders in place for HepB immunization of newborns. Standing orders could be employed

for influenza immunization of children ≥6 months of age who are hospitalized in the fall for any reason.

■ Immunization Information Systems

IISs, formerly known as *registries*, are confidential, population-based, centralized computerized systems that maintain information about immunizations. The ideal registry contains all persons in a geographic area and receives vaccination data from all regional providers. The need for registries is easy to see—an increasingly complex vaccine schedule must be administered to children who frequently relocate and change health care providers, and the number of vaccines being recommended for adults is increasing. For both children and adults, vaccination histories are often incomplete and fragmented, leading to both missed opportunities and unnecessary duplication. For these reasons, one of the *Healthy People 2010* (see *Chapter 3: Standards, Principles, and Regulations—Healthy People 2010 and 2020*) goals is for at least 95% of children <6 years of age to participate in a fully operational population-based IIS. As of 2008, 75% of US children in this age group participated in an IIS; 82% of programs had the capacity to track vaccinations for persons of all ages, and two-thirds of the data were entered within 30 days of vaccine administration.[14] However, many records were incomplete, particularly for core elements like vaccine manufacturer and lot number.

IISs can help ensure that patients remain current with immunization recommendations.[15] They can provide recalls and reminders; ensure timely vaccination after changes in location or provider; reduce unnecessary immunization; provide accurate documentation of immunization history; assess coverage rates; and facilitate monitoring of adverse events, among other benefits. There are also potential downsides, including the costs of data entry and retrieval; difficulties integrating into existing business practices; problems interfacing with other medical records and billing systems; concerns about confidentiality; and the perception of minimum value-added for participation.[16] Organizations such as the American Immunization Registry Association, in collaboration with the CDC, have worked on defining best practices to help overcome these barriers and ensure that IISs can support required core program activities at the state and local levels.[17]

The CDC has supported the development of state registries since 1993 through Section 317 Public Health Service grants.[18] Additional support has come from organizations such as the Robert Wood Johnson Foundation. In 1998, the National Vaccine Advisory Committee launched the Initiative on Immunization Registries to facilitate community- and state-based registries.[19] Four major challenges were identified:

- *Protecting confidentiality*—The need to gather and share information must be balanced with the family's right to privacy. Minimum specifications include executing written confidentiality policies, notifying parents of the existence of the registry and allowing them to opt out, and defining who has access and what can be done with the information.

- *Participation by providers and recipients*—Because the majority of vaccine delivery has shifted to the private sector, efforts to recruit private providers are essential. Part of what makes a registry attractive to providers is simplicity, minimization of administrative burden, high quality of data, and functionality (eg, ability to generate reminders).
- *Operational challenges*—The functional capabilities of registry hardware and software differ from community to community; this is not conducive to the overall goal of seamless information exchange. For this reason, the CDC developed minimum operational standards.[20]
- *Resources to maintain registries*—Registries are likely to result in cost savings by reducing the manual labor involved in pulling medical records for provider visits, managed care reporting, and school system review. Additional cost savings should accrue from eliminating duplicate immunizations and reducing disease burden. It costs about $5 or $6 per child per year to maintain a registry, and in 1999 only 40% of this cost was covered by federal sources. Since 2000, the Centers for Medicare and Medicaid Services (formerly the Health Care Financing Administration) has provided funding to state programs for the development of IISs in the context of the Medicaid Management Information System.

The AAP has strongly supported the development of IISs and has suggested that research be done into their cost-effectiveness in increasing immunization rates. In addition, the AAP has called for a critical examination of the cost and benefits for the practicing physician and has suggested that physicians be reimbursed for entering historical information into databases. Finally, it has cautioned that the data in IISs be used to improve quality, not to penalize poor performers.

■ Other Strategies

Parent and community education regarding the importance of immunizations can improve coverage rates by increasing demand. Physician and staff education is equally important, and it helps to designate an "Immunization Tsar" (or Tsarina) in the practice who can champion all issues related to vaccination, from decreasing missed opportunities to scanning for new recommendations to preparing talking points that address the latest parental concerns. Regular, systematic assessment and feedback can identify problem areas and evaluate the effectiveness of new interventions.

Along these lines, the CDC has developed a quality improvement methodology called AFIX, for Assessment (of a provider's vaccination coverage levels and practices), Feedback (of results to the provider along with suggestions for improvement), Incentives (to reward improved performance), and eXchange (of information and resources to facilitate improvement).[21] Traditionally used to evaluate immunization delivery systems for children, AFIX can be generalized to apply to any age group. The data used in AFIX assessments come from IISs or from chart reviews. A software application called CoCASA, for Comprehensive Clinic Assessment Software Application, is available from the CDC to assess immunization practices in clinics, private practices, or other sites where immunizations are given.[22]

Screening

Screening patients for contraindications, precautions, and other problems before every dose of a vaccine is an important part of preventing adverse events. This can be effectively accomplished by asking the simple questions shown in **Table 4.2**, which are applicable to both children and adults. The issues addressed by these questions are also indicated in the table. Standardized forms for screening can be downloaded from the Immunization Action Coalition web site free of charge.[23]

Administration

■ General Issues

During well care visits, it is probably most efficient to bring the vaccines to the examination room rather than have the patient move to a designated shot area. If reconstitution is needed, it should be done for each individual patient, rather than in batches, in order to reduce the risk of confusion and wastage. Young infants may do better if held on the parent's lap, while older children may prefer to sit on the edge of the examining table and hug their parent. Adolescents, who are at risk for syncope, may want to sit or lie down. Health care workers should wash their hands or use antiseptic hand gel before each patient, and sterile technique should be used, including swiping of the injection site with alcohol and allowing it to dry. Gloves are not required unless the individual administering the vaccine has open skin lesions and is likely to come in contact with body fluids.

The needle should not be changed after withdrawing vaccine from the vial and before injecting it into the patient. A direct, rapid plunge of the needle through the skin is recommended followed by a rapid withdrawal after delivering the vaccine. Aspirating back on the syringe after penetration in order to look for blood return is not necessary, although many nurses feel uncomfortable injecting before they can confirm that the needle is not resting in a vessel. Multiple vaccines can be given in the same limb but

TABLE 4.2 — Screening Questions

Question	Issues Addressed
Is the patient sick today?	Moderate-to-severe illness is a precaution for all vaccines
Does the patient have severe allergies to drugs, foods, or vaccines?	Severe allergy to vaccine components or previous doses is a contra-indication for future doses
	Severe egg allergy is a contraindication for influenza and YF vaccines
	Severe allergy to drugs (eg, neomycin) or other food ingredients (eg, gelatin, baker's yeast) may contraindicate certain vaccines
Has the patient had serious reactions to previous vaccinations?	Various contraindications and precautions for further doses
Has the patient had a seizure, brain, or neurologic problem?	Evolving neurologic disorder is a precaution for pertussis-containing vaccines
	Patients who are susceptible to febrile seizures may benefit from fever prophylaxis
	Guillain-Barré syndrome within 6 weeks of previous influenza vaccine or tetanus-containing vaccine is a precaution for further doses
	Personal history of Guillain-Barré syndrome is a precaution for MCV4-D[a]
Does the patient have asthma or another chronic medical condition (eg, lung, heart, kidney, or metabolic)?	LAIV may be contraindicated
	Certain nonroutine vacines may be recommended
If the patient is a child between 2 and 4 years of age, has a health care provider diagnosed wheezing or asthma in the past year?	LAIV may be contraindicated

114

Question	Comment
Does the patient have cancer, leukemia, a blood disorder, HIV infection, AIDS, tuberculosis, or any problem with the immune system?	Live vaccines are generally contraindicated in patients with immune impairment MMR can cause thrombocytopenia Active untreated tuberculosis is a precaution for MMR, VAR, and ZOS
In the last 3 months, has the patient received any treatments that might weaken his or her immune system, such as steroids, cancer chemotherapy, or radiation?	Live vaccines are generally contraindicated in patients with immune impairment Patient may respond poorly to vaccination
Are there any family members who have problems with their immune system?	The patient might be at risk for a heritable immune deficiency that would contraindicate live vaccines
Has the patient received blood transfusions or immune globulin in the past year?	Receipt of antibody-containing products is a precaution for MMR and VAR Undisclosed serious underlying illness may be discovered
Is the patient pregnant or is there a chance she could become pregnant in the next 3 months?	Live vaccines are generally contraindicated during pregnancy
Has the patient received any other vaccines in the last 4 weeks?	Live vaccines not given on the same day need to be separated by 1 month The AAP (but not the ACIP) recommends that if Tdap and MCV4-D are not given on the same day, they need to be separated by 1 month Violating the minimum interval between doses in a series may result in invalid doses

[a] Data are not available to evaluate the potential risk of GBS following administration of MCV4-CRM.

Adapted from Centers for Disease Control and Prevention. *Epidemiology and Prevention of Vaccine-Preventable Diseases*. 11th ed. Atkinson W, et al, eds. Washington, DC: Public Health Foundation; 2009:27-29, and Child screening questions and adult screening questions. Immunization Action Coalition Web site. http://www.immunize.org. Accessed January 27, 2010.

4

should be separated by 1″ to 2″. It has been suggested that multiple injections can be given simultaneously by different personnel in order to minimize anticipatory anxiety.

Smallpox vaccine is the only one that is given by an entirely unique method. This live vaccine is administered intradermally with a bifurcated needle that punctures the skin and draws a small amount of blood. As such, *gloves should be worn* and the site should be covered with gauze and a semipermeable dressing. Skin preparation is not required unless there is gross contamination, in which case soap and water should be used for cleansing. If alcohol is used, the skin must dry thoroughly before inoculation to prevent inactivation of the vaccine virus.

■ Intramuscular Administration

The needle should enter the skin at a 90° angle, penetrating deep enough to hit the muscle (**Figure 4.1**). Traction can be applied to the skin and subcutaneous tissue before injection and released after injection. Preferred sites, which differ by age, include the anterolateral aspect of the upper thigh (vastus lateralis muscle) and the upper, outer part of the arm above the armpit and below the acromion (deltoid muscle); the required needle length will also vary by patient age (**Table 4.3**). The buttocks should not be used because the fat layer is too thick and damage to the sciatic nerve is possible. An exception can be made for large-volume passive immunization (eg, immune globulin), but here the site should be the upper, outer mass of the gluteus maximus and the needle should be directed perpendicular to the table while the patient is lying prone. Alternatively, the injection can be given in the center of the triangle formed by the anterior superior iliac spine, the tubercle of the iliac crest, and the upper border of the greater trochanter. No more than 5 mL should be given to an adult at a single site.

■ Subcutaneous Administration

For subcutaneous injections, the skin and subcutaneous tissue should be pinched-up, and the needle directed at a 45° angle (**Figure 4.1**). The preferred sites and needle length again vary with age (**Table 4.3**).

■ Oral Administration

For infants, oral administration RV is best accomplished with the child lying in the feeding position in the parent's arms. The tip of the applicator is placed in the infant's mouth toward the inner cheek and slowly emptied until all of the liquid is dispensed. If the infant spits or regurgitates, the dose is counted and not repeated.

■ Intranasal Administration

LAIV is supplied in a sprayer that resembles a syringe. The recipient should be in the upright position. The tip of the sprayer is inserted just inside the nose and the plunger is rapidly depressed until the dose-divider clip stops the plunger. The clip is then removed and the remainder of the dose is given in the other nostril. Sneezing or leakage of some of the liquid from the nose is not a reason to repeat the dose.

■ Anxiety, Pain, and Fever

For infants, pain can be reduced by oral sucrose solution (50%) given directly into the mouth with a small syringe or administered on a pacifier; breastfeeding, non-nutritive sucking, and simply holding the baby also work well. For older children, stress and anxiety can be ameliorated by truthfully informing them what to expect before the visit occurs and by parental endorsement of vaccination as being valuable.[24] Parents should be allowed to comfort young children (rather than assist in restraining them) and should try to distract them by telling stories, playing music, or having them blow into pinwheels or imaginary candles. Technique is important: a quick "jab" into and out of the muscle is less painful than a slow injection with aspiration.[25] Stroking the adjacent skin before and during the injection may help, as may pressure applied to the site after withdrawal. For sequential injections, the least painful one should be given first.

Topical anesthetics, such as eutectic mixture of local anesthetic (EMLA cream) or vapocoolant sprays, should be considered for patients who are phobic or extremely anxious about the injection.[26] Administration of acetaminophen at the time of DTaP vaccination and over the course of the first day has been suggested for children with seizures, stable neurological disorders, and even a family history of seizures, with the aim to reduce fever that could trigger seizures.[27,28] In fact, prophylactic acetaminophen *does* reduce fever. In a randomized trial, fever ≥100.4°F (38°C) occurred in 42% of 226 infants in the prophylaxis group after at least one dose of a routine primary immunization series, as compared to 66% of 233 in the control group.[29] However, antibody responses to most of the vaccine antigens were lower in the prophylaxis group; one mechanism for this could be a reduction of inflammatory signals at the injection site. Fortunately, high fevers and medical attention for fever or other symptoms after vaccination are rare; given this, and the possibility of reduced immunogenicity, there is no role for routine fever prophylaxis with acetaminophen. Acetaminophen may be considered as needed for analgesia or antipyresis after immunization.

Emergencies

■ Preparation

Acute emergencies after vaccine administration are rare—the risk for children and adolescents is estimated at less than one episode per million doses.[30] The AAP suggests that when possible, patients should be observed in the office for 15 to 20 minutes

FIGURE 4.1 — Injection Technique

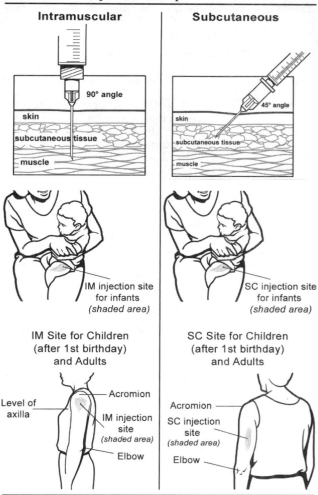

Adapted from Administering vaccines. Immunization Action Coalition
Web site. http://www.immunize.org/catg.d/p2020.pdf. Accessed January
24, 2010.

after vaccination; the ACIP has recommended this for HPV vaccination, where syncope appears to be a particular problem. Life-threatening emergencies such as anaphylaxis usually occur within minutes, when the patient is still likely to be within reach of medical personnel. The benefits of rapid, mass vaccination programs, such as drive-by influenza vaccine clinics, probably far outweigh the risks of curtailing any medical observation period.

Standing orders for emergencies should be in place in the office, and emergency supplies should be available in the event they are needed.[31]

■ Syncope

Vasovagal reactions are most common in adolescents and young adults, particularly females. About 60% occur within 5 minutes of vaccination and approximately 90% occur within 15 minutes. Between 1990 and 2001, slightly over 2200 reports of syncope were made to VAERS. Approximately 12% of cases resulted in hospitalization, and there are some reports of serious injury such as skull fracture. Since the advent of the adolescent vaccine platform—Tdap and MCV4 in 2005 and especially HPV vaccine in 2006—there has been a sharp increase in reported syncopal episodes related to vaccination.[32] However, the absolute number of reported episodes remains low—463 VAERS reports between 2005 and 2007, most of them in female adolescents. Health care personnel should be aware of predisposing conditions (eg, needle phobia) and presyncopal symptoms (eg, light-headedness or dizziness). At-risk individuals should be encouraged to sit or lie down, and consideration should be given to observing all patients for 15 minutes after vaccination. If syncope does occur, the patient should be protected as much as possible from fall injury and should be placed supine with the legs raised until symptoms abate.

■ Anaphylaxis

Anaphylaxis occurs rapidly and is a medical emergency. Signs and symptoms include:
- Flushing, warmth, urticaria, erythema, soft tissue edema, pruritus
- Dry mouth, swelling of the lips, tongue and throat, sneezing, congestion, rhinorrhea
- Hoarseness, stridor, cough, dyspnea, chest tightness, wheezing, cyanosis
- Tachycardia, hypotension, weak pulse, dizziness, shock, cardiovascular collapse
- Crampy abdominal pain, nausea, vomiting, diarrhea

For patients with mild symptoms, the initial approach is to administer epinephrine 1:1000 (aqueous) at a dose of 0.01 mL/kg intramuscular (the maximum dose is 0.5 mL). Injection should be

TABLE 4.3 — Needle Type and Injection Site

Age	Intramuscular[a] (22- to 25-gauge)		Subcutaneous[b] (23- to 25-gauge)	
	Site	Needle (inch)	Site	Needle[e] (inch)
0 to 28 days (including premature infants)	Anterolateral aspect of upper thigh	$5/8$[c]	Fatty part of upper anterolateral thigh	$5/8$ to $3/4$
1 to 12 months	Anterolateral aspect of upper thigh	1	Fatty part of upper anterolateral thigh	$5/8$ to $3/4$
1 to 2 years	Anterolateral aspect of upper thigh[d]	1 to $1\frac{1}{4}$	Fatty part of upper outer triceps area of arm or upper anterolateral thigh	$5/8$ to $3/4$
	Deltoid	$5/8$[c] to 1		
3 to 18 years	Deltoid[d]	$5/8$[c] to 1	Fatty part of upper outer triceps area of arm or upper anterolateral thigh	$5/8$ to $3/4$
	Anterolateral aspect of upper thigh	1 to $1\frac{1}{4}$		
≥19 years	Deltoid	Male or female <130 lbs (59 kg): $5/8$[c] to 1 Female 130-200 lbs (59 to 91 kg): 1 to $1\frac{1}{2}$ Male 130-260 lbs (59 to 118 kg): 1 to $1\frac{1}{2}$ Female >200 lbs (91 kg): $1\frac{1}{2}$ Male >260 lbs (118 kg): $1\frac{1}{2}$	Fatty part of upper outer triceps area of arm or upper anterolateral thigh	$5/8$ to $3/4$

[a] The needle is inserted at a 90° angle.

[b] Skin and subcutaneous tissue are bunched up and the needle is inserted at a 45° angle.

[c] When using a short needle, the skin should be stretched tight to ensure that the muscle is reached.

[d] Preferred site.

[e] CDC recommends a ⅝-inch needle; AAP recommends a ⅝- to ¾-inch needle.

Adapted from Centers for Disease Control and Prevention. *Epidemiology and Prevention of Vaccine-Preventable Diseases*. 11th ed. Atkinson W, et al, eds. Washington, DC.: Public Health Foundation; 2009:D-6, D-7, and American Academy of Pediatrics. *Red Book. 2009 Report of the Committee on Infectious Diseases*. 28th ed. Elk Grove Village, IL.: American Academy of Pediatrics; 2009:18-20.

in the lateral thigh. A dose can be repeated every 10 to 20 minutes if necessary for up to 3 total doses. In addition, an antihistamine such as diphenhydramine can be given at a dose of 1-2 mg/kg (maximum 100 mg per dose) PO, IM, or IV every 4 to 6 hours; an alternative antihistamine is hydroxyzine, 0.5-1 mg/kg (maximum 100 mg per dose) PO or IM every 4 to 6 hours. The patient should be observed for several hours, and if improved and stable, can be given a prescription for an autoinjector of epinephrine and sent home on an oral antihistamine for the next 24 hours. Additional therapies may include a short course of oral steroids and the addition of an H_2 blocker (cimetidine or ranitidine).

For more severe cases, the emergency medical system should be activated immediately. Patients may require intensive emergency management, including airway maintenance, oxygen, and blood pressure support with isotonic intravenous fluids and vasopressors. Biphasic reactions may account for up to 50% of fatal cases. Asymptomatic intervals vary widely and can be as long as 24 hours. All patients with mild or severe anaphylaxis reactions should be referred to an allergist prior to future vaccinations.

Coding, Billing, and Costs

Billing third-party payers for immunization services (and all other health services) is based on two systems[33]:

- *Current Procedural Terminology (CPT) Codes*—These describe the *procedures* or *services* performed during a visit. The *visit itself* usually falls under evaluation and management codes for preventive medicine services performed in the outpatient setting, provided the immunization occurs in the context of a comprehensive "checkup." These codes, which vary by age and whether the person is new to the practice or established as a patient, are given in **Table 4.4**. There are corresponding codes for the *vaccines themselves*, which are given in **Table 4.5** (this table includes the codes for selected immune globulin products as well). There are also codes for the *administration* of the vaccines and immune globulins, given in **Table 4.6**. If the visit is *only* for immunization (eg, before travel), most offices bill only for the vaccine and the administration, using the specific codes listed in **Tables 4.5** and **4.6**.

  If evaluation and management services unrelated to vaccination are performed during the vaccine visit, those services receive separate CPT and ICD-9-CM codes. Some payers may require that the modifiers be attached to the CPT code to indicate that the service was separate from immunization but delivered by the same physician on the same day. A relatively minor, incidental problem discovered by the nurse who is giving the immunizations could lead to use of CPT

TABLE 4.4 — CPT Codes for Preventive Medicine Services, 2010[a]

Age	New Patient[b] CPT	New Patient[b] ICD-9-CM	Established Patient[c] CPT	Established Patient[c] ICD-9-CM
<8 days	99381	V20.31	99391	V20.31
8 to 28 days	99381	V20.32	99391	V20.32
29 to 364 days	99381	V20.2	99391	V20.2
1 to 4 years	99382	V20.2	99392	V20.2
5 to 11 years	99383	V20.2[d]	99393	V20.2[d]
12 to 17 years	99384	V20.2[d]	99394	V20.2[d]
18 to 39 years	99385	V70.0	99395	V70.0
40 to 64 years	99386	V70.0	99396	V70.0
≥65 years	99387	V70.0	99397	V70.0

[a] If vaccinations are scheduled but not carried out, the following set of ICD-9-CM codes can be used to indicate the reason:
V64.00, vaccination not carried out, unspecified reason
V64.01, vaccination not carried out because of acute illness
V64.02, vaccination not carried out because of chronic illness or condition
V64.03, vaccination not carried out because of immune compromised state
V64.04, vaccination not carried out because of allergy to vaccine or component
V64.05, vaccination not carried out because of caregiver refusal
V64.06, vaccination not carried out because of patient refusal
V64.07, vaccination not carried out for religious reasons
V64.08, vaccination not carried out because patient had disease being vaccinated against
V64.09, vaccination not carried out for other reason.
[b] Initial comprehensive preventive medicine.
[c] Periodic comprehensive preventive medicine.
[d] If the visit is for a school physical, V70.3 (general medical examination for adoption, camp, school admission, etc) can be used.

Adapted from Abraham M, et al. *CPT 2010 Professional Edition.* Chicago, IL: AMA Press; 2010, and Hart AC, et al. *ICD-9-CM Expert for Physicians: International Classification of Diseases—9th Revision—Clinical Modification 2010 ed.* Salt Lake City, UT: Ingenix, Inc; 2009.

code 99211 (office or other outpatient services, established patient) along with the ICD-9 code describing the reason for the incremental service. To use this code, the presence of a physician is not required, but the presenting problem should be minimal and the time taken should be on the order of 5 minutes. Importantly, the service performed must be medically necessary and must be separate from the vaccine administration. An example is an incidental runny nose discovered during a routine vaccine visit and diagnosed as a mild upper respiratory viral infection.

TABLE 4.5 — Codes for Vaccines and Selected Immune Globulins, 2010

Drug Name		Manufacturer/	Codes	
Generic	Trade	Distributor	CPT	ICD-9-CM[a]
Vaccines				
Anthrax, SC	Biothrax	Emergent BioDefense Operations Lansing	90581	V03.89[b]
DT, <7 years, IM	Tetanus and Diphtheria Toxoids Adsorbed USP for Pediatric Use	Sanofi Pasteur	90702	V06.5
DTaP, <7 years, IM	Daptacel	Sanofi Pasteur	90700	V06.1
	Infanrix	GlaxoSmithKline		
	Tripedia	Sanofi Pasteur		
DTaP-HepB-IPV, IM	Pediarix	GlaxoSmithKline	90723	V06.8[c]
DTaP/Hib-T, IM	TriHIBit	Sanofi Pasteur	90721	V06.8[c]
DTaP-IPV, IM	Kinrix	GlaxoSmithKline	90696	V06.8[c]
DTaP-IPV/Hib-T, IM	Pentacel	Sanofi Pasteur	90698	V06.8[c]
HepA, adult, IM	Havrix	GlaxoSmithKline	90632	V05.3
	Vaqta	Merck		
HepA, pediatric/adolescent, 2 dose, IM	Havrix	GlaxoSmithKline	90633	V05.3
	Vaqta	Merck		
HepA, pediatric/adolescent, 3 dose, IM	Havrix	GlaxoSmithKline	90634	V05.3

HepA-HepB, adult, IM	Twinrix	GlaxoSmithKline	90636	V06.8[c]
HepB, adult, IM	Engerix-B	GlaxoSmithKline	90746	V05.3
	Recombivax HB	Merck		
HepB, dialysis or immunosuppressed, 3 dose, IM	Recombivax HB	Merck	90740	V05.3
HepB, dialysis or immunosuppressed, 4 dose, IM	Engerix-B	GlaxoSmithKline	90747	V05.3
HepB, adolescent, 2 dose, IM	Recombivax HB	Merck	90743	V05.3
HepB, pediatric/adolescent, 3 dose, IM	Engerix-B	GlaxoSmithKline	90744	V05.3
	Recombivax HB	Merck		
HepB-Hib-OMP, IM	Comvax	Merck	90748	V06.8[c]
Hib-OMP, 3 dose, IM	PedvaxHIB	Merck	90647	V03.81
Hib-T, 4 dose, IM	ActHIB	Sanofi Pasteur	90648	V03.81
HibMenCY, 4 dose, IM	MenHibrix[d]	GlaxoSmithKline	90644	V06.8[c]
HPV4, 3 dose, IM	Gardasil	Merck	90649	V04.89[e]
HPV2, 3 dose, IM	Cervarix	GlaxoSmithKline	90650	V04.89[e]
IIV, 6 to 35 months, IM	Fluzone	Sanofi Pasteur	90657	V04.81
IIV, preservative-free, 6 to 35 months, IM	Fluzone	Sanofi Pasteur	90655	V04.81
IIV, ≥3 years, IM[f]	Afluria	CSL Biotherapies/Merck	90658	V04.81
	Fluarix	GlaxoSmithKline		
	Flulaval	GlaxoSmithKline		
	Fluvirin	Novartis		
	Fluzone	Sanofi Pasteur		

Continued

4

125

TABLE 4.5 — *Continued*

Drug Name		Manufacturer/	Codes	
Generic	Trade	Distributor	CPT	ICD-9-CM[a]
IIV, preservative-free, ≥3 years, IM[f]	Afluria Fluarix Fluvirin Fluzone	CSL Biotherapies/Merck GlaxoSmithKline Novartis Sanofi Pasteur	90656	V04.81
IIV, cell culture-derived, preservative- and antibiotic-free, IM[d]	—	—	90661	V04.81
IIV, preservative-free, enhanced immunogenicity via increased antigen content, IM	Fluzone High-Dose	Sanofi Pasteur	90662	V04.81
Influenza, inactivated or live, pandemic formulation, H1N1, IM or IN	—	CSL Biotherapies/Merck ID Biomedical/ GlaxoSmithKline MedImmune (AstraZeneca) Novartis	90663	V04.81
IPV, SC or IM	IPOL	Sanofi Pasteur	90713	V04.0
JE-MB, SC	JE-Vax	Sanofi Pasteur	90735	V05.0
JE-VC, IM	Ixiaro	Novartis	90738	V05.0

LAIV	FluMist	MedImmune (AstraZeneca)	90660	V04.81
MMR, SC	M-M-R II	Merck	90707	V06.4
MMRV, SC	ProQuad	Merck	90710	V06.8[c]
MCV4-CRM, IM	Menveo	Novartis	90734	V03.89[b]
MCV4-D, IM	Menactra	Sanofi Pasteur	90734	V03.89[b]
MPSV4, SC	Menomune–A/C/Y/W-135	Sanofi Pasteur	90733	V03.89[b]
PCV7, IM	Prevnar	Pfizer (formerly Wyeth)	90669	V03.82
PCV13, IM	Prevnar 13	Pfizer (formerly Wyeth)	90670	V03.82
PPSV23, SC or IM	Pneumovax 23	Merck	90732	V03.82
RAB-HDC, IM	Imovax Rabies	Sanofi Pasteur	90675	V04.5
RAB PCEC, IM	RabAvert	Novartis		
RV5, 3 dose, PO	RotaTeq	Merck	90680	V04.89[e]
RV1, 2 dose, PO	Rotarix	GlaxoSmithKline	90681	V04.89[e]
Smallpox	ACAM2000	Sanofi Pasteur (formerly Acambis)	90749[g]	V04.1
	Dryvax	Pfizer (formerly Wyeth)		
Td, ≥7 years, IM	Tetanus and Diphtheria Toxoids Adsorbed for Adult Use	MassBiologics	90718	V06.5
Td, preservative-free, ≥7 years, IM	Decavac	Sanofi Pasteur	90714	V06.5

4

Continued

TABLE 4.5 — *Continued*

| Drug Name | | Manufacturer/ | Codes | |
Generic	Trade	Distributor	CPT	ICD-9-CM[a]
Tdap, ≥7 years, IM	Adacel	Sanofi Pasteur	90715	V06.1
	Boostrix	GlaxoSmithKline		
Tetanus Toxoid Adsorbed		Sanofi Pasteur	90703	V03.7
TT, adsorbed, IM				
Typhoid, live, PO	Vivotif	Crucell (formerly Berna Biotech)	90690	V03.1
Typhoid, Vi capsular polysaccharide, IM	Typhim Vi	Sanofi Pasteur	90691	V03.1
VAR, SC	Varivax	Merck	90716	V05.4
YF vaccine, SC	YF-Vax	Sanofi Pasteur	90717	V04.4
ZOS, SC	Zostavax	Merck	90736	V05.8[h]
Unlisted vaccine/toxoid	—	—	90749	—
Selected Immune Globulins				
Immune globulin, IM	GamaSTAN S/D	Talecris	90281	V05.3
Hepatitis B immune globulin, IM	HepaGam B	Apotex	90371	V05.3
	HyperHEP B S/D	Talecris		
	Nabi-HB	Nabi		
Rabies immune globulin, IM and/or SC	HyperRAB	Talecris	90375	V04.5
Rabies immune globulin, heat-treated, IM and/or SC	Imogam Rabies-HT	Sanofi Pasteur	90376	V04.5

RSV, monoclonal antibody, IM	Synagis	MedImmune (AstraZeneca)	90378	V04.82
Tetanus immune globulin, IM	HyperTET	Talecris	90389	V07.2
Varicella immune globulin, IM	VariZIG[d]	Cangene	90396	V05.4
Unlisted immune globulin	—	—	90399	V07.2

[a] The ICD-9-CM codes specify the reason for the vaccine or immune globulin. For example, the ICD-9-CM code that accompanies DTaP vaccination is V06.1, "need for prophylactic vaccination and inoculation against combinations of diseases, diphtheria-tetanus-pertussis." ICD-9-CM codes in addition to those listed may be submitted. For example, a visit for a DiGeorge syndrome patient for administration of varicella immune globulin might be coded as V05.4, "need for prophylactic vaccination and inoculation against single diseases, varicella", as well as 279.11, "disorders involving the immune mechanism, deficiency of cell-mediated immunity, DiGeorge's syndrome." In some cases, the diagnosis codes are sufficiently ambiguous as to allow several options. For example, although the table shows the code V05.8 ("need for other prophylactic vaccination and inoculation against single diseases, other specified disease") for ZOS, the code V04.89 ("need for other prophylactic vaccination and inoculation against certain viral diseases, other viral diseases") might also be appropriate.

[b] Need for prophylactic vaccination and inoculation against other specified single bacterial disease.

[c] Need for prophylactic vaccination and inoculation against other combination of diseases.

[d] Not licensed in the United States as of February 2010.

[e] Need for prophylactic vaccination and inoculation against other viral disease.

[f] See influenza vaccine tables in Chapter 15: Influenza for labeled age indications.

[g] Unlisted vaccine/toxoid (there is currently no specific CPT code for smallpox vaccine).

[h] Need for prophylactic vaccination and inoculation against other specified single disease.

Adapted from Abraham M, et al. *CPT 2010 Professional Edition*. Chicago, IL: AMA Press; 2010, and Hart AC, et al. *ICD-9-CM Expert for Physicians: International Classification of Diseases—9th Revision—Clinical Modification 2010 ed.* Salt Lake City, UT: Ingenix, Inc; 2009.

TABLE 4.6 — CPT Codes for Administration, 2010[a]

Procedure	Code	Example
Pediatric-Specific Codes[b,c]		
Immunization administration <8 years of age (includes percutaneous, intradermal, SC, and IM) when the physician counsels the patient/family; *first injection*[d] (single or combination vaccine/toxoid), per day	**90465** • Do not report in conjunction with 90467	DTaP given as the first injection of the day for an infant, where the physician performs face-to-face counseling
Immunization administration <8 years of age (includes percutaneous, intradermal, SC, and IM) when the physician counsels the patient/family; *each additional injection* (single or combination vaccine/toxoid), per day	**90466** • List separately in addition to code for primary procedure • Use in conjunction with 90465 or 90467	Hib given as the second injection of the day for an infant, where the physician performs face-to-face counseling
Immunization administration <8 years of age (includes IN and PO) when the physician counsels the patient/family; *first administration*[d] (single or combination vaccine/toxoid), per day	**90467** • Do not report in conjunction with 90465	RV5 given as the first immunization of the day for an infant, where the physician performs face-to-face counseling

Description	Code	Example
Immunization administration <8 years of age (includes IN and PO) when the physician counsels the patient/family; *each additional administration* (single or combination vaccine/toxoid), per day	**90468** • List separately in addition to code for primary procedure • Use in conjunction with 90465 or 90467	RV5 given as the second vaccine of the day for an infant, where the physician performs face-to-face counseling
2009 Influenza H1N1 Vaccine[e] Influenza H1N1 immunization administration (IM or IN), including counseling when performed	**90470**	IIV-2009 H1N1 given as the first or subsequent vaccine of the day
Non–Age-Specific Codes[f] Immunization administration (includes percutaneous, intradermal, SC, and IM); *one vaccine*[d] (single or combination vaccine/toxoid)	**90471** • Do not report in conjunction with 90473	VAR given as the first injection of the day
Immunization administration (includes percutaneous, intradermal, SC, and IM); each *additional* vaccine (single or combination vaccine/toxoid)	**90472** • List separately in addition to code for primary procedure • Use in conjunction with 90471 or 90473	MMR given as the second injection of the day
Immunization administration by IN or PO route; *one vaccine*[d] (single or combination vaccine/toxoid)	**90473** • Do not report in conjunction with 90471	LAIV-seasonal given as the first vaccine of the day

Continued

4

TABLE 4.6 — *Continued*

Procedure	Code	Example
Non-Age-Specific Codes[f]		
Immunization administration by IN or PO route; each *additional* vaccine (single or combination vaccine/toxoid)	**90474** • List separately in addition to code for primary procedure • Use in conjunction with 90471 or 90473	LAIV-seasonal given as the second vaccine of that day
Administration of Selected Immune Globulins		
IV infusion, for therapy, prophylaxis, or diagnosis (specify substance or drug); initial, up to 1 hour	**96365**	IV immune globulin given as prophylaxis against varicella
Each additional hour	**96366** • List separately in addition to 96365	Prolonged IV immune globulin infusion
Therapeutic, prophylactic, or diagnostic injection (specify substance or drug); SC or IM	**96372**	RSV mAB (palivizumab), IM

[a] Each code covers all administrative and clinical staff services associated with giving the vaccine, including making the appointment, preparing the chart, billing, filing, receptionist activities, taking vital signs, screening, reviewing the Vaccine Information Statement, answering questions, administering the vaccine, documenting the administration, and observing after administration. The CPT code for administration and the CPT code for the vaccine (listed in **Table 4.5**) are each reported along with the ICD-9-CM code corresponding to the vaccine (also listed in **Table 4.5**).

[b] These codes should be used (they are not "add-on" codes) when the patient is <8 years of age and the physician performs face-to-face counseling associated with administration of the vaccine. Vaccine counseling includes obtaining information related to contraindications, reviewing the

Vaccine Information Statement, discussing risks and benefits, obtaining consent, addressing parents' concerns, and entering information into immunization information systems (registries). The physician does not have to actually perform the administration. An advanced nurse practitioner who performs the counseling can report these codes as "incident to" a physician, provided the state allows this under the nurse practitioner's scope of practice. Medicare requires that in this situation, the patient must be an established patient and the service must be performed under the direct supervision of the physician (at the very least, he or she must be immediately available in the office suite).

c The RVUs assigned to these families of codes are the same; therefore, reimbursement is likely to be the same (except, perhaps, for some private payers). However, it is important to point out that the RVUs for all administration codes more than doubled between 2004 and 2007. In essence, the valuation of practice expenses and physician work that was inherent in the pediatric-specific codes was also incorporated into the non-age-specific codes.

d The idea here is that there can only be one "first" vaccine given during a particular visit. It does not matter which of the day's vaccines are reported as the first one (2009 influenza H1N1 vaccine is an exception—see below); all other vaccines given at that visit, however, must be reported using an "additional vaccine" administration code.

e 2009 influenza H1N1 vaccine is always considered the first vaccine of the day, regardless of when in sequence it was given. All other vaccines are considered subsequent.

f These codes should be used when neither of the requirements for pediatric-specific codes (90465-90468) are met.

Adapted from Comprehensive overview: immunization administration. American Academy of Pediatrics Web site. http://www.aap.org/moc/reimburse/codingrbrvsresources.htm. Accessed January 27, 2010.

- *International Classification of Diseases, Ninth Revision, Clinical Modification (ICD-9-CM) Codes*—These describe the *reason* for the service. The *visit itself* usually falls under V20.2 (health supervision of infant or child, routine infant or child health check beyond the first month of life) or V70.0 (general medical examination, routine general medical examination at a health care facility; adults). Most vaccines and immune globulins *themselves* have specific ICD-9-CM codes, given in **Table 4.5**. The compliance date for the tenth revision of these codes (ICD-10-CM) is October 2013.[34]

Many payers are now requiring that National Drug Codes (NDCs) for vaccines be submitted along with CPT and ICD-9-CM codes. The NDC is a unique 10-digit, 3-segment number. The first segment identifies the company that makes, repacks, or distributes the product. The second segment identifies the product, strength, dosage form, and formulation. The third segment identifies the package size and type. Sometimes an asterisk appears as a placeholder. NDCs can easily be found by searching the National Drug Code Directory[35] by proprietary name, active ingredient, or company name. It is also found on the package insert in the "How Supplied" section.

A routine visit for a 6-month-old infant might be coded as shown in **Table 4.7**. Remember, all components of all services should be clearly documented in the medical record. If the practice receives vaccines free-of-charge through the VFC Program, it cannot bill for the *vaccine itself*, but it can bill for *administration of the vaccine* and for the *visit itself*.

The vaccine tables in *Section B* contain information on the purchase price for commonly used vaccines. The public sector cost is the contracted price between the CDC and the manufacturer, which changes from year to year.[36] The listed private sector cost is based on the direct purchase price from the manufacturer and is most useful for highlighting relative differences between products. However, these data can be misleading. In a study conducted in 2007, 76 private practices in five states supplied data on their purchase price for vaccines for privately insured children.[37] Significant variation was seen—for example, some practices paid $8.77 per dose for Infanrix while others paid $21.60; some paid $8.25 for Recombivax HB while others paid $23.20; some paid $14.29 for IPOL while others paid $26.34. Variables associated with the price paid include the size of the practice, its location, use of purchasing cooperatives or buying groups, and the availability of discounts and rebates. Large variation was also seen in reimbursement—for example, some practices were reimbursed $59.02 per dose of M-M-R II, others $16.77; some were reimbursed $45.32 per dose of ActHIB, others $15.33. Reimbursement for first dose vaccine administration ranged from $0 to $26.55. In

TABLE 4.7 — Coding for a Routine Visit at 6 Months of Age, 2010[a]

Procedure	Visit		Vaccine		Vaccine Administration	
	CPT	ICD-9-CM	CPT	ICD-9-CM	CPT	ICD-9-CM
Checkup	99391[b]	V20.2[c]	—	—	—	—
DTaP-HepB-IPV	—	—	90723	V06.8	90465[d]	V06.8
Hib-T	—	—	90648	V03.81	90466	V03.81
PCV13	—	—	90670	V03.82	90466	V03.82
IIV	—	—	90655	V04.81	90466	V04.81
RV5	—	—	90680	V04.89	90468	V04.89

[a] The billing rules for particular insurance companies may vary.
[b] Established patient, periodic comprehensive preventive medicine, under 1 year of age.
[c] Routine infant or child health check.
[d] This series of codes is used if the requirements for pediatric-specific codes are met (see Table 4.5).

135

negotiating contract prices with private payers, physicians must consider all of the costs involved in providing vaccines, some of which are listed in **Table 4.8**.

TABLE 4.8 — Provider Costs for Vaccination Services

Direct Costs
- Vaccine purchase (includes excise tax)
- Sales or usage tax

Overhead
- Personnel time: order and inventory vaccines; negotiate prices, delivery, and payment terms; monitor stock; track unpaid claims
- Storage: refrigerator; freezer; locks; temperature monitoring devices and alarm systems; electricity; generators; associated monitoring and maintenance costs (some of these costs are depreciated)
- Insurance against vaccine loss
- Wastage: spills; expiration; damage; drawing up vaccine and having patient reconsider and not pay
- Nonpayment despite collection efforts
- Lost opportunity costs: occupied rooms that could have been used for other income-generating activities; money tied up in inventory that could have been gaining interest

Administration Expenses
- Physician work: time; technical skill and physical effort; mental effort and judgement; psychological stress associated with concerns about risks
- Staff work: time; technical skill and physical effort; mental effort and judgement; data entry into IISs
- Medical supplies: gloves; exam tables and paper; OSHA-compliant syringes with needles; alcohol swabs; band-aids; emergency response items; token patient rewards
- Professional liability insurance

Adapted from The Business Case for Pricing Vaccines and Immunization Administration. American Academy of Pediatrics Web site. http://practice .aap.org/content.aspx?aid=1808. Accessed January 23, 2010.

REFERENCES

1. Vaccine Storage and Handling Toolkit. Centers for Disease Control and Prevention Web site. http://www2a.cdc.gov/vaccines/ed/shtoolkit. Accessed February 10, 2010.

2. Briss PA, et al. *Am J Prev Med.* 2000;18(suppl 1):97-140.

3. Wood DL, et al. *Pediatrics.* 2003;112:993-996.

4. Szilagyi PG, et al. *JAMA.* 2000;284:1820-1827.

5. Jacobson VJC, Szilagyi P. Patient reminder and recall systems to improve immunization rates. Cochrane Review Web site. http://www.cochrane.org/reviews/en/ab003941.html. Accessed January 23, 2010.

6. CDC. *MMWR.* 1994;43:709-718.

7. Walton S, et al. *Arch Dis Child.* 2007;92:620-622.

8. Healy CM, et al. *Vaccine.* 2009;27:5599-5602.

9. Nation's first "cocoon strategy" vaccination program delivers 10,000th immunization. Texas Children's Hospital Web site. http://www.texaschildrens.org/AllAbout/News/2010/Cocoon.aspx. Accessed February 23, 2010.

10. Shah SI, et al. *Pediatrics.* 2007;120:e617-e621.

11. Dylag AM, et al. *Pediatrics.* 2008;122:e550-e555.

12. Walter EB, et al. *Academic Pediatr.* 2009;9:344-347.

13. McKibben LJ, et al. *MMWR.* 2000;49(RR-1):15-16.

14. Kelly J, et al. *MMWR.* 2010;59:133-135.

15. Committee on Practice and Ambulatory Medicine, et al. *Pediatrics.* 2006;118:1293-1295.

16. Turning barriers into opportunities: survey and best practice report. American Immunization Registry Association Web site. http://www.immregistries.org/pubs/index.phtml. Accessed January 23, 2010.

17. American Immunization Registry Association. Registry standards of excellence in support of an immunization program. http://www.immregistries.org/pdf/PROWstandardscomp1.pdf. Accessed January 23, 2010.

18. CDC. *MMWR.* 2008;57:289-291.

19. National Vaccine Advisory Committee. Development of community and state-based immunization registries: report of the National Vaccine Advisory Committee (NVAC). Atlanta, GA: US Department of Health and Human Services, CDC; 1999. Available at http://www.cdc.gov/vaccines/programs/iis/pubs/nvac.htm. Accessed February 4, 2010.

20. IIS: 2001 minimum functional standards for registries. Centers for Disease Control and Prevention Web site. http://www.cdc.gov/vaccines/programs/iis/stds/min-funct-std-2001.htm. Updated May 26, 2009. Accessed January 23, 2010.

21. Assessment, Feedback, Incentives, and Exchange (AFIX). Centers for Disease Control and Prevention Web site. http://www.cdc.gov/vaccines/programs/afix/default.htm. Accessed February 23, 2010.

22. Comprehensive Clinic Assessment Software Application (CoCASA). http://www.cdc.gov/vaccines/programs/cocasa/default.htm. Accessed February 23, 2010.

23. Screening questionnaires. Immunization Action Coalition Web site. http://www.immunize.org/printmaterials/topic_screening.asp. Accessed February 23, 2010.

24. Schechter NL, et al. *Pediatrics*. 2007;119:e1184-e1198.

25. Taddio A, et al. *Clin Ther*. 2009;31(suppl B):S48-S76.

26. Shah V, et al. *Clin Ther*. 2009;31(suppl B):S104-S151.

27. Kroger AT, et al. *MMWR*. 2006;55(RR-15):1-48.

28. General recommendations on immunization. In: Atkinson W, et al, eds. *Epidemiology and Prevention of Vaccine-Preventable Diseases*. 11th ed. Washington, DC: Public Health Foundation, 2009; 9-30.

29. Prymula R, et al. *Lancet*. 2009;374:1339-1350.

30. Bohlke K, et al. *Pediatrics*. 2003;112:815-820.

31. American Academy of Pediatrics Committee on Pediatric Emergency Medicine, Frush K. *Pediatrics*. 2007;120:200-212.

32. CDC. *MMWR*. 2008;57:457-460.

33. Tuck RH. *Pediatr Ann*. 2006;35:507-512.

34. Office of the Secretary, Department of Health and Human Services. Federal Register. 2009;74:3328-3362 (45 CFR Part 162).

35. National Drug Code Directory. US Food and Drug Administration Web site. http://www.accessdata.fda.gov/scripts/cder/ndc/default.cfm. Accessed January 27, 2010.

36. CDC Vaccine Price List. Centers for Disease Control and Prevention Web site. http://www.cdc.gov/vaccines/programs/vfc/cdc-vac-price-list.htm. Accessed January 20, 2010.

37. Freed GL, et al. *Pediatrics*. 2009;124:S459-S465.

5

General Recommendations

Vaccine recommendations have become very complex. The following general rules, derived from the CDC's *General Recommendations on Immunization*,[1] are offered as a guide to providers in day-to-day practice. Remember, however—there are exceptions to every rule.

■ **Any Vaccines Can Be Given at the Same Time**
   EXCEPTIONS: *1) VAR and smallpox vaccine; 2) LAIV-seasonal and LAIV-2009 H1N1.*
   Simultaneous administration of all vaccines for which a person is eligible at a given visit is encouraged for two reasons: achievement of optimal protection is not delayed and completion of all recommended vaccine series is more likely. There are no vaccines that cannot be given at the same time, considering both reactogenicity and immunogenicity, except for those listed above. In the case of VAR and smallpox, the concern is the potential for increased complications of smallpox vaccination. In the case of LAIV-seasonal and LAIV-2009 H1N1, the concern is potential competition between the vaccine viruses and decreased immunogenicity. Vaccines given on the same day must be given at separate sites and should never be mixed in the same syringe unless the products are specifically labeled for that purpose. Licensed combination vaccines can reduce the high number of shots that are now unavoidable at certain visits during childhood.
   Despite this rule, package inserts may warn against concomitant use of certain vaccines. For example, the ZOS package insert says not to administer the vaccine and PPSV23 at the same time because the antibody response to VZV might be impaired. CDC, however, considers simultaneous administration acceptable, because lower antibody levels do not necessarily mean reduced protection.

■ **Live Vaccines Not Given at the Same Time Should Be Separated by at Least 4 Weeks**
   EXCEPTIONS: *1) YF vaccine may be given at any time after single-antigen measles vaccine; 2) Live oral vaccines (RV and typhoid Ty21a) may be given at any time in relation to any other live vaccines.*
   Different live vaccines can be given simultaneously (except as above) at different sites. If live vaccines are to be given sequentially, they should be separated by at least 4 weeks so that

replication of the first vaccine does not interfere with replication of the second. Any timing sequence between live vaccines and inactivated vaccines is acceptable. LAIV, even though it replicates at a mucosal surface as do oral vaccines, is *not* an exception to this rule—if not given on the same day, live influenza vaccine and live parenteral vaccines should be administered at least 4 weeks apart.

■ **Different Inactivated Vaccines May Be Given at Any Time With Respect to Each Other**
 EXCEPTIONS: *None.*

Simultaneous administration, or better yet the use of combination vaccines, is preferred because of improved compliance. However, there is no evidence that sequential administration of *different* inactivated vaccines at any time interval interferes with immunogenicity or increases reactogenicity. The case of sequential administration of Tdap and MCV4-D is a little tricky. While these are ostensibly *different* vaccines, they both contain diphtheria toxoid (it is the carrier protein for the polysaccharide in MCV4-D). The AAP suggests a minimum interval of 1 month between Tdap and MCV4-D if the vaccines are not given on the same day—the concern is that too many doses of diphtheria toxoid in sequence can cause increased reactogenicity. The ACIP, however, does not recommend a minimum interval.

■ **There are Minimum Acceptable Intervals Between Doses of the Same Vaccine**
 EXCEPTIONS: *1) The 4-day grace period; 2) Early, accelerated, or compressed schedules in certain situations.*

Proper spacing of doses within a given vaccine series is essential for optimal immune responses. For this reason, doses of the same vaccine administered sooner than the specified minimum interval are considered invalid. The CDC suggests a "grace period" whereby a dose given up to 4 days before the recommended interval (or minimum age) should be counted as valid (exceptions include RAB and 2009 H1N1 influenza vaccine). However, some states and local jurisdictions may not accept this interpretation for school entry requirements, so the best advice is to give the vaccine at the recommended minimum age and interval. Invalid doses should be repeated, but the minimum interval should elapse between the invalid dose and the repeat dose. There are circumstances where early, accelerated, or compressed schedules can be used, such as for catch-up immunization or impending international travel. However, even here the minimum intervals should be followed. **Table 5.1** shows the recommended minimum ages and intervals for routinely used vaccines.

One other caveat: a minimum interval is a minimum interval except when it's not. So, for example, the minimum interval between doses 3 and 4 of DTaP is 6 months. However, if Dose 4 is given at least 4 months after Dose 3, it is considered valid. Similarly, the minimum interval between doses of VAR under 13 years of age is 12 weeks, but if Dose 1 is given ≥28 days after Dose 2, it is considered valid. One could legitimately ask why, then, are the respective minimum intervals not 4 months and 28 days? One explanation might be that the major studies leading to licensure of these vaccines used the longer interval, but that some studies attest to the safety and immunogenicity of the shorter interval.

The minimum interval between doses of modern combination vaccines is determined by the component antigen with the longest minimum interval.

■ **There Are Minimum Ages for Administration of All Vaccines**
  EXCEPTIONS: *BCG, HepB, and RAB.*

For live parenteral vaccines, the issue is inactivation of the vaccine by circulating maternal antibody, which can persist for as long as a year. Live oral vaccines such as RV have not been studied in children <6 weeks of age. For other vaccines such as Hib, the issue is that administration in the first 6 weeks of life might induce immunologic tolerance. HepB and BCG may be given at birth. During measles outbreaks when cases are occurring in infants under a year of age, and for impending travel outside the United States, measles vaccine can be given before the recommended minimum age of 12 months (and as early as 6 months). Doses given under 12 months of age, however, are not counted as part of the routine series.

■ **Partial or Fractional Doses of a Vaccine Should Never Be Used**
  EXCEPTIONS: *None.*

In the past, some practitioners gave "split" doses of vaccines (particularly DTwP) in order to minimize potential reactions. There is no support for this practice, even in premature infants. Less than full doses of vaccines should not be counted as valid.

■ **A Multidose Vaccine Series Should Not Be Restarted if the Recommended Dosing Interval Is Exceeded**
  EXCEPTION: *Oral typhoid Ty21a.*

If there is a lapse in the administration of sequential doses of a given series, simply begin where the series was suspended, keeping in mind the minimum intervals between doses. The only exception to this rule is the oral typhoid Ty21a vaccine, for which some experts recommend repeating the series if all 4 doses are not given within 3 weeks.

TABLE 5.1 — Minimum Ages and Intervals for Routine Vaccines

Vaccine	Dose Number	Age Recommended	Age Minimum	Interval to Next Dose Recommended	Interval to Next Dose Minimum
DTaP	1	2 months	6 weeks	2 months	4 weeks
	2	4 months	10 weeks	2 months	4 weeks
	3	6 months	14 weeks	6 to 12 calendar months	6 calendar months[a]
	4	15 to 18 months	12 months	3 years	6 calendar months
	5	4 to 6 years	4 years	—	—
HepA	1	12 to 23 months	12 months	6 to 18 calendar months	6 calendar months
	2	18 to 41 months	18 months	—	—
HepB	1	Birth[b]	Birth[b]	1 to 4 months	4 weeks
	2	1 to 2 months	4 weeks	2 to 17 months	8 weeks[c]
	3	6 to 18 months	24 weeks	—	—
Hib	1[d]	2 months	6 weeks	2 months	4 weeks
	2	4 months	10 weeks	2 months	4 weeks
	(3)[e]	6 months	14 weeks	6 to 9 calendar months	8 weeks
	4	12 to 15 months	12 months	—	—
HPV[f]	1	11 to 12 years	9 years	2 months	4 weeks
	2	11 to 12 years (plus 2 months)	109 months	4 months	12 weeks[g]

142

	3	11 to 12 years (plus 6 months)	114 months	—	—
IIV	1[h]	Annual	6 months[i]	1 month	4 weeks[j]
IPV	1	2 months	6 weeks[k]	2 months	4 weeks[k]
	2	4 months	10 weeks	2 to 14 months	4 weeks
	3	6 to 18 months	14 weeks	3 to 5 years	6 months
	4	4 to 6 years	4 years		(6 months)[l]
	(5)[l]	4 to 6 years	4 years		
LAIV	1[h]	Annual	2 years	1 month	4 weeks[m]
MCV	1	11 to 12 years	2 years	3 to 5 years[n]	3 to 5 years[n]
	2[n]	—	5 years	5 years	5 years
MMR	1	12 to 15 months	12 months	3 to 5 years	4 weeks[o]
	2	4 to 6 years	13 months	3 to 5 years	—
MPSV[p]	1	—	2 years	5 years[n]	5 years[n]
	2[n]	—	7 years	—	—
PCV	1[d]	2 months	6 weeks	2 months	4 weeks[q]
	2	4 months	10 weeks	2 months	4 weeks[q]
	3	6 months	14 weeks	6 months	8 weeks[q]
	4	12 to 15 months	12 months	—	(8 weeks)[r]
	(5)[r]	14 to 59 months	14 months	—	—

Continued

TABLE 5.1 — *Continued*

Vaccine	Dose Number	Age Recommended	Age Minimum	Interval to Next Dose Recommended	Interval to Next Dose Minimum
PPSV[s]	1	—	2 years	5 years	5 years
	2	—	7 years	—	—
RV[t]	1	2 months	6 weeks	2 months	4 weeks
	2	4 months	10 weeks	(2 months)	(4 weeks)
	(3)	6 months	14 weeks	—	—
Td	1	11 to 12 years[u]	7 years	10 years	5 years
Tdap	1	≥11 years	10 years[i]	—	—
VAR	1	12 to 15 months	12 months	3 to 5 years	12 weeks[o,v]
	2	4 to 6 years	15 months	—	—
Zoster	1	60 years	60 years	—	—

See *Conventions Used in This Book* for definitions of ages and time intervals.

[a] Dose 4 need not be repeated if given at least 4 months after Dose 3.
[b] Combination products cannot be used for the birth dose.
[c] Dose 3 should be given at least 16 weeks after Dose 1.
[d] Children receiving Dose 1 after 6 months of age require fewer doses.
[e] A dose at 6 months of age is not necessary if Hib-OMP (PedvaxHIB; Merck) is used for doses 1 and 2.
[f] This vaccine is only routinely recommended for females. HPV4 may be used in males for prevention of genital warts.
[g] Dose 3 should be given at least 24 weeks after Dose 1.

144

h For seasonal vaccines (IIV or LAIV), 2 doses separated by at least 4 weeks are required for children <9 years of age who are being immunized for the first time, as well as children <9 years of age who were immunized for the first time in the prior year and only received 1 dose. For 2009 H1N1 vaccines (IIV or LAIV), the age cut-off for 2 doses in the same season is <10. If a child turns 9 or 10, respectively, before the second dose, that dose becomes unnecessary.

i The minimum age differs by product.

j Whereas the minimum interval between 2 doses of IIV-2009 H1N1 is 4 weeks, doses given 21 to 27 days apart do not need to be repeated. The 4-day "grace period" does not apply to H1N1 vaccine intervals.

k Minimum age and minimum intervals during the first 6 months of life should only be used if the child is at risk of imminent exposure to poliovirus.

l Dose 5 is indicated if all 4 previous doses were given before 4 years of age (the final dose of IPV should be given at ≥4 years of age regardless of the number of previous doses). This would apply, for example, if a child received 4 doses of IPV as DTaP-IPV/Hib-T by 18 months of age.

m LAIV-seasonal and LAIV-2009 H1N1 should not be given at the same time. Whereas the minimum interval between 2 doses of LAIV-2009 H1N1, and between doses of LAIV-seasonal and LAIV-2009 H1N1, is 4 weeks, doses given 14-27 days apart do not need to be repeated. The 4-day "grace period" does not apply to H1N1 vaccine intervals.

n Revaccination is only recommended for persons who remain at high risk (college students without other risk factors who were appropriately immunized should not be revaccinated). Children who were vaccinated at 2 to 6 years of age (with MPSV or MCV) should be revaccinated with MCV 3 years after the first vaccination (as of February 2010, only MCV4-D is licensed for children 2 to 10 years of age). Persons who were vaccinated at ≥7 years of age (with MPSV or MCV) should be revaccinated with either MCV4-CRM or MCV4-D every 5 years (after 55 years of age, MPSV4 should be used).

o The minimum interval is 12 weeks if MMRV (ProQuad; Merck) is used.

p MCV is preferred for persons 2 to 55 years of age (as of February 2010, only MCV4-D is licensed for children 2 to 10 years of age).

q At <12 months of age, the minimum interval between doses of PCV is 4 weeks. At ≥12 months of age, the minimum interval is 8 weeks.

r PCV7 was routinely used from 2000 through 2009. PCV13 was licensed in February 2010. Children who started the series with PCV7 should switch to PCV13 at any point in the schedule. Those who have already received 4 doses of PCV7 and are ≤59 months of age should receive a single supplemental dose of PCV13 (for high-risk children, the single supplemental dose may be given up to 71 months of age).

s PPSV is recommended for children with high-risk conditions after the PCV series is completed. Dose 2 is recommended for children at highest risk.

Continued

145

TABLE 5.1 — *Continued*

t RV1 is given as a 2-dose and RV5 as a 3-dose series. The schedules in the package inserts differ from the ACIP recommendations; in this situation, the ACIP recommendations are usually followed in practice. According to the RV1 package insert, Dose 1 may be given between 6 and 20 weeks of age, and no dose should be given beyond 24 weeks. According to the RV5 package insert, Dose 1 should be given at 6 to 12 weeks of age, and no dose should be given beyond 32 weeks. ACIP recommendations call for Dose 1 of either vaccine to be given between 6 weeks and 14 weeks 6 days of age, and all doses should be given by 8 months 0 days. If any dose in the series is RV5 or unknown, a total of 3 doses should be given.

u Tdap is preferred for routine use at 11 to 12 years of age.

v If the second dose is given ≥28 days after the first dose, this should be considered valid and should not be repeated. The minimum interval is 4 weeks if the series is initiated after 12 years of age.

Adapted from Centers for Disease Control and Prevention. *Epidemiology and Prevention of Vaccine-Preventable Diseases*. 11th ed. Atkinson W, et al, eds. Washington, DC: Public Health Foundation; 2009: Appendix A, with modifications based on recommendations released since 2009.

■ **Similar Vaccines Made by Different Manufacturers Are Interchangeable**

EXCEPTION: *There is a preference for using the same DTaP, HPV and RV products for the entire series.*

Vaccines from different manufacturers differ in composition, formulation, and content. However, sufficient data exist to consider many of the vaccines made by different manufacturers interchangeable in a given series, including diphtheria toxoid, tetanus toxoid, HepA, HepB, and IPV. Hib vaccines are also interchangeable, but if ActHIB (Hib-T) is used as Dose 1 or Dose 2, the primary series should include 3 doses (an all-PedvaxHIB [Hib-OMP] schedule requires only 2 doses for the primary series). All types (inactivated and live) and brands of influenza vaccine are considered interchangeable, provided the products are used in the appropriate age groups. Because of limited data, the ACIP expresses a preference for the same DTaP product for the entire series. Practically speaking, however, this recommendation is difficult to implement, and vaccination *should not be deferred* if the same product is not immediately available or if the previous products are not known. Similarly, RV should not be deferred if the same product as the previous dose is not available; however, if any one of the doses in the series was RV5 or unknown, 3 total doses should be given (an all-RV1 schedule requires only 2 doses).

It should be mentioned that vaccines for the same disease are not strictly interchangeable if they are fundamentally different vaccines. For example, both MCV and MPSV protect against meningococcal disease. However, the former is a protein-polysaccharide conjugate and the latter is a pure polysaccharide, and the recommendations for each differ. The same is true for PCV and PPSV. VAR and ZOS contain the exact same live-attenuated VZV, although in differing amounts, and the two vaccines are used for entirely different purposes (respectively, prevention of varicella and herpes zoster). Likewise, DTaP and Tdap may contain the same antigens but are used for different purposes. Finally, recognize that if a mixed schedule of HPV vaccines is used, full protection against genital warts cannot be assumed, since only HPV4 protects against serotypes 6 and 11.

■ **There Is No Harm in Vaccinating a Person Who Has Already Had the Disease or the Vaccine**

EXCEPTION: *1) Administering too many doses of PPSV23, tetanus toxoid, or diphtheria toxoid can cause increased reactogenicity; 2) Anthrax vaccine in persons who have had anthrax disease.*

For some diseases, vaccination is actually *indicated* even if the person has had the disease. For example, infants <2 years of age who had invasive *H influenzae* infection should still be vaccinated because infection at that age does not confer effective immunity. ZOS is specifically designed to be given to people who have had VZV infection. For *S pneumoniae*, the vaccine protects against multiple serotypes, so prior infection with a particular serotype does not obviate the need for vaccination; similarly, completion of the 4-dose PCV7 schedule does not obviate the need for a dose of PCV13 in children ≤59 months of age, in order to confer immunity to the additional 6 serotypes. Along similar lines, HPV vaccine *should be given* to women who have already had HPV infection, not to alter the course of infection (which it does not do) but to protect against other serotypes. Influenza vaccine *must* be given each year whether or not the person has had influenza in the past. Some experts recommend pertussis vaccine for children who have had well-documented pertussis (culture positive or epidemiologically linked to a culture-positive case) because the duration of natural immunity is not known. Clinicians often wonder if a child with a questionable history of chickenpox or varicella vaccination should receive the vaccine. The motto here is—*when in doubt, vaccinate*! With chickenpox, as with most other diseases, there is no evidence of harm if a person who has had the disease or the vaccine receives another dose of the vaccine (one exception is anthrax—there is some evidence that vaccine adverse events are more severe in persons who have had the disease).

■ **Live Vaccines Should be Deferred After Receipt of Antibody-Containing Blood Products**
  EXCEPTIONS: *1) YF vaccine, oral typhoid Ty21a, LAIV, RV, and ZOS; 2) MMR and VAR should not be deferred in postpartum women who received antibody-containing blood products during pregnancy, including anti-Rho(D) globulin*

Antibodies contained in blood products can inactivate live vaccines and reduce effectiveness or "take." Several factors play into whether or not deferral is recommended and determine the time interval after which a vaccine can be given. One factor is the product itself—immune globulin intravenous is likely to contain more antibody than packed red cells, hence necessitating a longer delay. Another factor is the specific antibody content of the product; for example, blood products in the United States are unlikely to contain antibodies to yellow fever virus and *S typhi*, so these vaccines can be given at any time with respect to blood products. ZOS does not need to be delayed because it is *designed* to be given to persons with circulating antibody to VZV. Finally, passively transferred antibodies are unlikely to inactivate vaccines delivered at mucosal surfaces—hence the exception for LAIV and RV. **Table 5.2** shows the recommended intervals between blood product administration and certain live vaccines. Keep in mind that, in general, the antibodies in blood products do not interfere with inactivated vaccines (HepA may be an exception). Three other caveats deserve mention 1) if a child has already received MMR, VAR, or MMRV, 2 weeks should elapse before an antibody-containing blood product is given, because the vaccine viruses must still replicate in order to induce immunity; 2) if a pregnant woman receives a blood product, that should not result in deferral of her infant's first dose of RV; and 3) monoclonal antibody products such as RSV-mAB (Synagis) do not interfere with (heterologous) live vaccines.

5

■ Administration Errors

Sometimes, despite the best of intentions, mistakes are made in vaccine administration. **Table 5.3** lists some common administration errors and gives recommendations to remedy the situation.

■ More Vaccination Pearls

Here are some additional vaccination pearls:

- Serology is of limited utility in vaccine practice. Testing for varicella antibodies before vaccination might be cost-effective in adults who do not have a personal history of chickenpox. However, in most other circumstances vaccines should just be given without testing for immunity. This would include internationally adopted children with a questionable vaccination history—it is probably simpler just to reimmunize than to test for immunity to multiple antigens. For the most part, immunity is presumed to result from appropriate vaccine schedules and doses. Testing for seroconversion is indicated only rarely, such as in high-risk health care personnel or dialysis patients given HepB, laboratory workers receiving pre-exposure rabies vaccination, and in some cases where individuals received invalid doses.
- A physical examination is not required for vaccination of healthy persons.
- Gloves are not routinely needed to administer vaccines, but should be worn if the vaccinator may come in contact with body fluids or has open lesions on his or her hands.
- It is not necessary to change the needle after withdrawing a vaccine from the vial and before administering it to the patient. This only increases the risk of sharps injury and bacterial contamination.
- Aspirating back on the syringe after insertion but before injection is not necessary. There are no large vessels in the anatomic areas that are recommended for vaccine injection.
- There is no maximum number of vaccinations that can be given on a single day.
- While there is no specified limit to the number of injections that can be given in a single limb, injections in the same area should be separated by at least 1 inch.

149

TABLE 5.2 — Interval Between Receipt of Antibody-Containing Products and Administration of MMR, VAR, or MMRV[a]

Product (Route)	Indication	Usual Dose	Duration of Deferral
RSVmAB (IM)	Prevention of RSV disease	15 mg/kg	None[b]
IGIM	Pre- or postexposure prophylaxis for hepatitis A	0.02 (3.3 mg/kg) or 0.06 mL/kg (10 mg/kg)	3 months
	Postexposure prophylaxis for measles:		
	Standard	0.25 mL/kg (40 mg/kg)	5 months
	Immunocompromised[c]	0.5 mL/kg 80 mg/kg)	6 months
IGIV	Replacement therapy for immune deficiency[c]	400 mg/kg	8 months
	Postexposure prophylaxis for varicella	400 mg/kg	8 months
	Immune thrombocytopenic purpura	400 mg/kg	8 months
		1 g/kg	10 months
	Kawasaki disease	2 g/kg	11 months
Blood transfusion (IV)	Red blood cells:		
	Washed	—	None
	Adenine-saline added	10 mL/kg	3 months
	Packed	10 mL/kg	6 months
	Whole blood	10 mL/kg	6 months
	Plasma or platelet products	10 mL/kg	7 months
CMV-IGIV	Prevention of CMV disease in transplant patients[c]	150 mg/kg	6 months

HBIG (IM)	Postexposure prophylaxis for hepatitis B	0.06 mL/kg (10 mg/kg)	3 months
HRIG (IM and intrawound)	Postexposure prophylaxis for rabies	20 IU/kg (22 mg/kg)	4 months
RhoGAM (IM)	Prevention of maternal Rh isoimmunization	300 mcg	None[d]
TIG (IM)	Postexposure prophylaxis for tetanus	250 units (10 mg/kg)	3 months
VariZIG (IM)[e]	Postexposure prophylaxis for varicella	125 units/10 kg	5 months

[a] LAIV, RV, Ty21a, YF vaccine, and ZOS do not need to be deferred after receipt of antibody-containing blood products. Passively acquired antibodies would be unlikely to interfere with inactivate vaccines given at mucosal surfaces, like RV, LAIV, and Ty21a. In addition, blood products in the United States are unlikely to contain substantial amounts of antibody to *Salmonella typhi* and YFV, and antibody to last year's influenza viruses might not be effective against this year's strains. ZOS is normally given to people who already have circulating antibodies to VZV.

[b] This is a monoclonal product that contains no antibody to the vaccine viruses.

[c] Live viral vaccines may be contraindicated in these patients.

[d] Administration of live vaccines, if indicated, to postpartum women should not be delayed if antibody-containing products were given during the last trimester (this includes RhoGAM). Likewise, the infant's immunization with rotavirus vaccine should not be delayed.

[e] This product is licensed in Canada and is available in the United States under an investigational new-drug application expanded-access protocol.

Adapted from Centers for Disease Control and Prevention. *Epidemiology and Prevention of Vaccine Preventable Diseases.* 11th ed. Atkinson W, et al, eds. Washington, DC: Public Health Foundation; 2009: Appendix A, with modifications based on recommendations released since 2009.

5

TABLE 5.3 — Administration Errors and Corrective Actions

Vaccine Involved	Administration Error	Why This Is Incorrect	Corrective Action to be Taken
Any	Expired or damaged inactivated vaccine given	Vaccines should be used before their expiration date; damaged vaccines should not be used	Give nonexpired or undamaged vaccine as soon as the error is discovered
	Expired or damaged live vaccine given	Vaccines should be used before their expiration date; damaged vaccines should not be used	Give nonexpired or undamaged vaccine on the same day or 4 weeks later
	Less-than-full dose of inactivated vaccine given	Correct dose should be used	Give correct dose of the vaccine as soon as the error is discovered
	Less-than-full dose of live vaccine given[a]	Correct dose should be used	Give correct dose of the vaccine on the same day or 4 weeks later
	More-than-full dose of vaccine given	Correct dose should be used	None—dose is valid
	Subcutaneously-administered vaccine (VAR, ZOS, MMR, MMRV, YF vaccine, or MPSV4) given intramuscularly	These vaccines should be given subcutaneously	None—dose is valid
DTaP	Dose given to adolescent or adult	Tdap should be used	None—dose is valid[b]
DTaP-IPV (Kinrix)	Dose given to a child 15 to 18 months of age as Dose 4 of DTaP	DTaP-IPV is only indicated for Dose 5 of DTaP and Dose 4 of IPV in children 4 to 6 years of age	None—DTaP dose is valid

Vaccine	Error	Reason	Recommended action
DTaP-IPV (liquid component of Pentacel)	Dose given alone to a child as any dose of DTaP or IPV	The DTaP-IPV liquid component should only be used as part of Pentacel (after reconstitution of the lyophilized Hib component)[c]	None—dose is valid
HepB	Dose given subcutaneously	Should be given intramuscularly	Give HepB intramuscularly as soon as error is discovered
	Dose given to an adult in the gluteal muscle	Should be given in the deltoid muscle	Give HepB in the deltoid muscle as soon as the error is discovered
Hib-T (Hiberix)	Dose given as part of the primary Hib series	Hiberix is licensed only for the booster dose	None—dose is valid
LAIV	Dose given to individual receiving influenza antivirals within 48 hours before or 2 weeks after dose	Antivirals can inhibit immune response	Give IIV as soon as the error is discovered, or give LAIV 4 weeks later (if individual is not on antivirals at that time)
	Dose given <4 weeks after a dose of MMR, VAR, or MMRV	Replication of the first vaccine viruses could interfere with the immune response to the LAIV	Give IIV as soon as the error is discovered, or give LAIV 4 weeks later
LAIV-seasonal and LAIV-2009 H1N1	Doses given at the same time	Simultaneous replication of the different vaccine viruses could cause interference with the immune response	None—doses are valid
MCV	Dose given subcutaneously	Should be given intramuscularly	None—dose is valid

Continued

TABLE 5.3 — *Continued*

Vaccine Involved	Administration Error	Why This Is Incorrect	Corrective Action to be Taken
PPSV	Dose given to child <2 years of age	PCV should be used	Give PCV as soon as the error is discovered
RAB	Dose given to an adult or child in the gluteal muscle	Should be given in the antero-lateral thigh (infant) or deltoid (older child and adult)	Give RAB in the appropriate muscle as soon as the error is discovered
Tdap	Dose given to infant or child as part of the primary series	DTaP should be used	Give DTaP as soon as the error is discovered
	Dose given to infant or child as Dose 4 or 5 in the series	DTaP should be used	None—dose is valid
	Dose given to child 7 through 9 years of age	No diphtheria, tetanus, and diphtheria vaccine is licensed in this age group	None—dose is valid[b]
VAR	Dose given to an adult ≥60 years of age for prevention of shingles	ZOS should be used	Give ZOS at same visit or 4 weeks later
ZOS	Dose given to a child for prevention of varicella	VAR should be used	None—dose is valid

[a] Exceptions: sneezing or blowing nose after LAIV administration, and vomiting, spitting up, or regurgitating after RV administration.
[b] Counts as the one-time dose of Tdap.
[c] The remaining lyophilized Hib component of Pentacel can only be used if reconstituted with the DTaP-IPV liquid component of Pentacel or the 0.4% saline diluent for ActHIB.

- Syringes should not be prefilled by the end user. This increases the risk of administration error and raises stability and storage issues. The one exception is mass influenza immunization campaigns where only one vaccine type is being used. In this situation, a small number of syringes can be prepared and labeled in advance; they should be used soon after filling, and unused syringes should be discarded. Many vaccines are now supplied by manufacturers in single-use, prefilled syringes.

Contraindications and Precautions

A *contraindication* is a condition that *increases the likelihood of a serious adverse event*; when present, the vaccine in question should not be given. The only permanent contraindication for all routine vaccines is severe allergy or anaphylaxis to the vaccine or any of its components. Severe allergy is IgE-mediated, occurs in minutes to hours, and requires medical attention. Examples include generalized urticaria, facial swelling, airway obstruction, wheezing, anaphylaxis, hypotension, and shock. Delayed-type hypersensitivity occurs by different mechanisms and is generally not a contraindication to vaccination. Most vaccines contain buffers as well as excipients, which are substances other than the vaccine that are included in the manufacturing process or added to the final product (excipients are listed in the relevant vaccine tables in *Section B*, and the more common relevant allergies are listed as contraindications). In addition, there may be contaminating substances that carry over from early steps in processing, and some vial stoppers and syringes contain latex, which can carry over to the patient during injection. Both excipients and contaminants can be triggers for allergic reactions in sensitized patients.

Acute encephalopathy within 7 days of receipt of a pertussis-containing vaccine is a permanent contraindication for DTaP and Tdap, based on the theoretic possibility of exacerbation or recurrence of encephalopathy. Pregnancy is a contraindication for live vaccines based on theoretic risks to the fetus and the possibility that naturally occurring birth defects might be attributed to the vaccine (see *Chapter 6: Vaccination in Special Circumstances—Pregnancy*). However, there is no definitive evidence of fetal damage from any live vaccine except smallpox. In addition, in some circumstances, the benefits may outweigh the risks; for example, YF vaccine can be considered for pregnant women traveling to high-risk areas. Although live vaccines are generally contraindicated in persons with immune incompetence, there may again be situations where the benefits outweigh the risks (see *Chapter 6: Vaccination in Special Circumstances*). For example, natural varicella probably represents a greater risk to a DiGeorge syndrome patient with mildly impaired cellular immunity than does the live-attenuated vaccine.

A *precaution* is a condition that *might increase the risk of a serious adverse event, compromise the immunogenicity* of the vaccine, or *be mistaken for a vaccine reaction.* Moderate-to-severe acute illness with or without fever is a precaution for all vaccines because of the difficulty distinguishing natural illnesses from vaccine reactions. Understanding what to do when a precaution is noted is sometimes difficult. Technically speaking, the default position is to defer vaccination. However, the risks of deferral (susceptibility to disease) must be weighed against the risks of vaccination (largely theoretic). In making these judgments, the provider must take into account the prevailing epidemiology of the disease, the patient's personal circumstances, and the possibility that an opportunity for vaccination will be missed. Here is an example. A 2-month-old experiences 4 hours of inconsolable crying after receiving Dose 1 of DTaP. This would constitute a precaution to the administration of Dose 2 at 4 months of age. However, because the risk of a recurrence of inconsolable crying is low, the consequences of such an episode are not permanent, and the risk of pertussis is appreciable, the provider may elect to give Dose 2. Here is another example. A provider may elect to give the 6-month shots to an infant with a moderate febrile illness *if* there is substantial risk that the child will not return for vaccination after the illness resolves.

Sometimes it is difficult to know when a condition is a "contraindication" or a "precaution" (package inserts also contain "warnings," but it is not clear how these differ from "precautions" in terms of action). Here's an example: the ACIP states that HPV vaccine "is not recommended for use in pregnancy,"[2] and the CDC's Guide to Vaccine Contraindications and Precautions warns not to give the vaccine in pregnancy.[3] However, pregnancy is not listed under contraindications *or* precautions in the recommendations or in the package inserts. Here's another example: the ACIP classifies personal history of Guillain-Barré syndrome as a precaution to administration of MCV. The MCV4-D package insert lists GBS in the *Warnings* (not *Contraindications*) section but states that the vaccine should *not* be given (the MCV4-CRM package insert states that data are not available to assess the risk of recurrent Guillain-Barré syndrome, but does *not* say *not* to give the vaccine). All of this can be confusing. In *Section B*, each vaccine table lists contraindications and precautions, to be interpreted, respectively (and in good faith) as "do not vaccinate in these situations" and "defer vaccination in these situations, unless the benefits outweigh the risks."

Misconceptions about vaccine contraindications can result in missed opportunities. **Table 5.4** lists some erroneous contraindications; if present, vaccines can and should be given.

TABLE 5.4 — Erroneous Contraindications to Vaccination

- Mild acute illness, with or without fever
- Mild respiratory illness (including most cases of otitis media)
- Mild gastroenteritis
- Antibiotic or antiviral therapy[a]
- Low-grade fever and/or local redness, pain, and swelling after a previous dose
- Prematurity[b]
- Pregnant, unimmunized, or immunosuppressed household contact[c]
- Breast-feeding[c]
- Convalescent phase of illness
- Exposure to an infectious disease
- Positive tuberculin skin test without active disease[d]
- Simultaneous tuberculin skin testing[e]
- Allergy to penicillin, duck meat or feathers, or environmental allergens
- Fainting after a previous dose
- Seizures, sudden infant death syndrome, allergies, or vaccine adverse events in family members
- Malnutrition
- Lack of previous physical examination in a well-appearing individual
- Stable neurologic condition (eg, cerebral palsy, well-controlled seizure disorder, developmental delay)
- Allergy shots
- Extensive limb swelling after DTwP, DTaP, or Td that is not an Arthus-type reaction
- Brachial neuritis after previous dose of tetanus toxoid-containing vaccine
- Autoimmune disease
- Having had the disease that the vaccine is designed to prevent[f]

[a] Antibiotics could interfere with live bacterial vaccines (eg, Ty21a), and antivirals could interfere with live viral vaccines (eg, VAR).

[b] The birth dose of HepB should be delayed (because of poor immunogenicity) in infants weighing <2000 g whose mothers are HBsAg-negative.

[c] Pre-event smallpox vaccination is an exception.

[d] MMR, VAR and ZOS should not be given to patients with active, untreated tuberculosis.

[e] Measles vaccine could temporarily suppress tuberculin reactivity. Measles-containing vaccines can be given on the same day as a tuberculin skin test is placed; if not given on the same day, the measles-containing vaccine should be delayed at least 4 weeks.

[f] Immunity from natural infection may wane with time, as in the case of pertussis. Alternatively, the vaccine (eg, HPV vaccine, MCV, PCV, RV) might protect against serotypes to which the individual has not been previously exposed. Anthrax is an exception.

Continued

TABLE 5.4 — *Continued*

Adapted from *Guide to Vaccine Contraindications and Precautions to Immunizations, 2009*. American Academy of Pediatrics Web site. http://aapredbook.aappublications.org/cgi/content-nw/full/2009/1/6.6/TABLE6-6. Accessed March 6, 2010. More detail can be found in individual vaccine sections.

REFERENCES

1. Kroger AT, et al. *MMWR*. 2006;55(RR-15):1-48.

2. Markowitz LE, et al. *MMWR*. 2007;56(RR-2):1-24.

3. Guide to Vaccine Contraindications and Precautions. Centers for Disease Control and Prevention Web site. http://www.cdc.gov/vaccines/recs/vac-admin/contraindications.htm. Accessed March 6, 2010.

6

Vaccination in Special Circumstances

General Considerations for Patients With Impaired Immunity

Vaccination of patients with impaired immunity requires special consideration for a number of reasons[1,2]:

- *The balance between risks and benefits is complex*—Immunocompromised persons are at greater risk for complications and death from vaccine-preventable diseases. At the same time, they may be at increased risk for complications from live vaccines, and the response to all vaccines may be suboptimal. Decisions regarding vaccination are therefore more complicated than for healthy persons and must take into account the prevalence of disease and probability of exposure, the nature and degree of immunodeficiency, the type of vaccine and the likelihood of adverse effects, the efficacy of the vaccine when immunity is impaired, and the confounding effects of other interventions. Unfortunately, in many situations there are few data available to provide guidance.

- *Immunocompromised states differ qualitatively*—Qualitative differences dictate not only which vaccines are indicated but which vaccines represent a danger to the patient. Congenital immunodeficiencies may affect humoral immunity, cell-mediated immunity, phagocyte function, or complement function in different and interconnected ways. Humoral immune defects place patients at higher risk for invasive infection with encapsulated bacteria, demanding special consideration for vaccination against *H influenzae* type b, *S pneumoniae*, and *N meningitidis*. Whereas isolated humoral defects do not increase the risk of serious varicella per se, they may predispose the patient to bacterial complications of varicella. Therefore, VAR is indicated in patients with isolated humoral defects—as long as they are not receiving immune globulin replacement, in which case VAR is contraindicated (antibodies in immune globulin will inactivate the vaccine virus). Similarly, phagocyte dysfunction per se does not substantially weaken defenses against influenza virus, but it does increase the risk of bacterial superinfection. Thus patients with chronic granulomatous disease, whose neutrophils fail to undergo oxidative burst, should be on the high priority list to receive influenza vaccine yearly in order to prevent bacterial pneumonia. Complement deficiencies put patients at risk for bacterial infections but carry no implications for the safety of live or inactivated vaccines. Secondary immune deficiency states, such as those resulting from immunosuppressive medications, nephrotic syndrome, malnutrition, splenectomy, or bone marrow transplantation, also differ qualitatively from one another.

- *Immunocompromised states differ quantitatively*—In general, patients with cell-mediated immune defects should not receive live vaccines because of the risk of dissemination. However, cellular defects may range from mild to profound, and these differences affect the risk-benefit assessment for vaccination. For example, whereas VAR *should be avoided* in an HIV-infected individual with very low CD4 count, poor T-cell function, and a history of opportunistic infections, it *should be given* to a mildly symptomatic HIV-infected child whose CD4 percentages have consistently been ≥15%. In the former situation, the risk of vaccination is too great; in the latter, the risk of vaccination is small and is outweighed by the potential consequences of natural disease. Similarly, MMR may be given to HIV-infected children without severe immunosuppression as determined by CD4 counts. DiGeorge syndrome, a quantitative T-cell deficiency resulting from thymic dysplasia, is quite variable in expression. Whereas those patients with low CD4 and CD8 counts and abnormal T-cell function should not receive live vaccines, live vaccines are probably safe in those patients with normal T-cell studies.
- *Immune responses may be suboptimal*—Data on the immunogenicity of many vaccines in immunocompromised individuals are lacking. Some patients would not be expected to respond at all. For example, there is no point in giving inactivated vaccines to patients with X-linked agammaglobulinemia because they do not make antibody. On the other hand, patients with common variable immunodeficiency may or may not respond, and such vaccines are worth giving with the hope of some benefit. Some patients who have normal concentrations of antibody may *still* not respond appropriately to certain vaccines. In fact, this constitutes an operational definition of antibody deficiency with normal immunoglobulins or antibody dysfunction syndrome, most often diagnosed by failure to respond to PPSV23. In some cases, more intensive immunization regimens are necessary to achieve protective immunity. The immune globulin replacement therapy received by some patients with humoral defects protects them from disease but also limits the usefulness of live vaccines, which can be inactivated by passively acquired antibodies.
- *Immunization of close contacts is important but may carry some risks*—Immunocompromised patients can be protected by ensuring that close contacts, especially other household members, are appropriately immunized. For example, AIDS

patients may not respond well to influenza vaccine but can be protected from influenza by immunizing family members. Likewise, HepA should be given to contacts of immunosuppressed persons if the family resides in a high-incidence area. Live vaccines carry the theoretic risk of transmission from vaccinees to immunocompromised contacts, in whom they could cause disease. A historical example of this is vaccine-associated poliomyelitis resulting from transmission of OPV within the home. However, the risk of transmission varies by vaccine, and some live vaccines carry no risk of transmission at all. Likewise, the consequences of transmission range from demonstrably serious (eg, smallpox vaccine) to only theoretic (eg, RV). **Table 6.1** summarizes recommendations for use of live vaccines in household contacts of immunocompromised persons.

- *Official recommendations may differ from product labeling*—Many package inserts list immunodeficiency states as contraindications to vaccination. This labeling reflects allowable claims and mandated precautions that derive from data presented to the FDA at the time of licensure. Subsequent recommendations may be discordant with product labeling because of the availability of new data or reasoned re-evaluations of the pertinent risks and benefits. Practitioners should be aware of these discrepancies. For example, the package insert for VAR cautions against vaccinating persons who receive immunosuppressive therapy and those with cellular or

TABLE 6.1 — Use of Live Vaccines in Household Contacts of Immunocompromised Individuals

Vaccine	Recommendation
LAIV	Contraindicated if the household contact is profoundly immunosuppressed (eg, bone marrow transplant patient who requires specialized protective environment)
MMR	May be used
RV	May be used (use good hand hygiene)
Smallpox	Contraindicated
Ty21a	May be used (use good hand hygiene)
VAR	May be used (if vaccinee develops skin lesions, he or she should avoid contact with the immunocompromised person until the lesions resolve)
YF vaccine	May be used
ZOS	May be used (if vaccinee develops skin lesions, standard precautions should suffice to protect contacts)

humoral immunodeficiencies. The official recommendations, however, allow for vaccination of certain persons with these conditions.

- *Passive immunoprophylaxis may be indicated*—Immunocompromised individuals who receive intravenous immune globulin on a monthly basis are probably protected against measles and varicella, although in the case of exposure, consideration should be given to shortening the interval to the next dose by 1 or 2 weeks. Other immunocompromised individuals at risk for serious measles should receive intramuscular immune globulin (0.5 mL/kg, maximum 15 mL) within 6 days of exposure. The AAP recommends immune globulin prophylaxis for *all* HIV-infected children and adolescents exposed to measles, regardless of vaccination status, degree of symptoms, and level of immune suppression (the dose for asymptomatic HIV-infected persons is 0.25 mL/kg); the ACIP specifies prophylaxis only for *symptomatic* HIV infection.

Varicella zoster immune globulin (VariZIG) should be given within 96 hours of exposure to immunosuppressed individuals who are not immune to chickenpox (see **Table 25.2** for definition of immunity; persons with immunity who later become immunosuppressed are considered immune). The only product available in the United States is VariZIG, but this must be obtained under an investigational new drug protocol (FFF Enterprises, phone number 800-843-7477). Intravenous immune globulin can be used if VariZIG is not available. Chemoprophylaxis with acyclovir (20 mg/kg/dose given 4 times per day, maximum dose 800 mg) is another option. If used, it should be given for 7 days beginning about a week after exposure—this is intended to limit the primary viremia. Susceptible HIV-infected persons without evidence of immunosuppression do not need immunoprophylaxis.

Tetanus immune globulin should be administered to HIV-infected children with tetanus-prone wounds, regardless of their immunization status.

Specific Immune Deficiency States Other Than HIV Infection

Certain live vaccines, such as LAIV, MMRV, smallpox vaccine, and typhoid Ty21a are generally contraindicated in all patients with impaired immunity. Yellow fever vaccine should only be used in extraordinary, unavoidable circumstances. MMR, VAR and ZOS can be used in certain defined immunodeficiency states, and the guidelines for RV are generally permissive and dependent on the provider's assessment of the risks and benefits.

The following are general guidelines for use of common vaccines in persons with impaired immunity.

■ Humoral Deficiencies

- *Typical syndromes*: X-linked agammaglobulinemia, common variable immunodeficiency, IgA deficiency, IgG subclass deficiency, antibody deficiency with normal immunoglobulins (vaccine nonresponder state or antibody dysfunction syndrome), transient hypogammaglobulinemia of infancy
- *Safety issues*: VAR may be given and MMR may be considered. Patients with selective IgA deficiency can probably receive all vaccines safely because they have adequate serum IgG responses.
- *Special considerations*: Inactivated vaccines are not effective in patients with severe deficiencies of immune globulin synthesis. Since many of these patients receive monthly immune globulin, live viral vaccines are unlikely to be effective as they are neutralized by passively acquired antibodies. Less severely affected persons who are not receiving immune globulin may benefit from vaccination; in these cases, postimmunization antibody titers may be used to confirm responses.

■ Defects of Cell-Mediated Immunity

- *Typical syndromes*: severe combined immunodeficiency, DiGeorge syndrome, hyper-IgM syndrome (CD40 ligand deficiency), bare lymphocyte syndrome, autoimmune polyendocrinopathy-candidiasis-ectodermal dystrophy (chronic mucocutaneous candidiasis), Wiskott-Aldrich syndrome, ataxia-telangiectasia (humoral immunity is affected in most of these syndromes as well)
- *Safety issues*: Live vaccines are generally contraindicated.
- *Special considerations*: Live vaccines can be considered in some situations—for example, VAR may be considered in DiGeorge syndrome patients with minimal T-cell dysfunction. Inactivated vaccines may be given, but responses are variable.

■ Phagocyte Disorders

- *Typical syndromes*: chronic granulomatous disease, leukocyte adhesion deficiency, Chédiak-Higashi syndrome, myeloperoxidase deficiency, hyper-IgE/recurrent infection syndrome (Job's syndrome), secondary granule deficiency
- *Safety issues*: Live bacterial vaccines are contraindicated.
- *Special considerations*: Effective responses to all routine vaccines probably occur. Influenza vaccine is indicated to reduce the risk of secondary bacterial infection.

■ Complement Deficiencies

- *Typical syndromes*: deficiency of individual early (C1-C4) or late (C5-C9) components, properdin, mannose-binding lectin, Factor D, or Factor I, secondary deficiency due to complement consumption
- *Safety issues*: All vaccines can be used.

• *Special considerations*: Patients with early component deficiencies are particularly susceptible to infection with gram-positive organisms, such *S pneumoniae,* and should probably receive both pneumococcal and meningococcal vaccines. Those with late component deficiencies are uniquely susceptible to infection with *N meningitidis* and should be vaccinated against this pathogen. Influenza vaccine is indicated to reduce the risk of secondary bacterial infection.

■ Anatomic and Functional Asplenia

• *Typical syndromes*: congenital, traumatic, or surgical asplenia, sickle cell disease, polysplenia syndrome
• *Safety issues*: All vaccines can be used.
• *Special considerations*: Because of impaired clearance of opsonized bacteria, coordination of lymphocyte responses, and synthesis of IgM and phagocytosis-enhancing factors, these patients are at risk for life-threatening infection with encapsulated organisms, particularly *S pneumoniae*. The following guidelines are offered:
  – *All asplenic persons*: Yearly IIV should be given, beginning at 6 months of age, to prevent secondary bacterial infection. Family members should be immunized as well. Live vaccines, except for LAIV, may be given. Prophylactic antibiotics are indicated in certain individuals. Patients 2-55 years of age should receive MCV4 and should be revaccinated every 5 years. If the patient is 2 to 6 years of age at first receipt of any meningococcal vaccine, the first revaccination interval should be 3 years; as of February 2010, only MCV4-D is licensed for children 2 to 10 years of age. MPSV4 can be used for primary vaccination and revaccination after 55 years of age. Patients ≥2 years of age should receive PPSV23 (even if they have already received a complete course of PCV) and one-time revaccination should be considered in 3-5 years.
  – *Children who are anatomically or functionally asplenic from birth (including sickle cell disease) or are splenectomized in the first 2 years of life*: PCV and Hib should be given according to the routine schedule. At 2 years of age, MCV4-D and PPSV23 should be given. Revaccinate for meningococcal and pneumococcal disease as above.
  – *Elective splenectomy*: PCV (PPSV23 for adults), Hib, and age-appropriate MCV4 (if the patient is 2 to 55 years of age; beyond 55 years of age, MPSV4 should be used) should be given at least 2 weeks before surgery. Revaccinate for meningococcal and pneumococcal disease as above.
  – *Traumatic splenectomy beyond 2 years of age*:
    • *Patient has already received the routine PCV and Hib series*: The patient should receive 1 dose of PPSV23, a

booster dose of Hib, and age-appropriate MCV4 (beyond 55 years of age, MPSV4 should be used). Revaccinate for meningococcal and pneumococcal disease as above.

- *Patient never received PCV or Hib (this includes adults)*: Children 24 to 71 months of age should receive 2 doses of PCV followed by 1 dose of PPSV23, each separated by 2 months. They should also receive 2 doses of Hib 2 months apart. Persons ≥6 years of age should receive 1 dose of Hib and 1 dose of PPSV23, with a second dose of PPSV23 in 5 years. Age-appropriate MCV4 should be given if the patient is 2 to 55 years of age; beyond 55 years of age, MPSV4 should be used. Revaccinate for meningococcal disease as above.

■ Chronic Disease

Individuals with chronic underlying conditions may be unusually susceptible to infectious disease, whether or not they have immune deficiency in the classic sense. As a general rule, all routine vaccines should be given unless they are specifically contraindicated. Most of these patients are on the high priority list for yearly IIV (LAIV should not be used in patients whose conditions predispose to complications of influenza), including those with chronic cardiac (eg, congenital heart disease), respiratory (eg, cystic fibrosis), allergic (eg, asthma), hematologic (eg, sickle cell disease), metabolic (eg, diabetes), neuromuscular (eg, muscular dystrophy), hepatic (eg, cirrhosis), and renal (eg, chronic renal failure) disorders. Patients who are particularly susceptible to pneumococcal infection, such as those with nephrotic syndrome, should receive pneumococcal vaccine as well. Cochlear implants also represent a particular risk for pneumococcal meningitis. Patients with chronic liver disease are at risk for severe hepatitis and should receive HepA and HepB.

Medication-Induced Immunosuppression

■ Solid Organ Transplantation and Cancer Chemotherapy

- *Typical syndromes*: renal, heart, or liver transplant, leukemia, lymphoma, breast cancer, lung cancer, colon cancer
- *Safety issues*: Live vaccines are generally contraindicated during active therapy, but may be considered before and after treatment.
- *Special considerations*: Solid organ transplantation is usually a scheduled event; this affords the opportunity to optimize immunizations before patients receive immunosuppressive medications to prevent rejection; once transplanted, patients are likely to be chronically immunosuppressed, contraindicating live vaccines and increasing the risk of poor responses to inactivated vaccines.[3] To complicate matters, some conditions that lead to transplant—end stage renal disease, for instance—

can themselves lead to poor immune responses. As a general rule, patients should be caught-up on all age-appropriate immunizations in advance of transplantation. Serologic tests for IgG antibody against measles, mumps, rubella, and varicella can identify those patients who may need immunization; susceptible patients ≥12 months of age should be immunized with MMR and/or VAR (MMRV should not be used) at least 1 month before transplantation. Antibody titers should be measured 1 year after transplantation, as seronegative patients are candidates for passive immunization if exposed to disease. Routine yearly IIV can resume ≥6 months after transplantation; vaccination with other inactivated vaccines can resume about 1 year after transplantation, in order to ensure immunogenicity. Pneumococcal vaccination (PCV in children, PPSV23 in adults) should be included, but meningococcal vaccine is not routinely indicated (unless splenectomy has occurred). One dose of Hib should be considered for adolescents and adults.

In cancer patients, live vaccines are usually withheld for at least 3 months after immunosuppressive chemotherapy has been discontinued. This interval may vary with the type and intensity of immunosuppressive therapy, radiation therapy, underlying disease, and other factors. There is no harm in continuing routine inactivated vaccine schedules while on chemotherapy, although there is the risk of suboptimal response. As above, pneumococcal vaccine and Hib should be considered.

■ **Steroids**
- *Typical syndromes*: asthma, rheumatoid arthritis, other autoimmune disorders
- *Safety issues*: Live vaccines may be contraindicated in some patients.
- *Special considerations*: Because steroids may be immunosuppressive, they represent a potential problem in the use of live vaccines. Any patient receiving steroids in any form who has clinical or laboratory evidence of immunosuppression should not receive live vaccines. In addition, patients whose underlying disease itself is immunosuppressive should not receive live vaccines, except under special circumstances. The following guidelines are offered for live vaccines in other situations:
  - *Topical, inhaled, and compartmental depot injections*: Vaccination is acceptable.
  - *Physiologic replacement*: Vaccination is acceptable.
  - *Less than 2 mg/kg/day (<20 mg if >10 kg; daily or alternating days) of prednisone or equivalent*: Vaccination is acceptable.
  - *Greater than or equal to 2 mg/kg/day (≥20 mg if >10 kg; daily or alternating days) of prednisone or equivalent for <14*

days: Vaccinate right after stopping steroid therapy. Do not vaccinate if steroid therapy will extend to 14 days or more.

– *Greater than or equal to 2 mg/kg/day (≥20 mg if >10 kg; daily or alternating days) of prednisone or equivalent for ≥14 days*: Vaccinate 1 month after stopping therapy.

■ Disease-Modifying Antirheumatic Drugs (DMARDs)

- *Typical syndromes*: rheumatoid arthritis, spondyloarthropathies, other autoimmune disorders
- *Safety issues*: Live vaccines are generally contraindicated, although some patients may be able to receive ZOS.
- *Special considerations*: This class of drugs includes methotrexate, hydroxychloroquine, sulfasalazine, azathioprine, leflunomide, cyclosporine, tumor necrosis factor inhibitors (eg, etanercept, infliximab, adalimumab), interleukin-1 receptor antagonists (eg, anakinra), selective costimulation modulators (eg, abatacept), and anti-B-cell monoclonal antibodies (eg, rituximab).[4] Inactivated vaccines may be given, but effective responses are variable. Pneumococcal immunization is indicated and patients are high-priority for yearly IIV. There are no specific recommendations regarding the interval between dosing of these drugs and vaccination. Patients receiving low doses of methotrexate (≤0.4 mg/kg/week), azathioprine (≤3 mg/kg/day), or 6-mercaptopurine (≤1.5 mg/kg/day) may receive ZOS (this is considered safe because patients receiving ZOS have pre-existing immunity to varicella; patients on DMARDs should not receive MMR or VAR).

HIV Infection

Vaccine practice in HIV-infected persons depends on the degree of immunosuppression[5,6]:

- *Perinatally exposed infants whose HIV status is indeterminate*—These are infants who are born to HIV-infected mothers and are in the process of being evaluated for, but have no current evidence of, HIV infection. They should receive all routine vaccines, including RV in infancy and MMR and VAR at 12 to 15 months of age (by this age HIV infection will have effectively been ruled out in most of them). Influenza vaccine should be given beginning at 6 months of age; LAIV may be used beginning at 2 years of age if the child is otherwise healthy and household contacts are not profoundly immunosuppressed. All household contacts, including the mother, should receive influenza vaccine as well.
- *Perinatally exposed infants who are not infected with HIV*— HIV infection is reasonably excluded in at-risk infants who have negative virologic tests (eg, PCR) at ≥14 days and ≥1 month of age, or one negative virologic test at ≥2 months of

age, or one negative HIV antibody test at ≥6 months of age.[7] These infants should receive all routine vaccines.

• *HIV-infected infants and children*—Many children with HIV infection who receive highly active antiretroviral therapy or are natural long-term nonprogressors are relatively healthy and can be immunized according to the routine childhood schedule. The recommendations regarding RV are permissive—they essentially say that the risks of giving this live vaccine should be weighed against the benefits. The risks would appear to be very low in HIV-infected infants who are not severely immunosuppressed. Special attention should be paid to influenza immunization, not only to protect the child but to prevent spread of influenza to HIV-infected household members. MMR and VAR should be given to HIV-infected children who do not have evidence of *severe* immunosuppression, regardless of whether symptoms are present. For children up to 8 years of age, severe immunosuppression is indicated by a CD4 count <15%; beyond 8 years of age, severe immunosuppression is indicated by a CD4 count <200 cells/mcL. It is prudent to administer the 2 required doses of each vaccine as early as possible, as immune function may deteriorate before 4 to 6 years of age when the second doses are routinely administered. Given the minimum intervals of 1 month for MMR and 3 months for VAR, a simple approach would be to give both vaccines at 12 to 15 months of age and then again 3 months later. Remember, MMRV should not be used in HIV-infected persons.

HIV-infected children are at increased risk for invasive pneumococcal disease. The routine PCV schedule should be used (**Tables 23.2, 23.3,** and **23.4**), and 1 or 2 doses of PPSV23 should be considered after the first 2 years of life. For children 24 to 71 months of age who never received a pneumococcal vaccine, it would be reasonable to administer 2 doses of PCV followed by a dose of PPSV23, each separated by 2 months; a second dose of PPSV23 could be given 5 years later. Children 6 to 18 years of age may receive one dose of PCV, followed by PPSV23 with revaccination 5 years later. HIV-infected children are also at increased risk for invasive meningococcal disease, although to a lesser extent than for pneumococcal disease. It would be reasonable to give MCV4 at 2 years of age, with a second dose at 5 years of age (as of February 2010, only MCV4-D is licensed for children 2 to 10 years of age); thereafter, a dose of either MCV4-D or MCV4-CRM could be given every 5 years if the patient is considered sufficiently immunocompromised so as to increase the risk of disease.

• *HIV-infected adolescents and adults*—**Table 8**.6 summarizes vaccination recommendations for older persons with HIV infection. Note that if the CD4 count is ≥200 cells/mcL, the schedule is the same as for healthy adults, with three exceptions: 1) IIV should always be used instead of LAIV; 2) all nonimmune patients (not just high-risk patients) should be immunized with HepB; and 3) PPSV23 should be given soon after diagnosis (rather than waiting for routine vaccination at 65 years of age). If the CD4 count is ≥200 cells/mcL and there is no evidence of immunosuppression, ZOS may be given. For those with CD4 counts <200 cells/mcL, the same caveats hold true, but in addition MMR, VAR, and ZOS are contraindicated. Meningococcal vaccination is indicated only if other risk factors are present.

Hematopoietic Stem-Cell Transplantation (HSCT) and Leukemia

Allogeneic HSCT presents a complicated vaccination paradigm.[8] The underlying disease itself may be immunosuppressive, the therapy used to prepare for transplantation ablates existing immunity, immunosuppressive therapy may be given after the procedure (sometimes for life), patients may receive passive immunization with IGIV, and graft-versus-host disease may further compromise immune function and lead to end-organ failure. Moreover, the adopted immune system of the donor provides unreliable immunity of uncertain duration; fortunately, immune memory can be recalled by immunization after engraftment (it is not clear whether lasting benefits accrue from immunization of the donor prior to transplant, but there is evidence of benefit from donor immunization with Hib, tetanus and diphtheria toxoids, PCV and HepB). Although graft-versus-host disease is not an issue with autologous transplantation and the conditioning regimens may be less severe, studies show that vaccine-induced immunity may be lost after transplantation. Guidelines for vaccination of HSCT patients were published by the CDC in 2000[9] and by the European Group for Blood and Marrow Transplantation in 2005[10]; **Table 6.2** provides a summary protocol.

There are studies demonstrating loss of immunity to some vaccine antigens after successful treatment for acute leukemia.[11,12] However, official guidelines for revaccination are hard to come by. Some centers favor testing for antibodies once chemotherapy is completed, with selective revaccination using those antigens for which the patient's antibody levels have fallen below protective levels. The problem is that seroprotection correlates are not known for all diseases. Another approach is to routinely revaccinate with some or all antigens, using guidelines like those in **Table 6.2**.

TABLE 6.2 — Revaccination of Hematopoietic Stem-Cell Transplant Recipients

Disease/Infectious Agent[b]	Time After Transplant/Vaccine[a]	
	6-23 Months	≥24 Months
Diphtheria, tetanus, pertussis:		
Age <7 years	DTaP (3 doses)	
Age 7-9 years[c]	Td (3 doses)	
Age ≥10 years[c]	Tdap (1 dose) then Td (2 doses)	
Hepatitis A[d]	HepA (2 doses) if otherwise indicated	
Hepatitis B[e]	HepB (3 doses)	
H influenzae type b[f]	Hib (3 doses)	
Human papillomavirus[g]	HPV vaccine (3 doses) for females 9 to 26 years of age	
Influenza[h]	IIV (1 dose yearly)	
Measles, mumps, rubella[i]	MMR is contraindicated	MMR[j] (2 doses) if immunocompetent
N meningitidis[k]	MCV4 (1 dose) if 11 to 18 years of age or otherwise indicated	
Rotavirus	RV cannot be initiated beyond infancy	
S pneumoniae[l]	PCV and/or PPSV23	

Polio	IPV (3 doses)	
Varicella[i]	VAR is contraindicated	Consider VAR[j,m]
Zoster	ZOS is contraindicated	Consider ZOS[m]

[a] See **Table 5.1** for minimum ages and intervals between doses.

[b] For most of these diseases, HSCT patients are not at particular risk but they should be vaccinated if they fall under otherwise routine recommendations. Pneumococcal vaccine and Hib are indicated because of specifically increased risks. Influenza vaccination is universally indicated, but HSCT patients should receive high priority. There is no particular increased risk of measles, mumps, rubella, or varicella, but the consequences of infection are potentially severe. The same is true for hepatitis A and hepatitis B in patients with chronic liver disease due to GVHD.

[c] Tdap should be substituted 1 time for Td after the patient turns 10 years of age. Boostrix is licensed for use in persons 10 to 64 years of age; Adacel is licensed for persons 11 to 64 years of age.

[d] Patients with chronic liver disease should be immunized. Otherwise, HepA is recommended for all children in the second year of life, and catch-up immunization for older children should be immunized. Persons living in endemic areas who otherwise would qualify for routine vaccination, and persons living in areas experiencing outbreaks, should be immunized. IGIM in addition to vaccine is recommended for immunocompromised persons who are traveling.

[e] Patients with chronic liver disease should be immunized. HepB is recommended for all persons <18 years of age and for high-risk adults. Test for HBsAb 1 to 3 months after the third dose; if negative, repeat the 3-dose series one time.

[f] Hib should be given regardless of age.

[g] Vaccination is routinely recommended for females 9 to 26 years of age to prevent cervical cancer. HPV2 may be used for prevention of cervical cancer. HPV4 may be used for prevention of cervical cancer and genital warts. HPV4 may be used in males 9 to 26 years of age for prevention of genital warts but is not routinely recommended.

[h] IIV may be given as early as 4 months after transplantation. LAIV is contraindicated. Children 6 months to 9 years of age who are receiving influenza vaccine for the first time post-transplant, or who were vaccinated for the first time in the previous season and only received 1 dose, need 2 doses separated by 4 weeks. Chemoprophylaxis should be considered for all patients regardless of vaccination status.

Continued

TABLE 6.2 — *Continued*

i Passive immunoprophylaxis should be given to all measles- and varicella-exposed patients regardless of personal history of disease or vaccination.

j MMRV should not be used. Patients who are still considered immunocompromised or who have chronic GVHD should not receive MMR or VAR.

k MCV4 is routinely recommended for all persons 11 to 18 years of age. HSCT recipients with chronic GVHD should also be vaccinated or revaccinated with MCV4, and routine penicillin prophylaxis should be given (as if the patient were asplenic).

l Beginning in 2010, PCV13 will replace PCV7. Children 2 to 71 months of age should receive 2 doses of PCV (beginning 6 months post-transplant) followed by one dose of PPSV23. For persons ≥6 years of age, one dose of PPSV23 should be given at 12 months post-transplant. In both cases, one-time revaccination with PPSV23 in 5 years should be considered. Routine penicillin prophylaxis is recommended for patients with chronic GVHD (as if the patient were asplenic).

m Consider if there is no chronic GVHD or ongoing immunosuppression.

Adapted from CDC. *MMWR.* 2000;49(RR-10):1-128, and Ljungman P, et al. *Bone Marrow Transpl.* 2005;35:737-746. Practice varies from one transplantation center to another.

Whereas vaccination during pregnancy poses *theoretic* risks to the developing fetus, there is no evidence directly linking any routine vaccines, even live ones, to birth defects. Nevertheless, pregnant women should be vaccinated only when the risk for exposure to disease is high and the infection would pose a significant risk to the mother or fetus.[13] Delaying vaccination until the second or third trimester, when possible, is reasonable in order to minimize concerns about teratogenicity, despite the evidence against this. An exception is IIV, which should be given regardless of trimester to women who are or will be pregnant during influenza season.[14] Maternal influenza immunization is both safe[15] and cost-effective.[16]

In considering vaccination during pregnancy, clinicians should be aware of the following:

- Approximately 2% of all newborns have a major congenital malformation; it follows that some women who are vaccinated during pregnancy will have infants with birth defects. While a causal relationship with the vaccine may be lacking, there may be a tendency to attribute the birth defect to the vaccine. Pregnant women should be counseled about this before being vaccinated. Along the same lines, it stands that some children of women who receive thimerosal–containing vaccines (eg, some brands of IIV) during pregnancy will develop autism, even though thimerosal (which contains mercury) does not cause autism (see *Chapter 7: Addressing Concerns About Vaccines—Did the Thimerosal Used as a Preservative in Vaccines Cause Autism?*). Unfortunately, some states have banned the use of thimerosal-containing vaccines, which could jeopardize the supply of IIV for pregnant women.
- Very few vaccines have been tested for safety and efficacy in large numbers of pregnant women. For this reason, most vaccines are classified by the FDA as Pregnancy Category C (defined as: animal studies show adverse effects or have not been done *and* there are no adequate studies in pregnant women). Practically speaking, the official pregnancy classification has little impact on use. For example, Td is recommended during pregnancy if indicated, despite its category C designation. IIV is recommended during pregnancy, without brand preference, even though some brands are Pregnancy Category B and some are C (Pregnancy Category B is defined as: animal studies show no adverse effects but there are no adequate studies in pregnant women, *or* animal studies show adverse effects but adequate studies in pregnant women fail to demonstrate harm to the fetus). On the other hand, HPV vaccine is not recommended during pregnancy (albeit not specifically contraindicated), despite the fact that both HPV2 and

HPV4 are Pregnancy Category B. It is important to note that inactivated vaccines have never been demonstrated to harm the fetus. The only vaccines that carry a Pregnancy Category D designation (evidence of risk to the fetus but benefits might outweigh risks) are anthrax and smallpox.

- Live vaccines are generally contraindicated during pregnancy, with the exceptions noted in **Table 6.3**. However, inadvertent receipt of live vaccines is not a reason to terminate the pregnancy because there is no definitive evidence of maternal-fetal transmission or fetal harm. In the case of VAR, if a pregnant woman is known to be susceptible to varicella and a close contact develops a rash after vaccination, exposure should be avoided until the vaccinee's lesions are crusted over. Some manufacturers maintain registries of women inadvertently vaccinated during pregnancy in order to gather data on outcomes; the phone numbers for reporting are usually given in the package insert.
- The only live vaccine that is contraindicated in household contacts of pregnant women is smallpox.
- Theoretical concerns include the possibilities that the immune response in pregnant women will be suboptimal; that transplacental antibodies might interfere with the infant's ability to respond to vaccines; and that in-utero antigen exposure could lead to immune tolerance in the baby.
- The rationale for some official recommendations is difficult to understand. Here are some examples:
  - MPSV4 and PPSV23 are very similar vaccines in that both consist of pure polysaccharide. Yet MPSV4 falls under the "use-if-indicated" column and PPSV23 falls under the "special-language" column, wherein no specific recommendation is actually made.
  - HepA and IPV are very similar vaccines in that they consist of inactivated whole virions, and both carry a Pregnancy Category C designation. Yet the language regarding use in pregnancy differs—for HepA, the recommendations state that "the theoretical risk to the developing fetus is expected to be low," whereas for IPV, they state that "vaccination of pregnant women should be avoided on theoretical grounds...." It is not clear why the language is different and how it should be interpreted. In these situations, providers simply have to consider the risks and benefits and act accordingly.
- A tetanus toxoid booster is indicated for pregnant women who are unlikely to be immune to tetanus. See *Chapter 10: Diphtheria, Tetanus, Pertussis* for a discussion of the criteria for immunity and when Tdap may be substituted for Td.
- There are no known risks of passive immunization during pregnancy. In fact, VariZIG is *recommended* for susceptible

pregnant women who are exposed to varicella because the risk of complicated disease in the mother is high (it is not know whether passive immunization protects the fetus).
- Breast-feeding per se is not a contraindication to the use of any vaccines, including live ones, except for pre-event use of smallpox vaccine.

In April 2008, an ACIP working group offered guidance on the drafting of recommendations for vaccination during pregnancy and breastfeeding.[17] Hopefully, this will lead to more uniformity in future statements.

Preterm and Low Birth Weight Infants

Preterm (<37 weeks' gestation) and low birth weight (<2500 g) infants are at particular risk for vaccine-preventable diseases because of relatively immature immune systems.[18] Comorbidities contribute to this risk and cause delays in immunization. These infants should be vaccinated according to the routine schedule, using the routine doses, at the appropriate chronologic age. The only vaccine for which weight is relevant is HepB. Infants weighing <2000 g at birth whose mothers are HBsAg-negative should receive the first dose of vaccine at 1 month of age (rather than at birth) or at hospital discharge. Infants weighing <2000 g at birth whose mothers are HBsAg-positive or HBsAg-unknown should receive the first dose of vaccine within 12 hours of birth and should also receive HBIG 0.5 mL intramuscularly at a separate site from the vaccine. In these cases, the birth dose of vaccine does not count toward completion of the HepB series; 3 additional doses should be given as follows:
- *Mother HBsAg-positive*: doses at 1, 2, and 6 months of age. Test for HBsAg and HBsAb at 9 to 18 months of age. If HBsAg is negative and HBsAb is <10 mIU/mL, repeat 3-dose vaccine series.
- *Mother HBsAg-unknown*: doses at 1, 2, and 6 months of age and test the mother; if she is HBsAg-positive, proceed as above.
- *Mother HBsAg-negative*: doses at 1, 2, and 6 to 18 months of age.

RV should be given to preterm infants who are clinically stable and are being discharged from the nursery or who are already home, keeping in mind that the first dose should be given between 6 weeks and 14 weeks 6 days of age. Those who are remaining in the hospital should not receive RV—the vaccine virus strains are shed in the stool and there is the theoretic risk of transmission to other infants who may be acutely ill or ineligible for vaccination.
Preterm infants can experience cardiorespiratory events, such as apnea, bradycardia, and oxygen desaturation following vaccination and should be closely observed for at least 48 hours.[19]

175

TABLE 6.3 — Vaccine Use During Pregnancy

Administer Because of Pregnancy	Administer if Indicated for Other Reasons[a]	Contraindicated or Not Recommended[b]	Special Language Contained in the Recommendations[c]
IIV[d] Td or Tdap[e]	HepB MPSV4 RAB	HPV4 LAIV MMR VAR ZOS	Anthrax: Vaccinate only if the potential benefits outweigh the potential risks HepA: Theoretic risk is low; consider for women at high risk of exposure JE vaccine: Administer if travel to an endemic area is unavoidable and if there is increased risk for exposure IPV: Avoid on theoretic grounds but consider if risk of polio is increased and immediate protection is required MCV4: No data available in pregnant women; use only if clearly needed PPSV23: Safety during first trimester not evaluated Smallpox vaccine: Administer only to pregnant women who have been exposed to smallpox Typhoid (TViPSV and Ty21a): No data available in pregnant women YF vaccine: Administer if travel to an endemic area is unavoidable and if there is increased risk for exposure

[a] The recommendations for these vaccines are clear: give if indicated. Examples would include HepB for an unvaccinated pregnant injecting drug user; RAB for a pregnant woman who is bitten by a bat; and MPSV4 for an unvaccinated pregnant woman who has been diagnosed with a terminal complement component deficiency (MCV4 may be preferred in this situation; the package inserts for both MCV4-D and MCV4-CRM state that

the vaccines should be used in pregnancy only if clearly needed).

[b] LAIV, MMR, VAR, and ZOS are contraindicated because they are live and there is the theoretic risk of harm to the fetus. HPV vaccine is inactivated and is unlikely to cause harm; nevertheless, while not strictly contraindicated, it is not recommended during pregnancy. Inadvertent administration of MMR or VAR during pregnancy is not a reason to terminate the pregnancy. Pregnancy should be avoided for 1 month following MMR or VAR administration. ZOS is only indicated at ≥60 years of age and would therefore be unlikely to be used during pregnancy.

[c] The recommendations for these vaccines are less than clear-cut. Providers have to use their best judgment in balancing the risks and benefits.

[d] Pregnancy increases the risk of complications of influenza. Therefore, IIV should be given regardless of trimester to women who are or will be pregnant during influenza season.

[e] Babies born to mothers who are not immune to tetanus are at risk for neonatal tetanus. In addition, postpartum women can contract pertussis and give it to their infants. See *Chapter 10: Diphtheria, Tetanus, Pertussis* for discussion of use of Td and Tdap during pregnancy.

Modified from Guidelines for vaccinating pregnant women. Centers for Disease Control and Prevention Web site. http://www.cdc.gov/vaccines/pubs /downloads/b_preg_guide.pdf. Accessed August 15, 2008, and CDC. *MMWR.* 2008;57(RR-4):1-51.

6

The Immigration and Nationality Act requires all immigrants entering the United States to show proof of having received all ACIP-recommended vaccines before a visa is granted. In November 2009, CDC adopted the following criteria to determine which ACIP-recommended vaccines should be required: the vaccine must be age-appropriate and must either protect against a disease that has the potential to cause an outbreak or protect against a disease that has been eliminated or is in the process of being eliminated in the United States.[20] Based on these criteria, HPV vaccine and ZOS are not required. International adoptees <11 years of age can be exempted from this requirement but the adoptive parents must sign an affidavit indicating their intention to comply with immunization requirements within 30 days after the child arrives (children coming from Hague Convention countries such as China and the Philippines cannot be exempted). Refugees are exempted from immunization requirements at the time of entry, but must show proof of immunization at the time they apply for permanent residency.

The following issues are germane to the immunization management of persons from other countries, particularly international adoptees:

- Vaccination records are considered valid only if they are in written form and contain the vaccines, dates of administration, proper intervals between doses, and age at the time of immunization (influenza vaccine and PPSV23 are the only vaccines for which self-reported doses are considered valid[21]).
- Written records must be translated and interpreted correctly, and even then may be inaccurate or fraudulent.
- Even written records indicating adequate vaccination do not necessarily predict immunity.[22]
- Many immigrant adults are susceptible to vaccine-preventable diseases.[23]
- The immunization schedule in many countries differs from that in the United States. Some children will need additional vaccines to comply with the US schedule.
- Vaccines in some countries may have inadequate potency, especially because of handling issues. Country of origin predicts seroprotection, with the highest rates in children from Eastern Europe, then, in descending order, India, Latin America, China and Africa.[24]
- Serologic correlates of protection exist for some diseases but not for others. Testing may be expensive and the results require interpretation.
- There is no harm in revaccinating individuals who have already been vaccinated, although reactogenicity to DTaP

and pneumococcal polysaccharide vaccines may increase if too many doses are given within a short time frame.

- International adoptees may have subclinical vaccine-preventable diseases that are a risk to close contacts in the United States. For example, children from endemic countries may have hepatitis A without jaundice when they arrive. This is the basis for HepA vaccination of persons who will be in close contact with them during the first 60 days after arrival (the first dose should be given at least 2 weeks before arrival).[25]

It is desirable for all persons entering the United States permanently to receive all routinely recommended vaccines. For reasons mentioned, the simplest (and possibly least expensive) approach is to start over and revaccinate.[26] An alternative, although somewhat less practical, approach is to test for antibodies to the major vaccine antigens and administer those vaccines to which the child has no immunity. Young infants can be vaccinated according to the routine childhood schedule (**Table 8.1**); older children can be vaccinated according to catch-up schedules (**Tables 8.4 and 8.5**), with attention paid to the minimum allowable intervals between doses (**Table 5.1**). For adults who immigrate to the United States, consideration should be given to vaccination with MMR, Tdap, HepB, and VAR. Individuals from hepatitis B-endemic areas should be screened for HBsAg; if positive, vaccination is not necessary.

Health Care Personnel (HCP)

HCP, as well as persons who work in residential institutions, may be exposed to vaccine-preventable diseases and may transmit them to patients or residents, as well as their own families.[27] Individuals who fit into this category include staff, physicians, nurses, students, and ancillary personnel; in essence, anyone who might have contact with patients. The risk of infection might be particularly high for people working in emergency departments or ambulatory care settings, especially if the facility serves underimmunized populations. The consequences of transmission to patients might be particularly high wherever there are vulnerable patients, such as intensive care units, newborn nurseries, obstetric wards, chronic care facilities, and oncology or transplant units. HCP should be up-to-date on all routinely recommended vaccines.

Hospitals and other facilities may develop policies that require documentation of immunization or immunity, and these should be part of a comprehensive occupational health program. Immunizations should be provided at no cost to the worker. Studies have shown that this preventative strategy is more cost-effective than treating patients and their contacts for vaccine-preventable diseases. The extent to which these recommendations are carried out varies considerably from institution to institution.

Importantly, vaccination cannot be forced upon HCP who are reluctant to be vaccinated, although some institutions have developed strategies wherein individuals must sign a release form in order to opt out. In these situations, it should be emphasized that exposure to a vaccine-preventable disease could result in leave without pay during the period of potential communicability, and worker's compensation benefits would not apply unless the disease actually developed.

Diseases that deserve particular attention include the following:

- *Measles, mumps, and rubella*—All HCP should be immune to these diseases (see **Table 17.2** for criteria for evidence of immunity). HCP who are not immune should receive 2 doses of MMR separated by at least 1 month.

- *Hepatitis B*—HepB is recommended for all HCP who are likely to be exposed to blood or blood-containing body fluids.[28] In fact, the Bloodborne Pathogens Standard (see *Chapter 3: Standards, Principles, and Regulations— Occupational Safety and Health Administration [OSHA]*) mandates that vaccination be made available at no cost to all employees with potential blood contact. Personnel should be tested for HBsAb 1 to 2 months after Dose 3, and those who test negative (<10 mIU/mL) should receive another 3-dose series (one time only). If they remain seronegative after this, they should be tested for HBsAg, since chronic carriage could explain failure to respond to the vaccine. Persons who do not respond to a total of 6 properly administered doses should also be counseled about precautions to prevent hepatitis B infection and the need for HBIG if there is an exposure. Individuals who received the HepB series in the past need not be tested for HBsAb when they enter a health-care related job, but they should be tested at the time of an exposure and, if they are seronegative, managed accordingly.

- *Varicella*—All HCP should be immune to varicella (see **Table 25.2** for criteria for evidence of immunity). HCP who are not immune should receive 2 doses of VAR separated by 4 to 8 weeks. Vaccinated persons can return to work immediately, but if a rash develops (for example, vesicles at the inoculation site), the worker should not have contact with immunocompromised patients—he or she can continue to work with patients who are immunocompetent as long as the lesions are kept covered. Those who develop a generalized rash after vaccination should be furloughed until the rash resolves. Vaccinated HCP who are exposed to chickenpox or shingles should be observed carefully during days 10 to 21 postexposure; symptoms suggestive of varicella should prompt a medical leave, and if varicella develops, the worker should remain on leave until all the lesions are crusted or faded and there are no new lesions within a 24-hour period. HCP who have had only one dose of VAR and are exposed to the virus should receive a second dose within 5 days of exposure (as long as it has been at least 4 weeks since the first dose) and should be observed carefully as above.

- *Influenza*—All HCP should be immunized against influenza in the fall of each year.[29] In 2009, immunization against both seasonal influenza and novel H1N1 (the vaccines were separate) was recommended. Either IIV-seasonal or LAIV-seasonal (if age appropriate) was used for seasonal influenza, and either IIV-2009 H1N1 or LAIV-2009 H1N1 was used for the 2009 pandemic influenza. For the 2010-2011 season, the 2009 H1N1 strain will replace the previous H1N1 strain in the 3-valent vaccine, so only one vaccine will be necessary. HCP who are in close contact with severely immunosuppressed patients (the equivalent of HSCT patients who are in protective environments) should only receive IIV; HCP who receive LAIV should avoid contact with such patients for 7 days postvaccination. HCP who work in the neonatal intensive care unit may receive LAIV. Incidentally, HCP who themselves are too old to receive LAIV or have medical contraindications may nevertheless administer LAIV to others.

Nationally, less than half of HCP receive influenza vaccine every year. In 2007, responding to this dismal statistic, the Joint Commission on Accreditation of Health Care Organizations approved a standard that requires accredited organizations to offer influenza vaccination to staff and even volunteers with close patient contact. In that same year, the Infectious Diseases Society of America called for mandatory influenza vaccination of HCP, and, in 2008, the Association for Professionals in Infection Control and Epidemiology followed suit. The ethical framework for mandatory HCP immunization continues to be debated.[30] Several things, however, are clear. For one, HCP may be leary of mandates because of misperceptions about vaccine safety and their risk of acquiring influenza at work.[31] For another, when HCP do get vaccinated, they do so for their own benefit and not for the benefit of their patients.[32] Finally, influenza vaccine coverage rates among HCP should be followed as an integral part of all health care facility patient safety programs.

- *Tetanus, diphtheria, pertussis*—All HCP should have completed a primary series of tetanus and diphtheria vaccines and should receive a Td booster every 10 years. For those <65 years of age, one dose of Tdap should be given as soon as possible (a minimum interval of 2 years between the last Td and Tdap is safe, and shorter intervals may be used). The dose of Tdap "resets the clock" for subsequent 10-year Td boosters.

Travelers going to Canada, Western Europe, Australia, and New Zealand are probably at no higher risk for illness than those traveling within the United States, although the United Kingdom is now considered a measles-endemic region. For other destinations, however, consideration may need to be given to specialized vaccines or to accelerated schedules for routine vaccines, depending to some extent on what circumstances the traveler will encounter.[33] Travel to certain areas may require other measures, including malaria chemoprophylaxis, insect avoidance, food hygiene, and the availability of emergency medical services. Moreover, certain persons may be at higher risk than others for particular diseases.

Travel medicine clinics, which may be available at local health departments, academic medical centers, or in private practice settings, maintain up-to-date information and provide vaccination services for travelers. Primary care physicians who choose to provide travel vaccines to their patients should be aware of the following:

- *Planning*—Consultation should take place *at least* 4 to 6 weeks before departure in order to allow for the development of protective immunity after vaccination. More time may be required if certain vaccines will need to be ordered.

- *Itinerary*—It is not enough to know where the person will be traveling. The duration of stay and the particular activities in which the person will be engaged can help determine risk. For example, a 2-day stay in a sophisticated urban hotel carries different risks than extended field work in rural areas.

- *Routine vaccines*—All travelers should be up-to-date on routinely recommended vaccines. Some special considerations are listed below:

  - *Childhood vaccination schedule*: The routine childhood schedules (**Tables 8.1** and **8.3**) provide some flexibility in the timing of doses. For example, Dose 3 of HepB and IPV can be given as early as 6 months of age and Dose 4 of Hib and PCV as early as 12 months of age. Dose 4 of DTaP can be given as early as 12 months of age provided that at least 6 months have elapsed since Dose 3. VAR and HepA can be given as early as 12 months of age. The first dose of MMR should be given to all infants 6 to 12 months of age who will be traveling outside the United States (reimmunization with 2 doses after the first birthday is necessary). For children in the second year of life, Dose 2 of MMR can be given as early as 4 weeks after Dose 1, and Dose 2 of VAR as early as 3 months after Dose 1. Physicians should be aware of flexibility in the schedule and administer all eligible vaccines before the anticipated date of travel.

- *HepA*: For most travelers to endemic areas, vaccination is now preferred over administration of immune globulin and should be initiated as soon as travel is considered. One dose of HepA at any time before departure is likely to provide protection for most healthy people (only monovalent HepA should be used for this purpose). For older adults, immunocompromised individuals, and persons with chronic liver disease or other chronic medical conditions, immune globulin intramuscular (0.02 mL/kg) should be given (at a separate site) in addition to vaccine *if* there are <2 weeks before departure. Immune globulin alone should be given to infants <12 months of age and to persons who cannot be or do not want to be vaccinated.
- *HepB*: For those travelers who might have missed universal immunization, HepB should be given if the person might be exposed to blood, have sexual contact with the local population, stay >6 months, or be exposed through medical treatment.
- *Influenza*: Yearly influenza vaccine is now recommended for everyone. High priority should be given to persons traveling to areas with influenza activity. This includes the southern hemisphere during April through September and the tropics at any time of year. Travel with organized tourist groups that include persons from the tropics or southern hemisphere is also a risk factor. Individuals who were vaccinated during the preceding fall or winter *do not* need to be revaccinated before summer travel; however, those who are vaccinated only before summer travel *do* need to be revaccinated the next fall. Vaccine should be given at least 2 weeks before travel, but can be given up to the day of travel if this is not possible. Priority should also be given to persons at risk for complicated influenza (see *Chapter 15: Influenza*). Patients should understand that the vaccine strains used in the northern hemisphere during the fall may not optimally match the strains circulating in the southern hemisphere during April through September.[34]
- *Polio*: Previously immunized adults traveling to endemic areas should receive one dose of IPV (this does not need to be given again for subsequent travel). If travel of an infant to an endemic area is imminent, 3 doses of IPV can be given at 4-week intervals.
- *PPSV23*: All adults ≥65 years of age and adult smokers and asthmatics should be immunized.
- *Td*: Although boosters are recommended only every 10 years in adults, consideration should be given to a dose if >5 years have elapsed and the person will be working in situations where dirty wounds might be incurred or traveling to regions where diphtheria outbreaks have occurred. If

6

the person has not yet received a dose of Tdap, this should be substituted for Td.

- *Mandatory vaccines*—The only vaccine covered by international health regulations at the present time is YF vaccine, for which travelers to certain countries must have a valid International Certificate of Vaccination or Prophylaxis. However, some countries have their own regulations. For example, Saudi Arabia requires meningococcal vaccine for pilgrims visiting Mecca for the Hajj, and some countries may require the vaccine for persons returning from the Hajj.
- *Recommended vaccines*—**Table 6**.4 gives some general guidelines regarding vaccines for travel to certain parts of the world. Specific information about the vaccines is contained in the referenced sections of this book. Since disease outbreaks are always occurring and guidelines frequently change, the best advice is to check updated resources before traveling. The following web sites are useful for this purpose (Accessed March 30, 2010):
  - *Centers for Disease Control and Prevention: Travelers' Health*: http://wwwn.cdc.gov/travel/default.aspx
  - *World Health Organization: International Travel and Health*: http://www.who.int/ith/en
  - *International Society of Travel Medicine*: http://www.istm.org

Other Special Circumstances

Table 6.5 covers other situations and groups that deserve special attention for certain vaccines.

REFERENCES

1. CDC. *MMWR*. 1993;42(RR-4):1-18.
2. Abzug MJ. *Pediatr Infect Dis J*. 2009;28:233-236.
3. Chow J, et al. *Clin Infect Dis*. 2009;49:1550-1556.
4. Glück T, et al. *Clin Infect Dis*. 2008;46:1459-1465.
5. Mofenson LM, et al. *MMWR*. 2009;58(RR-11):1-166.
6. Kaplan JE, et al. *MMWR*. 2009;58(RR-4):1-207.
7. Working Group on Antiretroviral Therapy and Medical Management of HIV-infected Children: Guidelines for the use of antiretroviral agents in pediatric HIV infection. http://aidsinfo.nih.gov/Content Files/PediatricGuidelines.pdf. Accessed March 30, 2010.
8. Singhal S, et al. *Bone Marrow Transplant*. 1999;23:637-646.
9. CDC. *MMWR*. 2000;49(RR-10):1-125.
10. Ljungman P, et al. *Bone Marrow Transpl*. 2005;35:737-746.
11. Nilsson A, et al. *Pediatrics*. 2002;109:e91.
12. Patel SR, et al. *Clin Infect Dis*. 2007;44:635-642.

TABLE 6.4 — Particular Vaccine-Preventable Diseases by Region[a]

Region	Hepatitis A[b]	Japanese Encephalitis[c]	Meningococcus[d]	Polio[e]	Typhoid[f]	Yellow Fever[g]
Caribbean	√				√	√
Central Africa	√		√	√	√	√
East Africa	√[h]		√	√	√	√
East Asia	√	√			√	
Eastern Europe and Northern Asia	√				√	
Indian Ocean Islands	√					
Mexico and Central America	√				√	√[i]
Middle East	√		√[j]		√	
North Africa	√				√	
North America						
South Asia	√	√		√	√	
Southeast Asia	√	√		√[k]	√	
Southern Africa	√			√	√	
Southern and Western Pacific	√[l]	√[m]		√		

Continued

TABLE 6.4 — *Continued*

Region	Hepatitis A[b]	Japanese Encephalitis[c]	Meningococcus[d]	Polio[e]	Typhoid[f]	Yellow Fever[g]
South America						
Temperate	√				√	√[n]
Tropical	√				√	√
West Africa	√		√	√	√	√
Western Europe	√[o]					

[a] Vaccination might not be indicated for every country in the region. Specific recommendations can be found at http://wwwn.cdc.gov/travel/regionList.aspx. Accessed March 30, 2010. Two diseases are not listed but deserve special comment:

Hepatitis B: HepB is recommended for all unvaccinated persons traveling to or working in countries with intermediate to high levels of endemic transmission, which includes much of the world. Since exposure to blood or body fluids (through, for example, sexual contact or emergency medical treatment) may not be predictable, immunization should be strongly considered for all travelers.

Rabies: RAB should be considered in most parts of the world if exposure to animals is expected. At particular risk are travelers spending a lot of time outdoors, especially in rural areas, or who are involved in activities such as bicycling, camping, hiking, or outdoor work. Children are considered at higher risk because they tend to play with animals and may not report bites. Spelunkers are also at risk because of potential exposure to bats.

[b] Risk increases with duration of travel and is highest for those who live in or visit rural settings, trek in back-country areas, or frequently eat or drink in areas with poor sanitation.

[c] The risk to short-term travelers and those staying in urban centers is very low. Risk increases with prolonged visits to rural settings, and with extensive outdoor, evening, and nighttime exposures such as bicycling, camping, working outdoors, or sleeping in unscreened structures without bed nets.

[d] Risk is increased for travelers to sub-Saharan Africa (the "meningitis belt") during the dry season, especially if there is prolonged contact with local populations. Saudi Arabia requires that Hajj and Umrah visitors have a certificate of meningococcal vaccination before entering.

186

e Adult travelers to endemic or epidemic areas who have had a primary immunization series in the past should receive a dose of IPV before departure. Saudi Arabia requires polio vaccination for those attending the Hajj.

f Risk is higher for those visiting relatives or friends and those who will not have access to cooked foods and safe beverages.

g Check marks indicate a risk of acquiring YF in at least some countries in the region. Even if there is no YF in the country, vaccination may be required of travelers coming from endemic areas, even if they are just in transit (for example, there is no risk of acquiring YF in Haiti, but the country requires travelers from endemic areas to have been vaccinated so that YF is not introduced into the country). Vaccination must occur at a certified center and vaccinees must receive an *International Certificate of Vaccination or Prophylaxis* that carries a Uniform Stamp. Some countries with endemic YF may waive the requirements for travelers coming from uninfected areas and staying <2 weeks. Vaccination is also recommended for travel to countries that lie in YF-endemic zones but do not officially report the disease.

h Except Japan.

i Panama only.

j Saudi Arabia only.

k Myanmar only.

l Except Australia and New Zealand.

m Torres Strait, far northern Australia, Papua New Guinea.

n Northern and northeastern forested areas of Argentina only.

o Greenland only.

TABLE 6.5 — Vaccination in Other Special Circumstances[a]

Condition or Circumstance	Particular Risks and Considerations
Animal workers and veterinarians	Anthrax vaccine and RAB may be indicated
Bleeding diathesis	Use IM vaccines with caution; patients who receive clotting factors should receive HepA and HepB
Children and adolescents on long-term aspirin therapy	At risk for Reye syndrome if they get influenza or varicella; do not give VAR or LAIV while on aspirin because of theoretic risk of Reye syndrome
College students living in dormitories	Should receive MCV4; high priority for influenza
Foreign field personnel	Should receive travel-related vaccines
Food handlers	HepA not routinely recommended, but could be considered on a local basis
Foresters	RAB may be indicated
Injecting illegal drug users	Should receive HepA and HepB
Laboratory workers	Should be immunized against laboratory pathogens for which vaccines are available (eg, *N meningitidis*)
Men who have sex with men	Should receive HepA and HepB
Military personnel	Special immunizations may include MCV4, anthrax vaccine, smallpox vaccine, and travel vaccines; high priority for influenza
Morticians	Should receive HepB
Native Americans and Alaskans	Special attention to timely immunization against pneumococcus and *H influenzae* type b
Patients with cochlear implants or CSF leaks	Should receive PCV13 and/or PPSV23

Providers of essential community services	High priority for influenza
Public safety workers	Should receive HepB
Residents of long-term care facilities	High priority for influenza
Sewage workers	Not at increased risk for typhoid or hepatitis A in the United States
Spelunkers	RAB may be indicated
Staff of correctional facilities	Should receive HepB; high priority for influenza
Staff of day care centers	High priority for influenza
Staff of institutions for developmentally disabled	Should receive HepB; high priority for influenza

[a] This table assumes that all routinely recommended vaccine series and boosters have been given.

13. Guidelines for vaccinating pregnant women. Centers for Disease Control and Prevention Web site. http://www.cdc.gov/vaccines/pubs/downloads/b_preg_guide.pdf. Accessed March 31, 2010.

14. Mak TK, et al. *Lancet Infect Dis*. 2008;8:44-52.

15. Munoz FM, et al. *Am J Obstet Gynecol*. 2005;192:1098-1106.

16. Beigi RH, et al. *Clin Infect Dis*. 2009;49:1784-1792.

17. Advisory Committee on Immunization Practices Workgroup on the Use of Vaccines During Pregnancy and Breastfeeding. Guiding principles for development of ACIP recommendations for vaccination during pregnancy and breastfeeding. Centers for Disease Control and Prevention Web site. http://www.cdc.gov/vaccines/recs/acip/downloads/preg-principles05-01-08.pdf. Accessed January 25, 2010.

18. Saari TN, et al. *Pediatrics*. 2003;112:193-198.

19. Pourcyrous M, et al. *J Pediatr*. 2007;151:167-172.

20. Centers for Disease Control and Prevention Web site. Notice of revised vaccination criteria for U.S. immigration. http://www.cdc.gov/immigrantrefugeehealth/laws-regs/vaccination-immigration/revised-vaccination-criteria-immigration.html. Accessed March 30, 2010.

21. Immunization Action Coalition. *Needle Tips*. 2008;18:18.

22. Verla-Tebit E, et al. *Arch Pediatr Adolesc Med*. 2009;163:473-479.

23. Greenaway C, et al. *Ann Intern Med*. 2007;146:20-24.

24. Cilleruelo MJ, et al. *Vaccine*. 2008;26:5784-5790.

25. CDC. *MMWR*. 2009;58:1006-1007.

26. Cohen AL, et al. *Pediatrics*. 2006;117:1650-1655.

27. CDC. *MMWR*. 1997;46(RR-18):1-42.

28. CDC. *MMWR*. 2001;50(RR-11):1-52.

29. Pearson ML, et al. *MMWR*. 2006;55(RR-2):1-16.

30. van Delden JJM, et al. *Vaccine*. 2008;26:5562-5566.

31. Douville LE, et al. *Arch Pediatr Adolesc Med*. 2010;164:33-37.

32. Hollmeyer HG, et al. *Vaccine*. 2009;27:3935-3944.

33. Travelers' Health— Yellow Book. Centers for Disease Control and Prevention Web site. http://wwwnc.cdc.gov/travel/content/yellowbook/home-2010.aspx. Accessed January 25, 2010.

34. CDC. *MMWR*. 2009;58:312.

7

Addressing Concerns About Vaccines

Vaccines have saved more lives than virtually any other public health intervention, and they are safer now than ever before. Despite this, providers face the daily challenge of convincing parents and patients that vaccines are safe, effective, and necessary. It is true that good things have come from public concern about vaccines—the replacement, for example, of DTwP with the less reactogenic DTaP. However, the sensational claims made by antivaccination activists, celebrities, wealthy financiers, and rogue (largely discredited, if not outright debarred) scientists have not held up to scientific scrutiny. Despite this, these claims receive airtime in the lay press and make their way to the Internet. As a result, some well-meaning parents are either refusing to have their children vaccinated or asking for negotiation on the schedule, and adults who should be vaccinated are opting out. This has translated directly into personal and public harm, and many fear an impending public health crisis. This section provides tips on communicating the true risks and benefits of vaccination and gives some background on the concerns that people have.

Communicating Risks and Benefits

■ The Meaning of Safety

What do we mean when we say that vaccines are *safe*? One definition of the word safe is *harmless*. This definition would imply that any negative consequence of vaccines would make them *unsafe*. But we know that all vaccines have side effects. For example, shots can cause pain, redness, swelling, and tenderness. Some vaccines cause more concerning side effects—DTaP, for example, can very rarely cause persistent, inconsolable crying, and MMRV can double the risk of febrile seizures. While these symptoms do not result in permanent damage, they can be frightening. There are historical examples of more serious side effects—for example, OPV caused paralytic polio, but only one case for every 2.3 million doses distributed. The recommendation to change to IPV in the year 2000 was based on the occurrence of this extremely rare side effect, which had by then become more of a risk than natural polio itself in the United States.

Few things in life meet the definition of harmless. Even everyday activities contain hidden dangers. For example, each year in the United States, 350 people are killed in bath- or shower-related accidents and 200 people are killed when food lodges in their windpipe. Just being outdoors can be dangerous—100 people are killed each year by lightning. By the harmless criterion, even routine daily activities could be considered unsafe.

Another definition of the word safe is *having been preserved from a real danger*. Using this definition, the danger (*the disease*) must be significantly greater than the means of protecting against the danger (*the vaccine*). To put it another way, a vaccine's benefits must clearly and definitively outweigh its risks. For all routinely recommended vaccines, the benefits clearly outweigh the risks.

■ Probabilistic and Heuristic Thinking

Scientists, public health officials, and providers tend to think (subconsciously, if not consciously) about vaccines in terms of probability and expected utility. The health value of getting a vaccine, and presumably the basis for decision making, can simplistically be seen as the difference between two things: 1) the probability of avoiding the disease multiplied by the *utility*, or value, of avoiding the disease; and 2) the probability of a vaccine side effect multiplied by the *disutility* of that side effect. For example, the probability of avoiding measles through vaccination is nearly 100%, and the utility of avoiding measles for any given individual is very high (because 1 in 100 patients develop pneumonia and 1 in 1000 die). Thus, the first part of the equation has a high value. On the other hand, the probability of getting fever and rash from MMR is low, say 5%, and the disutility of fever and rash is low, since these side effects are self-limited. Thus, the second part of the equation does not detract appreciably from the value of the first part. In other words, the overall mental model overwhelmingly favors vaccination.

At the societal level, the value of vaccines paradoxically decreases as their effectiveness increases; when disease is eliminated, the public perceives no benefit from vaccines. The truth is, when vaccines work, *nothing* (as opposed to *disease*) happens. This fact, combined with widespread attention given to rare adverse events, leads to the perception that vaccines do more harm than good. At the individual level, several thought processes might be operative in a person's reluctance to be vaccinated or have his or her child vaccinated. Some of these are heuristics, shortcut ways of thinking or rules of thumb that we use (subconsciously or consciously) to simplify complex decision-making.[1] In order to communicate effectively, physicians should understand these thought processes and be prepared to address them, armed with information. The goal of communication is not to convince doubtful individuals to accept vaccination, but rather to listen to their concerns, provide accurate information, and facilitate their informed decision-making.

Here are some examples of heuristic thinking, along with some suggested responses:

- **Availability**—The ease with which a person remembers something correlates with the perceived probability that it will occur.
  - *Example*: A vivid, frightening news story about a child who has an anaphylactic reaction to a vaccine might make a parent think that anaphylaxis is more common than it really is.
  - *Response*: The risk of anaphylaxis after vaccination is estimated to be less than 1 in a million.[2]
- **Avoidance of ambiguity**—A *known* risk is more acceptable than an *unknown* risk.
  - *Example*: The serious sequelae of chickenpox (a disease with which people are familiar) seem more acceptable than the potential risks of the vaccine (with which people are not familiar).
  - *Response*: There is a side to chickenpox that many people have not seen—but health professionals have (eg, hemorrhagic varicella, necrotizing fasciitis, encephalitis, etc). Convert the unknown risk of the vaccine to a known risk by reviewing the safety data (*Section B: Diseases and Vaccines*) and describing the rigorous pre- and postlicensure evaluation process that ensures safety (see *Chapter 2: Vaccine Infrastructure in the United States—Vaccine Development and Licensure*)
- **Do no harm**—A bad outcome is more tolerable if it occurs from *inaction* rather than *action*.
  - *Example*: Hospitalization with influenza (something that just *happens*) is more tolerable than side effects of the vaccine (something that a person *causes* by choice).
  - *Response*: Nothing in medicine (or life for that matter) has zero risk, and not taking a vaccine is actually an *action* to accept vulnerability to the disease.
- **Framing**—The context in which a decision is made affects the decision.
  - *Example*: A parent may be reluctant to take on the risks of vaccination because it involves making a decision on behalf of the child.
  - *Response*: Reframe the vaccination discussion around the viewpoint of the child, who would likely choose protection from disease if given the chance. In fact, there are studies showing that school-aged children who have had chickenpox would rather have had the shot.
- **Freeloading**—Herd immunity protects unvaccinated people.
  - *Example*: Since other children get the MMR, my child will not get measles and there is no reason for him or her to take the risk of the vaccine.
  - *Response*: The risk of measles is actually 35-fold higher in exemptors, even in communities where >90% of children are immunized.[3] In truth, freeloaders *are* protected—that

is, until enough people in a population are also freeloading. Then everyone is unprotected, and all it takes is a case of measles to arrive on an international flight for an outbreak to ensue.

- **Maintaining the status quo**—There is an aversion to taking on one risk to reduce another.
  - *Example*: We're more comfortable just taking the risk of the disease since that's how things are now and so far we've been fine.
  - *Response*: The status quo, ie, susceptibility to disease, is not the optimal position to be in because protection from disease is available.
- **Representativeness**—The probability that something will occur correlates with similarity of circumstances.
  - *Example*: A vaccine side effect is likely because it happened to a child just like mine who lives in the same community.
  - *Response*: Again, this is where the cold hard facts on adverse events can be helpful. Sometimes we identify so strongly with individuals in similar circumstances that we feel we actually *know* them. For example, in a 2009 survey,[4] 40% of parents said they personally knew of someone who experienced a harmful adverse event from MMR, something that would be impossible given the established rarity of serious adverse events.[5]

Vaccine hesitancy may be driven by other though processes as well. For example, there is *confirmation bias*, our tendency to seek out confirmatory evidence for what we already believe and to ignore contradictory evidence (we begin with the *belief* that vaccines must be harmful, then seek *validation* for this belief). And there is *folk numeracy*, our intuitive sense of numbers that upholds small, anecdotal experiences and makes it difficult for us to see the big picture.[6] So, for example, we intuitively "get" 3 kids with diabetes in the same school but we have difficulty conceptualizing a prospective cohort study with 4.7 million person-years of follow-up. Likewise, we have trouble coming to terms with background rates of adverse events. According to one study, if 10 million people were given a shot, 22 would develop Guillain-Barré syndrome and 6 would die suddenly within 6 weeks.[7] If all 10 million were women, 86 would develop optic neuritis, and if all 10 million were pregnant women, 16,684 would have a spontaneous abortion. All of this would happen—*if the shot were a placebo*!

There is also *patternicity*, our tendency to find meaningful patterns in meaningless noise ("Almost all children with autism have received the MMR, so there must be a connection"). And there is *agenticity*, our belief that something or someone must be behind things (there *must* be a conspiracy to cover up the dangers of vaccines, otherwise we would know about them).[8] Each of these is part of our evolved psychology, and understanding this is a starting place for shepherding parents and patients from ill-founded beliefs to rock-solid science. The task is all the more difficult in an age of consumerism, pop culture, and celebrity, where likeable actors and sports figures are entrusted as anti-establishment heros and truth-seekers.[9]

■ Communication Strategies

People will not undertake a risk-control measure like vaccination unless they believe they can effectively control the risk. In other words, they need to understand that the vaccine really does prevent the disease. In addition, the risk should be personally relevant and serious. While there are heuristics that tend to favor vaccination, such as *bandwagoning* (the tendency for people to choose the decision of the majority as what might be wise for themselves) and *altruism* (a willingness to take on personal risks if it is for the benefit of others), nothing substitutes for a straightforward discussion about risks and benefits.

There is a disconnect between what physicians do and what patients want. For example, people want personal verbal communication from their physicians that conveys a sense of trust and respect. Time-motion studies, however, show that physicians spend <2 minutes discussing vaccines with their patients.[10] Physicians are sometimes reluctant to mention risks for fear of "opening a can of worms," but patients are interested in relevant, practical information that can be easily understood.[11] Here are some tips on getting to the point of what parents want to know about routine childhood vaccinations[12]:

- Describe which vaccines the child will receive today.
- Give the pertinent Vaccine Information Statements (VISs) to the parent (see *Chapter 3: Standards, Principles, and Regulations—Vaccine Information Statements [VISs]*)
- Explain why these vaccines are important.
- Review contraindications to each vaccine.
- Give a detailed account of the common, mild side effects and how to manage them.
- Give a brief account of any severe risks.
- Place today's vaccinations in the context of the overall schedule.

In addition, here are some suggestions regarding communication in the office setting:

- *Begin the discussion early*—One of the advantages of the birth dose of HepB is that it opens the door to discussing vaccines immediately after parenthood has begun (similarly, a postpartum dose of Tdap is a good way to emphasize the importance of adult immunization, especially as this relates to protecting kids). In those initial discussions before hospital discharge, vaccines should be portrayed as part of the routine care the child will receive as he or she grows up. Parents who express doubt or concern should be targeted for further discussion and should receive printed materials and other resources well before the 2-month visit. The discussion can even begin before the baby is born, in the setting, for example, of prenatal classes (and, similarly, when pregnant women receive the influenza vaccine).

• *Use a team approach*—Communication should be a coordinated effort between doctors, nurses, and other office personnel. Even the receptionist can provide an introduction to the vaccination visit, give VISs, and direct the parent or guardian to informational materials in the waiting room. Office nurses (who are often trained in risk-benefit communication) are accessible, highly invested in immunization, and can have a great impact on parents. Each member of the team should be empowered and should know his or her function during the vaccination visit.

• *Be consistent*—Try to reach consensus on how the practice will handle specific issues. Communication is that much more difficult when some providers in the practice endorse "alternative schedules" while others do not.

• *Organize the visit effectively*—Face-to-face time with the doctor can be increased by building efficiencies into the visit, beginning with a preparatory phone call to remind the parent or guardian to bring the child's shot record and perhaps introducing the vaccines that are scheduled for the visit. Use of a screening questionnaire for contraindications (**Table 4.2**) can be helpful. Development of simple, direct messages and easy-to-understand printed materials can eliminate some questions and help focus the discussion. Ultimately, the use of newer combination vaccines may increase office efficiency and allow more time for communication. DVDs, books, and other printed materials that can be taken home may solidify concepts that were initiated during the visit.

• *Understand individual backgrounds*—Many factors affect risk perception, including educational, emotional, religious, psychological, spiritual, philosophical, and intuitive foundations. Families differ in their orientation toward the medical establishment—some are traditional and trusting, others are cautious, challenging, and oriented toward alternative practices. Vaccine messages should be delivered with these differences in mind.

• *Layer information appropriately*—Information should be presented with sensitivity to individual needs. Providers should be aware of the patient's cognitive foundation and begin with information appropriate to that level. Parents who want to know more will ask.

- *Engage patients in a decision-making partnership*—Research repeatedly shows that parents trust their physicians more than anyone else for accurate, honest information. Building on this trust, the approach should be nonjudgmental, empathetic, and mutually respectful. That said, a physician's direct, personal advocacy ("My kids have received all of their immunizations", or "I get a flu shot every year") may carry the most weight.
- *Remove barriers*—Insufficient time is the most important barrier to effective communication. Consider scheduling vaccination visits at off-peak hours.
- *Be aware of pitfalls*—Avoid the tendency to extrapolate from limited data and to fit equivocal data into preconceived notions. Consciously avoid being paternalistic and belittling.
- *Check for understanding*—Make sure parents and patients understand what you have told them and ask if they have any questions.

Vaccine Refusal

More and more parents are requesting alternative schedules, agreeing to only selected formulations and antigens, or refusing to have their children vaccinated altogether—despite the best efforts of providers and public health agencies to allay their concerns. Surveys show that the majority of pediatricians and family practitioners have had at least one family in their practice that has refused vaccination.[13,14] In 2004, it was estimated that slightly more than 1% of the birth cohort in the United States was underimmunized due to parental concerns about safety.[15] Ironically, *unvaccinated* children are more likely to come from backgrounds with ready access to health care—they have white, married, college-educated mothers and their household income is >$75,000 (2001 dollars).[16] In contrast, *undervaccinated* children—those who might be vaccinated if they had better access—tend to be black, have single mothers without college educations and live near the poverty level in the inner city. In a study published in 2008, about 28% of a national sample of parents had significant concerns about vaccinating their children.[17] The largest proportion (nearly 40%) of those who changed their mind about delaying or refusing vaccination did so based on information or assurances from their health care provider; other reasons included having had more time to think about it (20%), information from other sources (15%), and the possibility of dismissal from the provider's practice or concerns about admission to day care (10%). The most recent data come from 2009—in a national survey, 11.5% of parents reported refusing at least one vaccination for their children.[4] The good news was that 90% still believed that vaccines are a good way to protect their children and that the vast majority trusted their doctors' recommendations. The disturbing news was that over half were concerned about serious adverse effects, and 25% believed that vaccines cause autism.

How should vaccine refusal be handled? First, listen to what the parent is saying. Providers may mistake the need for information or reassurance for flat-out refusal. Some parents may be refusing a single vaccine; others may be refusing all the vaccines that are due at a single visit. Few parents refuse all vaccines at all visits. Second, it must be recognized that whereas the decision not to vaccinate goes against the best medical advice, it rarely puts a child directly in harm's way. Ironically, this is due to the success of vaccination programs. The truth is that indigenous polio has been eliminated from the Western Hemisphere; therefore, any given unvaccinated child in the United States is, on the whole, unlikely to get polio. In this context, refusing to allow a child to receive the polio vaccine can hardly be interpreted as actionable medical neglect. On the other hand, there are some situations where vaccine refusal could bring immediate harm to a child—during an epidemic, for example, or after a tetanus-prone injury. In such situations, it would be appropriate to involve governmental agencies or the courts to force action in the child's best interest. While states may be reluctant to act unless there is immediate and substantial danger, it is notable that the courts have repeatedly upheld compulsory immunization laws as a reasonable exercise of the state's power, even in the absence of an epidemic (see *Chapter 3: Standards, Principles, and Regulations—School Mandates and State Legislation*).

Third, parents need to understand that the decision not to immunize their children places other children at risk. Outbreaks are spread by unvaccinated persons, and even vaccinated children whose parents have diligently tried to protect them can still get the disease—this is due to the (fortunately unusual) phenomenon of primary vaccine failure. In addition, some children cannot be immunized for medical reasons and can therefore only be protected by herd immunity. Thus, immunization can be construed as a *civic duty*, and failure to immunize can be seen as indirectly bringing the possibility of harm to others. Interestingly, some religious traditions may see immunizations as an imperative—Judiasm, for example, where immunizations may be seen to fulfill the obligation to guard one's own health and to prevent others from becoming sick.[18] If parents understood the scientific facts about the safety of vaccines—and that is a big "if"—it is hard to imagine that most parents would not agree to have their children immunized on the basis of altruism alone. Many parents, however, fear things that have not been, and may not ever be, studied—side effects that could appear decades down the road, for example.

Yet there are still parents who will not agree to vaccination. For these situations, the American Academy of Pediatrics developed a *Refusal to Vaccinate* form[19] that can be signed by the parent.

The form is not intended to be a legal document and it is not clear what legal protection it would afford the practitioner in the case of a bad outcome from a vaccine-preventable disease (nevertheless, it should be placed in the permanent medical record). Its main purpose is to encourage parents to rethink the issue and to document the provider's efforts to communicate the true risks and benefits of immunization. By signing the form, the parent acknowledges that he or she understands the purpose of the vaccine, why it is recommended, what the risks of vaccination are, and what the consequences of infection may be, including disease, death, permanent impairment, transmission to others, and exclusion from school during outbreaks. Some providers place an expiration date on the form in order to encourage readdressing the issue in the future.

Some parents want a modified schedule for their children, one that spreads the shots out over time, minimizing what they perceive to be a bolus of "toxins" and an assault on the child's immune system. Whereas the end of negotiation in this case—namely that the child receives all recommended vaccines—might justify the means, it also places a burden on the provider to prioritize the immunizations. If the parent will only allow two shots on a given day, which ones should be given and which ones deferred? The decision should be made based on the epidemiology and potential consequences of infection. So, for example, given the above discussion about polio, it might make sense to defer IPV in favor of DTaP, since pertussis is still prevalent and the consequences of infection include a high probability of hospitalization and the possibility of death. Deferral prolongs the period of vulnerability to disease, which in the case of polio may not be consequential; however, it also increases the likelihood that the vaccine series will not be completed.

In a 2005 clinical report (reaffirmed in 2009), the AAP took the position that negotiation is in the best interest of the child, and that physicians should avoid discharging patients from their practices because of vaccine refusal.[20] However, there is no law that says a provider must acquiesce to a parent's wishes. Some providers may not be willing to accept the potential exposure to liability that is inherent in negotiating a modified schedule, and they worry about unimmunized kids in their waiting rooms. Others may feel that negotiation is a slippery slope—what if the next request is for half doses, or worse yet homeopathic ones? Still other providers may feel that drawing a hard line behind the recommended schedule is the best way to send the message that vaccinations—at the proper time, in the proper doses, and according to the proper schedule—are a critical component of preventive medicine; this alone might be enough to change some parents' minds. Unfortunately, there are no controlled trials comparing "hard-line" and "soft-line" approaches, and the provider is left to his or her best judgment in terms of how to proceed.

Ultimately, failure to come to terms about immunization may predict a poor therapeutic relationship in general, which could affect the care of the child. In this situation, the AAP suggests that families may be encouraged to find another physician or practice. It should be noted that the American Medical Association Code of Ethics, Section E-8.115, states that physicians have the option of withdrawing from a case, so long as notice is given far enough in advance as to permit another medical provider to be secured.[21] Ultimately, physicians need to decide whether to retain patients in their practice who refuse all immunizations. Bear in mind that despite the risks, retention allows continued opportunities to break down barriers and protects the child from seeking care from chiropractors and alternative medicine practitioners.

Many studies suggest that the most trusted person in this whole debate is you—the provider. Personally advocating for vaccination, tempered by compassionate engagement and recognition of a shared, firm commitment to the child's well-being, underpinned by unequivocal scientific data, is the most important thing you can do to ensure the protection of children. Parents should be part of the decision-making process, but many parents will want to know what you have done or would do with your own children.

Antivaccinationism

A simple Internet search using terms such as vaccines or immunization yields a multitude of web sites that contain non-peer-reviewed data, frightening anecdotes, and pseudoscientific arguments intermingled with legitimate concerns for adverse events such as fever, redness, and swelling. Parents may have trouble separating the *information* from the *misinformation*. In fact, in a study published in 2010, 71% of Google "hits" using the term "vaccination" were opposed to vaccination.[22] Many of these web sites are sponsored by organizations that claim authority, credibility, and scientific rigor, which, along with some lay people, vocal celebrities, and rogue investigators, collectively constitute a modern antivaccination movement.[23,24] In truth, antivaccinationism is as old as vaccination itself. It is rooted in a host of underlying sentiments, from libertarianism to distrust of government and science to naturopathy and even religious fundamentalism; it is fueled by sensationalistic and irresponsible journalism, easy access to unfiltered analyses, and a pervasive cultural lack of critical thinking and understanding of science. Superb books on antivaccinationism and its consequences have been published.[25-27]

Antivaccinationists offer strong emotive or political appeals, make explicit claims about vaccines that are unsupported or even contradicted by published data, and they call people to action in opposing vaccine policy. Examples of explicit claims include the following: vaccines cause idiopathic diseases; adverse reactions are underreported; vaccines erode immunity; vaccine policy is motivated by profit; vaccines are ineffective, diseases declined without vaccines; and vaccination is a violation of civil liberties.[22,28] **Table 7.1** summarizes some of the rhetorical appeals that are used.

Table 7.2 lists some web sites (and their sponsoring organizations) that have an antivaccination orientation. Providers should remain informed about the content of these sites in order to be better prepared to address issues that patients may raise. Some of the claims made on these sites are patently false, if not ridiculous—claims, for example, that smallpox is harmless and not very infectious; that diseases are caused by imbalanced bodily

7

TABLE 7.1 — Rhetorical Appeals Made by Vaccine-Protest Organizations on the Internet

Authoritative and Scientific
- Present their organization as a legitimate, official body with scientific credibility
- Reference self-published works and alternative medicine literature
- Use indiscriminate citations (eg, letters to newspapers, television interviews)
- Draw alternative conclusions from peer-reviewed studies
- Claim to present "both sides"
- Provide links to provaccine sites

Emotive Appeals
- Paint an "us" (the organization, concerned parents) vs "them" (the medical establishment, government, pharmaceutical industry) picture
- Describe physicians as willing conspirators or manipulated pawns
- Pit parents' love and compassion against cold, analytical science
- Feature anecdotal accounts of purported vaccine injury
- Suggest that responsible parenting means refusing vaccination
- Urge parents to resist coercion
- Warn the public about conspiracy
- Characterize vaccines as "unnatural" and suggest that a natural lifestyle will prevent disease

Search for Truth
- Depict their struggle as a search for truth against a backdrop of cover-up
- Highlight excavated "facts" that were hitherto neglected
- Portray rank-breaking doctors as enlightened heroes

Adapted from Davies P, et al. *Arch Dis Child*. 2002;87:22-25.

TABLE 7.2 — Web Sites With a Vaccine-Protest Orientation

URL	Sponsor or Name of Web Site
http://www.ageofautism.com/	Age of Autism
http://avn.org.au	Australian Vaccination Network
http://www.autism.com/	Autism Research Institute
http://www.cryshame.co.uk/	Cryshame!
http://generationrescue.org/	Generation Rescue
http://www.gval.com	Global Vaccine Awareness League
http://www.ias.org.nz/	Immunization Awareness Society of New Zealand
http://www.informedchoice.info/index.php	Informed Choice
http://www.jabs.org.uk/	Justice Awareness and Basic Support (JABS)
http://www.know-vaccines.org	Kids Need Options With Vaccines (KNOW Vaccines)
http://mvvic.org	Medical Voices Vaccine Information Center
http://www.nvic.org/	National Vaccine Information Center
http://goodlight.net/nyvic/default.htm	New Yorkers for Vaccination Information and Choice
http://vaccineinfo.net	Parents Requesting Open Vaccine Education (PROVE)
http://www.vaccineeducation.org/	People Advocating Vaccine Education (PAVE)
http://safeminds.org/	Safe Minds
http://www.shirleys-wellness-cafe.com/vaccines.htm	Shirley's Wellness Cafe
http://thinktwice.com/	Thinktwice Global Vaccine Institute
http://www.vaccination.co.uk/	Vaccination

http://www.whale.to/vaccines.html	Vaccination
http://www.vaclib.org/sites/debate/index.html	Vaccination Debate
http://www.vaccinationnews.com	Vaccination News
http://vran.org/	Vaccination Risk Awareness Network (VRAN)
http://www.nccn.net/~wwithin/vaccine.htm	Vaccination Information & Choice Network
http://www.vaccination.inoz.com	Vaccination Information Service
http://www.vaclib.org	Vaccination Liberation

Accessed January 24, 2010.

7

conditions and lifestyle choices rather than microorganisms; that polio is caused by sugary foods; and that rabies might be psychosomatic.[22]

Individuals and organizations that oppose immunization or argue for "alternative" approaches share common sentiments. **Table 7.3** lists some of those ideas and the reasons why they represent flawed thinking.

The Costs of Public Concern

It is one thing to understand that unvaccinated persons are at increased risk of disease. This makes common sense and has been repeatedly demonstrated, even in the era when most people are vaccinated and many vaccine-preventable diseases are less common. In addition to the elevated risk of measles among exemptors,[3] the risk of pertussis is also high,[29] and a study from Michigan demonstrated that the highest risk of pertussis was in areas with the highest rates of nonmedical exemption.[30]

It is another thing to connect the dots between public fear of vaccination and public harm; **Table 7.4** represents an attempt to do this. The best example is what happened in the United Kingdom in the late 1970s. Anecdotal case series claiming that the whole-cell pertussis vaccine caused encephalopathy, popularized in the lay press, led to widespread fear of the vaccine and to a dramatic decline in immunization rates. The result was a tragic increase in pertussis cases and many infant deaths.[31] Not surprisingly, the same scenario played out in other countries where antivaccination movements gained traction, but not in countries that had sustained vaccine use.[32] Similarly, claims that MMR vaccine causes autism led to dramatic declines in MMR uptake in the United Kingdom in the late 1990s—predictably resulting in outbreaks of measles. In fact, the United Kingdom had been declared free of endemic measles in 1994; in 2008, that declaration was reversed, the direct result of parents refusing to vaccinate their children.[33] More recent studies have shown alarming increases in the rates of philosophical or personal-belief exemptions. States granting such exemptions have higher rates of pertussis, and the incidence of pertussis correlates directly with the ease with which such exemptions are obtained.

To understand the impact of vaccine refusal, one need go no further than Indiana, where in 2005 an unvaccinated teenager returned from a mission trip to Romania, unknowingly incubating measles.[34] The next day she attended a gathering of approximately 500 church members, and the result was 33 cases of measles among church members and 1 case in a hospital phlebotomist (who was not a church member). Three people were hospitalized and one spent 6 days on a ventilator. The vast majority of cases occurred in unvaccinated persons. Several important things can

TABLE 7.3 — Flawed Thinking About Vaccines

Claim	Why This is Incorrect or Misleading
Doctors do not understand vaccines.	Doctors may not always review the primary data, but the advisory committes that do are composed of experts whose historical record has been spot-on.
Government and pharmaceutical companies conspire to misrepresent data.	There is no evidence of a conspiracy.
Vaccine-preventable diseases are rarely seen in practice.	This is evidence of the success of vaccine programs. Some diseases (like pertussis) are not rare. National surveillance data trump antecdotal experiences.
Natural immunity is better than vaccine-induced immunity.	The cost of natural immunity is the risk of serious disease.
Vaccines are not adequately tested for safety.	Vaccines are among the most thoroughly tested pharmaceuticals. The post-licensure safety net is robust.
Vaccines protect the public but not individuals.	Individuals benefit by becoming immune and, *as long as others are immunized*, by having less chance of exposure.
Reports in VAERS and language in the package insert constitute accurate profiles of vaccine side effects.	VAERS reports do not establish causality and the package insert lists *any* reported events, whether or not they are causally related to vaccination.
There is a middle ground between causality and coincidence.	Either vaccine *do* or *do not* cause certain adverse events.
Science fails because it cannot prove there is no connection between vaccines and certain adverse events.	Science works by rejecting or failing to reject the null hypothesis.

Adapted from Offit PA, Moser CA. *Pediatrics* 2009;123:e164-e169.

TABLE 7.4 — Fear of Vaccines Leads to Public Harm

Vaccine[a]	Event or Finding	Evidence that Event Resulted From Willful Refusal to Vaccinate
DTwP	Outbreaks of pertussis in the United Kingdom, late 1970s	Intense media coverage of anecdotal reports of neurological reactions resulted a drop in vaccination rates from 81% to 31%. Outbreaks were not seen in countries without antivaccine movements.[b]
DTaP	Higher risk of pertussis in certain states	Risk correlates with availability of personal belief exemptions and the ease with which such exemptions are granted.[c]
	Pertussis cases and controls in Colorado	Odds of vaccine refusal 23-times higher among cases. Virtually all cases among refusers, and 11% of cases in the whole population, were due to refusal itself.[d]
MMR	Measles eliminated from the United Kingdom in 1994 but endemic again in 2008[e]	Immunization rates fell dramatically after Wakefield's 1998 article that suggested a causal link with autism.[f]
	33 cases of measles among members of a church in Indiana, 2005	31 cases occurred among members who refused vaccination because they feared adverse reactions.[g]
	Measles outbreaks in the United States, 2008	The vast majority of cases were unvaccinated or vaccination status unknown. Of eligible persons, 66% not vaccinated because of religious or personal beliefs.[h]
Hib	*H influenzae* disease in Minnesota in 2008—highest number of cases since 1992	3 of the 5 cases were intentionally not immunized, including one who died.[i]
VAR	Varicella cases and controls in Colorado	Odds of vaccine refusal 9-times higher among cases. Virtually all cases among refusers, and 5% of cases in the whole population, were due to refusal itself.[j]

[a] In some cases, the concern may have been about all vaccines, or multiple vaccines, rather than the one cited.
[b] Gangarosa EJ, et al. *Lancet*. 1998;351:356-361.
[c] Omer SB, et al. *JAMA*. 2006;296:1757-1763.
[d] Glanz JM, et al. *Pediatrics*. 2009;123:1446-1451.
[e] Measles once again endemic in the United Kingdom. Eurosurveillance Web site. http://www.eurosurveillance.org/viewarticle.aspx?articleid=18919. Accessed January 24, 2010.
[f] Jansen VAA, et al. *Science*. 2003;301:804.
[g] Parker AA, et al. *N Engl J Med*. 2006;355:447-455.
[h] CDC. *MMWR*. 2008;57:893-896.
[i] CDC. *MMWR*. 2009;58(3):58-60.
[j] Glanz JM, et al. *Arch Pediatr Adolesc Med*. 2010;164(1):66-70.

7

be gleaned from the Indiana outbreak. First, fear of adverse events was the main reason people refused vaccination. In testament to the prevalence of misinformation, some families feared MMR because of the preservative thimerosal, which has *never* been part of the vaccine. Second, the church was largely white, middle class, and well educated, reflecting the demographic of unvaccinated children mentioned earlier. Third, the church itself had no official position on immunization—vaccine refusal was a subcultural phenomenon (20 of the 28 affected children were home-schooled, suggesting that there are other sociodemographic correlates of vaccine refusal). Fourth, even though the attack rate was much higher in unvaccinated persons, some vaccinated people still got measles. This illustrates the real issue of primary vaccine failure and the fact that unvaccinated people place vaccinated people at risk. Fifth, the outbreak was almost entirely confined to church members—vaccination-coverage rates in the surrounding community were high enough to prevent spread. Finally, the case could not be made more clearly that diseases such as measles are only a plane flight away, and that all it takes to ignite an outbreak is for the virus to land in a community with enough susceptible individuals.

Specific Concerns

Here are some specific questions about vaccines that are on the minds of parents and patients. The information provided should serve as a foundation for effective communication of the true risks and benefits. Some of these issues were addressed by the Institute of Medicine (IOM) Immunization Safety Review Committee (**Table 2.3**).

■ Are Vaccines Still Necessary?

Everyone agrees that vaccine-preventable diseases are less prevalent now than they were before vaccines were introduced (see **Table 1.5**). However, the myth still circulates that the diseases were disappearing before we had the vaccines. Nothing could be farther from the truth, to which anyone whose medical career has spanned the demise of *H influenzae* type b can testify. In the early 1980s, 1 in 200 children, year in and year out, were affected by invasive *H influenzae* disease. Call nights in the hospital were replete with cases of bacteremia, meningitis, periorbital cellulitis, and the like. Today's pediatric residents have never seen a case—and the change occurred in the early 1990s, after the institution of universal infant Hib immunization. There is an undeniable association between the introduction of new vaccines and the beginning of the end of the respective diseases, as has been seen in the last 2 decades with varicella, hepatitis A, and *S pneumoniae*.

Now that many of these diseases are rare, it is hard for parents and patients to understand why vaccines are still important. Here are a few reasons.

- *Some diseases are still prevalent*—Despite our successes, many vaccine-preventable diseases are still around. The choice not to vaccinate against pertussis, for example, is a choice to take a significant risk of getting the disease. The same is true for *S pneumoniae*. Influenza still kills 36,000 people every year in the United States, and HPV is still highly prevalent.

- *Diseases could easily re-emerge*—Some diseases continue to circulate at very low levels. If immunization rates decrease, outbreaks are likely to occur. This is exactly what happened between 1989 and 1991 in the United States, when 55,622 cases of measles and 123 deaths from the disease were reported.[35] The single most important contributing factor was low vaccine coverage, especially among preschoolers in inner cities. By 2003, after renewed efforts to achieve universal vaccination and the implementation of a 2-dose schedule, measles was no longer endemic in the United States. This means that there was enough population immunity to prevent sustained transmission, but the situation could change dramatically if coverage rates fall. The outbreak of >6000 cases of mumps in the Midwest in 2006 is further evidence that diseases can re-emerge.[35]

- *Infections can easily be imported from other parts of the world*—Diseases such as polio and diphtheria still occur in other countries. Tourism, immigration, and international business travel contribute to the ease with which these diseases can be imported into the United States. The outbreaks of measles that occurred in the United States in 2008 were probably due to importation from Europe.

- *Some diseases cannot be eradicated or extinguished*—Tetanus, which is acquired from the environment as opposed to person-to-person transmission, is a good example.

■ Is Natural Infection Better at Inducing Immunity?

Natural infection may induce stronger and longer-lasting immunity than vaccines. Whereas immunity from disease often follows a single natural infection, immunity from vaccines usually occurs only after several doses and, in some cases, can wane with time. A notable example of waning immunity occurs with the pertussis vaccine—by the time children are teenagers, they have lost the protective immunity imparted by the childhood DTaP series (it is important to understand that even natural immunity to pertussis also wanes with time). As a result, teenagers account for a large proportion of reported cases and serve as a reservoir for transmission in the community. Fortunately, there are now vaccines that can boost immunity in adolescents and adults.

There *are* some diseases for which vaccines are actually better at inducing immunity than natural infection. Infants who are infected with *H influenzae* do not develop effective antibody responses due to an inherent maturational defect in recognizing polysaccharide antigens (see *Chapter 1: Introduction to Vaccinology—Active Immunization*). Hib vaccines, on the other hand, are very effective in young infants because, in coupling the polysaccharide to proteins, they are capable of enlisting T-cell help in driving antibody production by B-cells.

The difference between vaccination and natural infection is the price paid for immunity. For chickenpox, the price paid for natural immunity might be pneumonitis, respiratory failure, encephalitis, or necrotizing fasciitis. For *S pneumoniae*, it might be mental retardation from meningitis—and that would only buy you immunity to the one serotype that caused the infection. Likewise, for HPV the price might be cervical dysplasia—and if you are lucky enough to resolve the dysplasia without progression to cancer, you are left with immunity to only one HPV type (the vaccines protect against 2 of the many cancer-causing serotypes). The price of immunity to shingles is a case of shingles, and, in some cases, postherpetic neuralgia, which can be intractable. The cost of vaccine-induced protection against shingles is the cost of the vaccine, plus minor reactogenicity.

■ Can Multiple Vaccines Overload the Immune System?

One hundred years ago, children were routinely vaccinated against one disease—smallpox. Forty years ago, it was 5 diseases—diphtheria, pertussis, tetanus, polio, and smallpox, necessitating as many as eight shots by 2 years of age. The routine childhood immunization schedule in 2010 calls for as many as 53 separate vaccine doses by 18 years of age. The good news is that through all of this, 16 different diseases are prevented; the bad news is that some people wonder if it is just too much.

The possibility of immune overload must be put into perspective. Every day, people are bombarded by antigens to which their immune systems must respond. This includes viruses and bacteria from the external environment as well as organisms from within, particularly those in the mouth, nasopharynx, and gut. Most people are not sick most of the time—this speaks to the robustness of the immune system's ability to meet these challenges. Even the most vulnerable people—neonates—seem to do just fine. Within a matter of hours of birth, the initially sterile gastrointestinal tract becomes heavily colonized with a wide variety of bacteria, some of which are potentially harmful. Yet the specific secretory IgA responses that are stimulated by colonization are, by and large, adequate to prevent invasion.

Even though children receive more vaccines today than they did 40 years ago, the number of separate immunologic challenges (ie, bacterial and viral proteins and bacterial polysaccharides) represented by the routine childhood schedule has drastically decreased (**Table 7.5**). The main reason for this is the elimination of smallpox vaccine, which contained about 200 antigens, and the whole-cell pertussis vaccine, which contained about 3000 antigens. In this context, the vaccine schedule is "purer" than it used to be.

TABLE 7.5 — Maximum Number of Separate Antigens Represented by Vaccines Routinely Recommended for Children and Adolescents

Vaccine	1960	1980	2000	2010
Smallpox[a]	200			
Diphtheria	1	1	1	1
Tetanus	1	1	1	1
Pertussis	3000[b]	3000[b]	5[c]	5[c]
IPV	15	15	15	15
MMR[a]		24	24	24
Hib			2	2
VAR[a]			69	69
PCV			8	14[d]
HepB			1	1
HepA				4
HPV vaccine				4[e]
RV[a]				20[f]
MCV4				5
IIV[g]				12[h]
Total	~3217	~3041	126	177

[a] These are live vaccines. Estimates are given of the number of different proteins expressed during infection. Not all of these proteins necessarily represent an antigenic challenge to the host.

[b] Estimate of the number of proteins contained in DTwP.

[c] DTaP contains anywhere from 2 to 5 separate pertussis antigens.

[d] In 2010, PCV13 replaced PCV7.

[e] Routinely recommended only for girls. HPV2 contains 2 separate antigens and HPV4 contains 4.

[f] Rotavirus codes for 12 proteins, 6 structural and 6 nonstructural. RV1 therefore expresses 12 separate antigens and RV5, because it contains a mixture of reassortants, expresses a total of 20 separate antigens (some proteins expressed by each reassortant are the same).

[g] Contains 3 different strains of influenza virus.

[h] The influenza virion contains 8 structural proteins, 3 of which (hemagglutinin, neuraminidase, and M2) are embedded in the lipid envelope and one of which, M1, is closely associated with the envelope. Vaccines are made from the solubilized lipid envelope and therefore are estimated to contain as many as 4 antigens from each strain. However, only the hemagglutinin and neuraminidase are immunologically relevant.

Adapted from Offit PA, et al. *Pediatrics*. 2002;109:124-129.

People fear that vaccines might weaken the immune system and thereby increase susceptibility to infectious agents not contained in the vaccines (so-called *heterologous infections*). Vaccines may cause temporary suppression of delayed-type hypersensitivity skin reactions or transiently alter certain lymphocyte function tests. MMR may decrease the immune response to VAR if the latter is administered within 30 days (and not given on the same day). However, the short-lived immunosuppression caused by certain vaccines does not result in an increased risk of heterologous infections. In fact, just the opposite has been seen. For example, a study from California showed a *decrease* in invasive heterologous infections in the few months following immunization.[37] Similarly, a study from Germany found that children who received the diphtheria, pertussis, tetanus, Hib, and polio vaccines in the first 3 months of life actually had *fewer* infections with vaccine-related as well as vaccine-unrelated pathogens.[38] A study in Denmark that included 2,900,463 person-years of follow-up found no causal association between any of the childhood vaccines and hospitalization for any of seven different infectious diseases unrelated to the vaccine-preventable diseases themselves.[39] Other studies also refute the notion that vaccines increase susceptibility to infection.[40,41]

Bacterial and viral infections, on the other hand, often *do* predispose children and adults to severe, invasive infections with other pathogens. For example, influenza infection clearly predisposes patients to pneumococcal and staphylococcal pneumonia. Similarly, varicella infection increases susceptibility to group A beta-hemolytic streptococcal infections including necrotizing fasciitis, toxic shock syndrome, and bacteremia. Thus if susceptibility to heterologous infection is the concern, vaccination makes more sense than no vaccination.

■ Are Adjuvants Dangerous?

Adjuvants, substances that enhance the immune response to vaccine antigens, are discussed in detail in *Chapter 1: Introduction to Vaccinology—Basic Vaccine Immunology*. Aluminum salts have been used as adjuvants for over 80 years, and hundreds of millions of people have received vaccines containing them.[42] Whereas local reactions such as erythema, nodules, hypersensitivity, and granuloma formation have been reported, serious or persistent adverse events have not. A meta-analysis published in 2004 included studies that compared alum-adjuvanted DTP vaccines to their nonadjuvanted counterparts.[43] In children ≤18 months of age, vaccines containing aluminum hydroxide caused nearly twice as much erythema and induration but there was no increase in collapse, convulsions, or persistent screaming or crying. In older children, aluminum-containing vaccines caused more localized, persistent pain, but not erythema, induration or fever. In some sense, the pain is part of the gain—the irritation or inflammation (and hence pain) caused by the adjuvant also drives the immune response.

Large quantities of aluminum can cause neurologic disease.[44] However, the burden of aluminum exposure through vaccines is far less than the guidelines for safe exposure established by the Agency for Toxic Substances Disease Registry. In fact, infants are exposed to much more aluminum through their diets than through vaccines. Whereas the total aluminum exposure from vaccines in the first 6 months of life is <5 mg, breast-fed infants ingest 7 mg and formula-fed infants as much as 38 to 117 mg over the same period of time, depending on the type of formula.[45]

The newest adjuvant on the block, AS04 (used in HPV2), contains a derivative of lipopolysaccharide, a major component of bacterial cell walls. Parents may cite this when they say that vaccines "contain toxins". However, they need to understand that exposures to toxins like lipopolysaccharide occur continuously given our symbiotic relationship with bacteria.[46] The truth is that anything (even water!) can be dangerous if taken in large amounts. The amount of lipopolysaccharide in AS04-adjuvanted vaccines is just enough to stimulate a robust antibody response but not nearly enough to cause major problems. This is borne out by many studies demonstrating excellent tolerability and no association with serious adverse events. Even more insidious events have been carefully studied; for example, in an integrated analysis of randomized controlled trials involving nearly 70,000 vaccinees, autoimmune events occurred in about 0.5% of both AS04-exposed and nonexposed individuals after a mean follow-up period of 21 months.[47]

■ Are the Additives in Vaccines Harmful?

We think of vaccines as antigens, but in truth vaccines contain additional ingredients that have functions ranging from stabilizing the antigens to preventing them from sticking to the vial. The nature of these substances varies widely and includes the following: proteins; sodium and potassium salts; buffers; sugars; antibiotics; preservatives; amino acids; inactivating agents; and detergents. Some of these are added purposefully in measurable, albeit small, quantities—gelatin or sucrose, for example, added as stabilizers. Others "leak through" from the manufacturing process and are present in only trace amounts—formaldehyde and sodium deoxycholate, for example, used to inactivate and disrupt viruses. All of the "extra" substances contained in each vaccine are listed in the tables in *Section B: Diseases and Vaccines* under "Excipients and contaminants" (technically, an excipient is an inert substance used as a diluent or vehicle for a drug, but here it has a broader meaning, something along the lines of "everything added except the antigen").

Some vaccine ingredients can trigger allergic reactions in sensitized individuals. A classic example is the residual egg protein in influenza vaccines, which can trigger anaphylaxis in those who are egg-allergic. Other examples include the gelatin and neomycin in MMR. To some extent, these reactions can be avoided through proper screening (see *Chapter 4: Vaccine Practice—Screening*).

None of the other ingredients in vaccines have been demonstrated to be harmful in the quantities used. For example, influenza vaccines may contain at most 100 mcg of residual formaldehyde (see **Tables 15.1a** and **15.1b**); for a 10 kg child, that would amount to 10 mcg/kg of exposure *on one day*. The (oral) reference dose for formaldehyde, which is an estimate of *daily* exposure that is likely to be without appreciable risk of deleterious effects *during a person's lifetime*, is 200 mcg/kg.[48] Moreover, a 10 kg child would be expected to have more than 2000 mcg of formaldehyde circulating in blood at any given time, the result of normal biosynthetic processes.[42]

■ Are "Alternative Schedules" a Good Idea?

Many parents are leery of a "one size fits all" vaccine schedule and are interested in "alternative" schedules that "spread the vaccines out" over time. One of their main concerns, addressed above, is that too many vaccines in one visit could overwhelm the immune system. They also worry about the potential for serious reactions and the cumulative effects of chemical additives (also addressed above) and "toxins" derived from pathogens. Sympathetic voices, which make many of the arguments found in **Table 7.3**, are easily found.[49] Alternative schedules are seductive—they reduce the cognitive dissonance between wanting to remain "pro-vaccine" and "pro-protection" and the fear that vaccines are harmful. The problem is that alternative schedules do not provide optimal protection. Moreover, there is no scientific basis for their implementation; in fact, the "basis" for alternative schedules, like so many other antivaccination positions, is anecdotal experience, conjecture (hyperbole), false assumptions, misinterpretation of published data, and a failure to understand the workings of science.[50]

Here are some take-home points:

• *Tailor-made schedules violate an implicit social contract.* This is perhaps the most egregious aspect of schedules that delay vaccinations. Any given individual has the personal luxury of delaying certain vaccines because the diseases are uncommon. But *the diseases are uncommon because the other children are immunized on time.* To put it another way, the other children and their families have taken on the personal risk of immunization (eg, sore arms and low-grade fevers) so that all children are protected; in this context, delaying vaccinations in your own child exploits the goodwill of others. What proportion of the population would need to delay vaccinations such that the diseases would come back in force? What if everyone chose to delay?

- *Alternative schedules necessitate prioritizing some vaccines over others*. None of the vaccines in the routine childhood schedule have priority over the others. This is because the occurrence, by importation or otherwise, of any of these diseases is completely unpredictable.
- *Spreading out vaccines requires more visits*. The routine childhood schedule accomplishes series completion in 4 or 5 visits by 15 or 18 months of age. Some alternative schedules require as many as 15 visits to accomplish the same goal, with series completion delayed until 42 months of age. At a time when health care costs are under scrutiny, it seems wrong to spend money on unnecessary visits. In addition, the more scheduled visits there are, the more visits that will be missed, leading to further delays and costs.
- *Delaying vaccines creates risk without benefit*. Here's an example. Some advocate delaying the birth dose of HepB until the third year of life. As we learned in 1999, when hospitals deferred the birth dose because of the thimerosal scare, this practice will inevitably result in some infants who should have been protected by vaccination but were not (the issue is that many women have unknown HBsAg status at delivery, and even when the maternal record says "HBsAg-negative," that might not be true).[51] Given the safety and immunogenicity of the birth dose of HepB, there is no benefit to delay. Likewise, given the safety and efficacy of all routine vaccines, the only accomplishment of delayed vaccination is susceptibility to the diseases, which are still out there (see **Table 7.4**). In fact, a study published in 2010 showed no adverse effect of on-time infant vaccination on long-term neurophysiological outcome.[52]

■ Do Vaccines Cause Allergies and Autoimmune Disease?

The Hygiene Hypothesis

Developed countries have seen an increase in the incidence of allergic diseases during the same time that many new vaccines have been introduced, leading some to believe there is a relationship. The theoretical basis for this belief has to do with the *hygiene hypothesis*, which holds that "clean living" brought on in part by the elimination of vaccine-preventable diseases creates an immunologic environment during ontogeny that is replete with Th2-cells and deficient in T regulator cells (see *Chapter 1: Introduction to Vaccinology—The Germinal Center Reaction*), an environment that promotes allergy and autoimmunity.[53] However, several large epidemiologic studies favor rejection of this hypothesis.[54] For vaccines to cause allergies by this mechanism, unimmunized children would have to receive the "benefit" of vaccine-preventable diseases; few studies, however, offer data on this. There's also an inherent inconsistency in the idea that by preventing infections, vaccines cause allergies—for live vaccines, anyway, vaccination *is* infection!

Asthma

A well-controlled study in the United States identified 18,407 children with asthma who were born between 1991 and 1997 and compared them with a control group without asthma.[55] Relative risks of asthma in vaccinated compared to unvaccinated children were 0.92 for DTwP, 1.09 for OPV, and 0.97 for MMR. In children who had at least two medical encounters during their first year of life, the RR for asthma following receipt of Hib was 1.07, and for HepB it was 1.09. Another large, population-based cohort study was performed in Leicestershire, United Kingdom.[56] A total of 6811 children were enrolled between 1993 and 1997 and questioned about respiratory symptoms repeatedly until 2003. Data on pertussis vaccinations were independently acquired, and the study included 23,201 person-years of follow-up. No association between vaccination and wheezing or asthma was seen. In a subsequent analysis, it was shown that delaying the first immunization beyond the first 2 months of life did not protect against wheezing at 5 to 10 years of age.[57] Other studies also refute an association between vaccinations and the development of asthma.[58]

Other Forms of Atopy

A well-controlled study of over 600 children prospectively evaluated the risk of allergies following receipt of the pertussis vaccine.[59,60] Infants were randomized to receive a 2-component DTaP vaccine, a 5-component DTaP, DTwP, or DT beginning at 2 months of age. They were followed for the first few years of life and the presence of allergies at 7 years of age was determined by parent questionnaires. The disorders studied included asthma, atopic dermatitis, allergic rhinoconjunctivitis, urticaria, and food allergies. No difference in the incidence of allergic diseases was observed in children who did or did not receive pertussis vaccine. Of interest, children with natural pertussis infections were more likely to develop allergic diseases than children not infected with pertussis.

A cohort study from Tasmania published in 2007 showed small and inconsistent associations between receipt of diphtheria toxoid and asthma, eczema, and food allergies.[61] The authors, however, acknowledged the problems with this and other similar studies: the possibility of recall bias (wherein parents of children with allergies may falsely recall immunizations that were not actually given), difficulty ascertaining the timing of vaccination and types of vaccines that were given, inaccurate reporting of allergies by parents, and health care-seeking behavior on the part of parents (certain parents may seek both immunizations and diagnoses of allergy). Many of these factors could have led to an increased association between immunizations and atopic conditions.

One of the strongest studies to date was the PARSIFAL (Prevention of Allergy-Risk Factors for Sensitization in Children Related to Farming and Anthroposophic Lifestyle) study, conducted in five European countries and involving over 12,000 children born between 1987 and 1996.[62] No association between measles vaccination and allergy was seen (interestingly, measles *infection* was associated with a *reduced* risk of allergy). One strength of this study was the inclusion of allergen-specific serum IgE levels as a marker of allergic sensitization in a subset of children.

Diabetes

Several uncontrolled observational studies claimed that the introduction of vaccines, particularly Hib, into certain populations caused an increase in the incidence of type 1 diabetes. The purported link is vaccine-induced enhancement of preexisting subclinical islet cell autoimmunity. Once again, the data do not support an association. One study from the VSD compared 252 cases of type 1 diabetes with 768 matched controls without diabetes.[63] The odds ratio was 0.28 for the association between diabetes and DTwP, 1.36 for MMR, 1.14 for Hib, 0.81 for HepB, 1.16 for VAR, and 0.92 for DTaP. For children vaccinated at birth with HepB, the odds ratio for diabetes was 0.51 and for those vaccinated at 2 months of age or later was 0.86. In another study, 21,421 children who received Hib between 1988 and 1990 in the United States were followed for 10 years and the risk of type 1 diabetes was 0.78 when compared with a group of 22,557 children who did not receive the vaccine.[64] Several other well-controlled retrospective studies also found that immunizations are not associated with an increased risk of developing type 1 diabetes.[65-67]

Figure 7.1 shows a representative result from the Danish Cohort Study of childhood vaccination and type 1 diabetes.[68] A total of 739,694 children were included and there were 4,720,517 person-years of follow-up. Not surprisingly, the risk of diabetes was much higher in children who had at least one sibling with diabetes. None of the childhood vaccines, however, in any number of doses, was associated with diabetes.

■ Are Vaccines Made From Fetal Tissue?

Some vaccines—rubella, HepA, RAB-HDC, VAR, ZOS, and one form of IPV (the Poliovax contained in Pentacel)—are grown in cultured human embryo fibroblast cell lines (WI-38 or MRC-5) because these are the only cells that replicate the viruses in high enough titer for mass production (the rubella vaccine strain itself was originally isolated from an aborted fetus with intrauterine infection). Each of these cell lines was first obtained from an aborted fetus in the early 1960s.[69] These very same embryonic cells have been passaged in tissue culture in the laboratory since then. Whereas no new fetal material has ever been involved, this situation does represent a moral dilemma for some people.[70,71]

218

FIGURE 7.1 — Danish Cohort Study of Vaccines and Diabetes

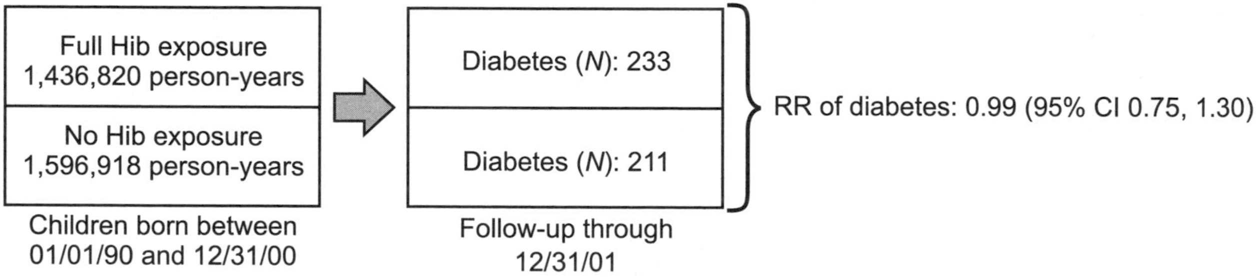

Full Hib exposure
1,436,820 person-years

No Hib exposure
1,596,918 person-years

Children born between
01/01/90 and 12/31/00

Diabetes (N): 233

Diabetes (N): 211

Follow-up through
12/31/01

RR of diabetes: 0.99 (95% CI 0.75, 1.30)

A cohort of children was retrospectively assembled and exposure or nonexposure to various vaccines was ascertained. The occurrence of type 1 diabetes among cohort children was determined, and the rates of outcome in the exposed and nonexposed groups were compared. Shown here are the data pertaining to 3 doses of Hib versus no Hib among all children in the cohort. The study also looked at children at higher risk for diabetes because of family history and found similar resultsts. In addition, no associations were seen with other vaccines.

Adapted from Hviid A, et al. *N Engl J Med*. 2004;350:1398-1404.

In helping patients work through this, it may be worth emphasizing that the original abortions were not done with the intent to produce vaccines (they were done for therapeutic reasons, and the intent of culturing the cells was to understand immortalization and oncogenesis), that they occurred in the distant past, that the modern day vaccine producers never intended for fetuses to be aborted, and that the moral imperative to save lives through vaccination might outweigh their objection to a singular, distant moral transgression. Many religious organizations, including the United States Conference of Catholic Bishops, have used these arguments to support vaccination, despite their opposition to abortion.[72]

■ Does MMR Cause Autism?

In 1998, Wakefield and colleagues in London described 12 children with chronic enterocolitis and regressive developmental disorder.[73] Ten of these children had autism, and in eight, the onset of regression was linked by the child's parent or physician to receipt of MMR. The authors suggested that replication of the three vaccine viruses in gut tissues caused a unique form of intestinal inflammation. They speculated that this led to the absorption of toxins that affected the brain, resulting in regressive autism.

Since a control group that was never exposed to the vaccine was not included in the study, a causal relationship between MMR and autism could not be established. Moreover, many questions about the integrity of the work were raised, spurred by the discovery that Wakefield had been commissioned by a group of lawyers to investigate a putative relationship between MMR and autism. At the very least, this raised the possibility that some of the patients in the 1998 study made their way to Wakefield *because* of his interest in this—in other words, the study population might have been biased toward patients who already thought their symptoms were brought on by the vaccine. By 2004, these and other concerns prompted 10 of the 13 original authors to retract their previous interpretation of the study.[74] In 2010, the United Kingdom's General Medical Council found evidence of serious professional misconduct by Wakefield and colleagues Walker-Smith and Murch[75]; on February 2, 2010, *The Lancet* formally retracted the original paper and struck it from the published record.[76]

Unfortunately, this imperfect paper rekindled a new wave of antivaccinationism. The notion that MMR causes autism fed directly into the public's natural tendency to assume causality when two events are temporally associated—children get MMR at 1 year of age and the signs of autism become apparent right around the same time.

MMR does not cause autism. Here is a summary of the evidence:
- *Persistent measles virus infection is not found in inflammatory bowel disease (IBD) or autism*—Studies range from

219

attempts to find the viral genome in bowel tissues using molecular amplification techniques to rigorous case-control studies. For example, one study of 30 patients with IBD, all of whom had had either natural measles infection or MMR vaccination, found no measles genomic sequences in bowel biopsies or blood lymphocytes using a sensitive nested PCR technique.[77] A 2006 study found no differences in antimeasles antibody titers between 54 autistic children (51 had received MMR) and 34 controls (31 had received MMR), and no study subjects had detectable measles virus DNA sequences in their peripheral blood mononuclear cells.[78] The final blow came in 2008, when investigators studied 25 children with autism and gastrointestinal disturbances and 13 children with gastrointestinal disturbances without autism.[79] Ileal and cecal tissues were obtained and probed for measles virus sequences using molecular amplification techniques in three blinded laboratories, including the one wherein the original association between persistent measles virus and autism was reported. The results were unequivocal—only one case and one control had positive results, directly refuting Wakefield's hypothesis.

- *Case-control studies show no association between MMR vaccine and IBD*—One such study done through the Vaccine Safety Datalink (VSD) showed no more risk of exposure to MMR among 142 cases with IBD compared with 432 controls without IBD.[80]
- *There is no relationship between MMR uptake at the population level and the increased incidence of autism*—Most studies show that autism cases are increasing, but many epidemiologists believe this is a reflection of expanded case definitions, diagnostic substitution for other neurodevelopmental conditions, and more public awareness rather than a true increase in incidence.[81] In any event, studies done in very different settings—the United Kingdom,[82] California,[83] and Montréal,[84] to name a few—consistently show that the incidence of autism over time does not parallel the uptake of MMR, as it would if MMR caused autism. **Figure 7.2** shows the data from the Montréal study. Another study from the United Kingdom showed no increase in cases of autism after introduction of MMR, which occurred in 1988.[85] In addition, there was no clustering of cases of autism after receipt of MMR vaccine, even when the observation period was extended to many years.[86]
- *There is no new form of gastrointestinal disease or autism that appears with the introduction of MMR*—One study in the United Kingdom found that the proportion of children with developmental regression or bowel symptoms did not change significantly between 1979 and 1998, a period that

FIGURE 7.2 — Birth Cohort Study in Montréal, Quebec: MMR

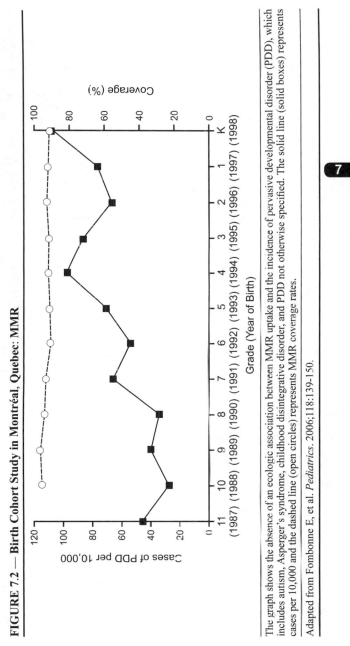

The graph shows the absence of an ecologic association between MMR uptake and the incidence of pervasive developmental disorder (PDD), which includes autism, Asperger's syndrome, childhood disintegrative disorder, and PDD not otherwise specified. The solid line (solid boxes) represents cases per 10,000 and the dashed line (open circles) represents MMR coverage rates.

Adapted from Fombonne E, et al. *Pediatrics*. 2006;118:139-150.

included introduction of MMR.[87] Similarly, a study of 262 patients with autism found no evidence for the emergence of a new form of the disease that included intestinal symptoms following widespread use of MMR. Other studies confirm that there is no distinct MMR-induced autism syndrome or "autistic enterocolitis."[88]

• *Case-control studies show no association between MMR and autism*—One study done in the United Kingdom found that 78.1% of 1010 cases had received MMR before being diagnosed with autism, as compared with 82.1% of 3671 controls without autism, for an adjusted odds ratio of 0.86 (95% CI 0.68, 1.09).[89] This means that the odds of being diagnosed with autism among persons who had received MMR were essentially the same as those who had not received MMR. Another study, done in Atlanta, showed there was no difference in the proportion of children vaccinated with MMR before 18 or before 24 months of age among 624 case children and 1824 matched controls.[90]

• *Cohort studies provide strong evidence against an association between MMR and autism*—Cohort studies are among the most rigorous epidemiologic investigations. The methodology is simple—a group of subjects is assembled, exposure or nonexposure to the risk factor is determined, and the subsequent development of the outcome is ascertained. The rate of the outcome is then compared between exposed and nonexposed persons; the ratio of the two is called the relative risk (RR), and an RR of 1 means there is no association between the exposure and the outcome. The beauty of retrospective cohort studies, wherein the cohort is identified in the past and followed to the present, is that the exposure and outcomes have already taken place, so that measurement of the exposure (in this case, receipt of MMR) cannot be biased by knowledge of the outcome (autism); therefore, robust inferences can be made. **Figure 7.3** shows the results of the Danish Cohort Study, which involved 537,303 children.[91] The outcomes of autism or autistic-spectrum disorder were no more common in 1,647,504 person-years of exposure to MMR than they were in 482,360 person-years of nonexposure. The study further showed no association with age at vaccination, interval since vaccination, or the date of vaccination. This study provided very strong evidence against MMR as a cause of autism.

There is no scientific rationale for giving the monovalent components of MMR in lieu of the combination, and, in fact, as of 2008 the separate components were no longer available in the United States. Finally, the US Court of Federal Claims addressed the MMR-causes-autism theory as part of the Omnibus Autism Proceedings—see discussion of thimerosal below.

FIGURE 7.3 — Danish Cohort Study of MMR and Autism

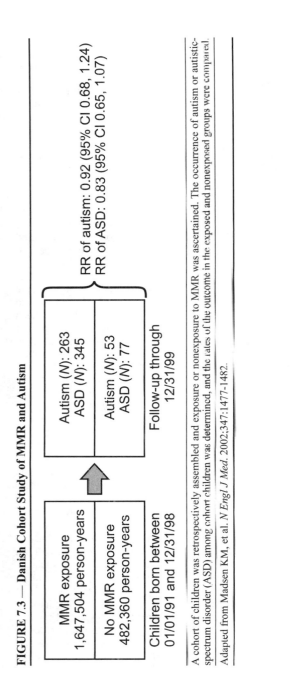

MMR exposure
1,647,504 person-years

No MMR exposure
482,360 person-years

Children born between
01/01/91 and 12/31/98

Autism (*N*): 263
ASD (*N*): 345

Autism (*N*): 53
ASD (*N*): 77

Follow-up through
12/31/99

RR of autism: 0.92 (95% CI 0.68, 1.24)
RR of ASD: 0.83 (95% CI 0.65, 1.07)

A cohort of children was retrospectively assembled and exposure or nonexposure to MMR was ascertained. The occurrence of autism or autistic-spectrum disorder (ASD) among cohort children was determined, and the rates of the outcome in the exposed and nonexposed groups were compared.

Adapted from Madsen KM, et al. *N Engl J Med.* 2002;347:1477-1482.

■ Did the Thimerosal Used as a Preservative in Vaccines Cause Autism?

High levels of mercury are known to damage the nervous system and kidneys. In addition, studies in the Faroe Islands, the Seychelles, and Iraq showed that fetuses might be harmed when pregnant women ingest large quantities of mercury. For these reasons, the FDA Modernization Act of 1997 required the FDA to compile a list of drugs and foods that contain mercury. At that time (and really since the beginning of the modern vaccine era), some vaccines used thimerosal, which contains *ethylmercury* as a preservative, so these vaccines were included in the FDA list. Preservatives were necessary in multidose vials to prevent contamination with bacteria or fungi.

The cumulative level of mercury represented by the routine vaccine schedule for infants was within the acceptable range published by the FDA, the Agency for Toxic Substance and Disease Registry, and the WHO. However, it slightly exceeded the level considered to be safe by the Environmental Protection Agency (EPA). To determine safe levels of mercury, the EPA evaluated a study performed in Iraq where pregnant women were accidentally exposed to large quantities of *methylmercury* (a more toxic organic compound than *ethylmercury*) that had been used to disinfect grain. The EPA then estimated the lowest dose of mercury that was found to cause neurodevelopmental delay in infants as a result of fetal exposure. From this, the lowest dose of methylmercury that could possibly harm an unborn child was calculated and then divided by ten, yielding a very conservative estimate of the lowest acceptable dose of mercury.

There are many problems with using the study in Iraq to determine levels of thimerosal in vaccines that would be safe in children. Among them is the fact that the mercury contained in thimerosal is in the form of *ethylmercury*, which behaves in the body much differently than *methylmercury*. In addition, vaccines are administered to children after, not before, they are born, when the nervous system is more mature and, therefore, much less likely to be susceptible to harmful effects.

Nevertheless, the Public Health Service and the AAP issued a joint statement on July 9, 1999, calling for manufacturers to eliminate thimerosal from vaccines as a precautionary measure, stating the following: "The current levels of thimerosal will not hurt children, but reducing those levels will make safe vaccines even safer."[92] One might wonder how safe vaccines can be made safer, particularly by removing a component that had not been shown to be harmful in the first place. The consequences of this statement ranged from confusion on the part of providers, dismantling of the machinery that had been put in place to deliver the birth dose of HepB, failure to give HepB to many high-risk infants, an onslaught of litigation, and a loss of public confidence.[51,93,94] The effects were still evident in 2010, with a barrage of celebrities on television talk shows claiming that thimerosal is responsible for the "epidemic" of autism, op-ed pieces in newspapers, and nearly 5000 thimerosal injury claims pending under the National Vaccine Injury Compensation Program (VICP; see *Chapter 3: Standards, Principles, and Regulations—National Vaccine Injury Compensation Program [VICP]*). The issue reached a penultimate climax in early 2008, when the special federal court for the VICP ruled that multiple vaccinations received in a single day had aggravated an underlying mitochondrial disorder in a child, ultimately manifesting as regressive encephalopathy with features of autistic spectrum disorder.[95] This reignited the controversy, even though the ruling was strictly applicable only to this case of a child with a previously undiagnosed and very rare metabolic defect.

The climax itself occurred in early 2009. Because of the overwhelming burden of petitions before the VICP claiming that vaccines cause autism, the vaccine court asked the petitioners to put forward three test cases for each of three theories, in what became known as the Omnibus Autism Proceedings.[96] The theories were that 1) MMR and thimerosal-containing vaccines combine to cause autism; 2) thimerosal-containing vaccines alone cause autism; and 3) MMR alone causes autism (this theory was subsequently dropped because the evidence was presented as part of the first theory). On February 12, 2009, the court handed down its decision in the first theory.

A typical case that is heard in the vaccine court involves a review of 10 medical articles and the testimony of 2 to 6 expert witnesses. The proceedings for the first theory generated 5,000 pages of transcript, more than 700 pages of post-hearing briefs, 50 expert reports, and involved the testimony of 28 experts and a review of 939 medical articles. The first case (Cedillo vs Secretary of Health and Human Services, No. 98-916V) was heard in June 2007, the second (Hazlehurst vs Secretary of Health and Human Services, No. 03-654V) in October 2007, and the third (Snyder vs Secretary of Health and Human Services, No. 01-162V) in November 2007. The petitioners only had to prove their case by a "preponderance of the evidence." Despite this, their claims for compensation were denied, and the judges did not mince words. In essence, they stated unequivocally in each case that the theory was incorrect and that the evidence presented was marginal, paling in comparison to the validated, reproducible, rigorous scientific evidence that had been generated over the years in many parts of the world. Each of the decisions was appealed, and each appeal was denied.

On March 12, 2010, the decisions for the three test cases of the second theory were handed down (Dwyer vs Secretary of Health and Human Services, No. 03-1202V; King vs Secretary of Health and Human Services, No. 03-584V; Mead vs Secretary of Health and Human Services, No. 03-215V). Once again, the court unequivocally rejected the petitioners claims that thimerosal caused autism in these children. And, once again, the judges did not mince words. Special Master Vowell, for example, wrote in the Dwyer case, "The witnesses setting forth this improbable sequence of cause and effect were outclassed in every respect by the impressive assembly of true experts in their respective fields who testified on behalf of respondent."

Thimerosal in vaccines did not cause autism or any other neurodevelopmental problem. Here is a summary of the evidence:

- *Toxic levels of mercury are not found in infants receiving thimerosal-containing vaccines*—In a pilot study published in 2002, 40 full-term infants ≤6 months of age were given vaccines containing thimerosal and 21 were given thimerosal-free vaccines.[97] No infants had blood mercury concentrations exceeding 29 parts per billion, the level thought to be safe in cord blood. Stool concentrations were high, suggesting elimination through the gastrointestinal tract. A follow-up study looking at 216 infants was published in 2008.[98] The blood half-life of mercury after administration of thimerosal-containing vaccines was 3.7 days. The highest levels of mercury were seen in the first 24 hours after vaccination, and all were ≤8 ng/mL (some infants received as much as 57.5 mcg of mercury at one time through the vaccinations). Inorganic mercury was detected in stools within days. The results suggest rapid elimination of ethylmercury from the body after vaccination with thimerosal-containing vaccines.
- *Autism rates continued to increase after thimerosal was removed from vaccines*—Whether one looks in Denmark[99] and Sweden,[100] where thimerosal was removed from vaccines in 1992, or Canada,[84] where no vaccines contained thimerosal after 1996, the data are remarkably consistent—continued increases in reported cases of autism (data from the Canadian study are shown in **Figure 7.4**). A study from California published in 2008 showed no decrease in autism prevalence by age or birth cohort several years after the last lots of thimerosal-containing vaccines would have expired.[101] As discussed earlier, epidemiologists do not uniformly agree that there is a *true* increase in the incidence of autism. However, there *are* many cases being diagnosed, and while the causes remain elusive, the ecologic data argue very strongly against thimerosal being one of them.
- *Cohort studies provide strong evidence against an association*—A retrospective cohort study involving 109,863 children in the United Kingdom born between 1988 and 1997 found no convincing associations between thimerosal exposure and developmental disorders.[102] **Figure 7.5** shows the results of the Danish Cohort Study, which involved 467,450 children.[103]

FIGURE 7.4 — Birth Cohort Study in Montréal, Quebec: Thimerosal

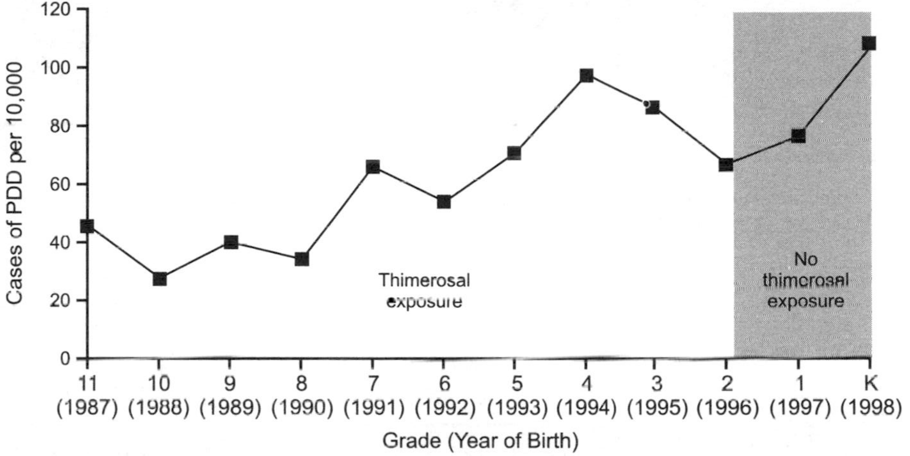

The graph shows the absence of an ecologic association between thimerosal exposure from vaccines and the incidence of pervasive developmental disorder (PDD), which includes autism, Asperger's syndrome, childhood disintegrative disorder, and PDD not otherwise specified. The solid line (solid boxes) represents cases per 10,000 and the shaded box represents the period of time when exposure to thimerosal in vaccines did not occur.

Adapted from Fombonne E, et al. *Pediatrics.* 2006;118:e139-e150.

227

FIGURE 7.5 — Danish Cohort Study of Thimerosal and Autism

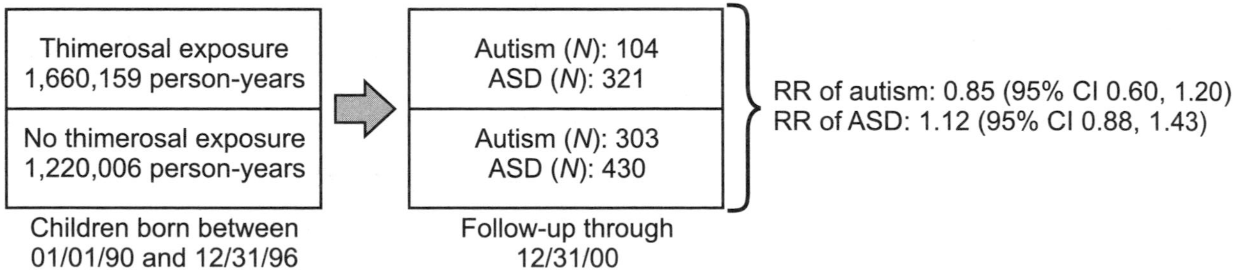

Children born between 01/01/90 and 12/31/96

Thimerosal exposure 1,660,159 person-years

No thimerosal exposure 1,220,006 person-years

Autism (*N*): 104
ASD (*N*): 321

Autism (*N*): 303
ASD (*N*): 430

Follow-up through 12/31/00

RR of autism: 0.85 (95% CI 0.60, 1.20)
RR of ASD: 1.12 (95% CI 0.88, 1.43)

A cohort of children was retrospectively assembled and exposure or nonexposure to thimerosal in vaccines was ascertained. The occurrence of autism or autism spectrum disorder (ASD) among cohort children was determined, and the rates of the outcome in the exposed and nonexposed groups were compared.

Adapted from Hviid A, et al. *JAMA*. 2003;290:1763-1766.

The outcomes of autism or autistic-spectrum disorder were no more common in 1,660,159 person-years of exposure to thimerosal than they were in 1,220,006 person-years of nonexposure. The study further showed no evidence of a dose-response relationship between cumulative amounts of ethylmercury exposure and autism. A prospective cohort study in the United Kingdom (children were enrolled at birth and behavioral data were collected regularly thereafter) involving over 14,000 children showed that poor prosocial behavior at 47 months of age was correlated with ethylmercury exposure by 3 months of age.[104] However, the same study showed that ethylmercury exposure was associated with *better* outcomes in eight other areas, including conduct, fine motor development, reported tics, and the need for special education. A 2-phase retrospective cohort study in the United States involving over 100,000 children also found no consistent associations with neurodevelopmental outcomes.[105] Finally, in a 2007 study, 1047 children were given a 3-hour assessment involving 42 different neuropsychologic tests; no consistent associations were seen between earlier exposure to thimerosal-containing vaccines and the test results.[106]

Authoritative bodies are virtually unanimous in rejecting the purported link between thimerosal and autism. As of 2010, the only routine childhood vaccines that still contain thimerosal as a preservative are some brands of IIV (although preservative-free formulations for children are available). Thimerosal activists argue, however, that vaccines labeled *preservative-free* are still not safe because they contain trace amounts of thimerosal, levels that are essentially below the limit of detection. Since a product cannot be labeled *thimerosal-free* if thimerosal is used anywhere in the manufacturing process, companies have either dropped out of the market or scrambled to revise their protocols and package their products in single-dose vials or prefilled syringes. The public has paid the price in dollars as well as in vaccine availability.

Some autism advocacy groups have urged that we turn our attention away from vaccines and towards more promising lines of research.[107] In fact, there is a growing body of evidence that genetic abnormalities play a role in the development of autism.[108,109]

■ Does Pertussis Vaccine Cause Brain Damage?

In 1974, an uncontrolled case series was published describing children who allegedly developed mental retardation and epilepsy following receipt of the whole-cell pertussis vaccine.[110] Over the next several years, fear of the pertussis vaccine generated by media coverage of this report caused a decrease in pertussis immunization rates in British children from 81% to 31%; the decrease in vaccine use resulted in >100,000 cases and over 600 deaths from pertussis.

Decreased immunization rates and increased pertussis deaths also were seen in Japan, Sweden, and Wales.[32]

The National Childhood Encephalopathy Study (NCES), conducted in the United Kingdom from 1976 to 1979, suggested the possibility of a relationship between the vaccine and encephalopathy, although methodologic problems with this study were quickly highlighted.[111,112] For example, the study included only a small number of cases that had been exposed to the vaccine. The IOM independently analyzed the NCES data in 1991 and concluded that there was a rare but causal relationship with encephalopathy in the immediate postvaccination period, even though there was no evidence that permanent brain damage occurred.[113] A reanalysis by the IOM in 1994 reached a different conclusion—whole-cell pertussis vaccine did not cause encephalopathy.[114]

Other studies also refuted the initial findings of the NCES. For example, another UK study compared over 130,000 children who had received DTP with a similar number who had received only DT and found no association with encephalopathy.[115] In Denmark, a shift to administration of pertussis vaccine earlier in life was not followed by a shift in diagnosis of neurological disorders.[116] A study in Tennessee found 2 cases of encephalitis among 38,171 children who had received 107,154 DTP shots; in both cases, the onset of symptoms was >2 weeks following immunization.[117] Finally, in a case-control study conducted in Washington and Oregon states involving 218,000 children, 424 cases with neurological illness were each matched with 2 controls.[118] No association was seen with DTP administration, even when the analysis was restricted to encephalopathy or complicated seizures and adjusted for factors that might have affected vaccine administration.

In a study published in 2006, the records of four large US health maintenance organizations were used to address this issue once again.[119] A total of 452 children with encephalopathy diagnosed between 1981 and 1995 were compared with matched controls without encephalopathy. Exposure to pertussis vaccine in any postvaccination time period was no more common among cases than controls. The maximum possible all-cause incidence of encephalopathy after pertussis immunization was 1 in 370,000, which is no different from the background rate of encephalopathy in young children.

The availability of new tools has shed light on the issue of pertussis vaccine and brain damage. In a landmark study, de novo mutations in the gene encoding a neuronal sodium channel protein were found in 11 of 14 patients who allegedly had suffered vaccine encephalopathy.[120] These individuals were born with a molecular defect that would cause seizures and regression, *vaccines or no vaccines*. Despite this finding, and despite the fact that acellular pertussis vaccines have replaced whole-cell vaccines, encephalopathy remains an injury that can be compensated through the Vaccine Injury Table under the VICP.

■ Do Vaccines Cause Guillain-Barré Syndrome (GBS)?

GBS is an acute, immune-mediated, demyelinating peripheral neuropathy characterized by progressive symmetric weakness. Most cases occur after an infectious event, most notably *Campylobacter jejuni* enteritis. In 1976, a new H1N1 influenza strain caused severe respiratory illness in 13 soldiers at Fort Dix, New Jersey; ultimately, approximately 230 soldiers were infected.[121] The virus, dubbed A/New Jersey/76 (Hsw1N1) and known to be closely related to the deadly 1918 pandemic strain, had circulated in pigs for years and had apparently jumped to humans. Fearing the start of a new pandemic, the US government responded with a mass immunization campaign. In retrospect, this event may have been an anomaly—an animal virus introduced into a stressed, crowded, closed population that actually had little potential to spread in normal communities. In fact, the virus never spread beyond the military installation. Unfortunately, the mass immunization campaign was not benign. Over 45 million people were immunized over a 3-month period of time, resulting in more than 500 cases of GBS; the attributable risk of GBS to swine flu vaccination was estimated at around 1 in 100,000.[122] The mechanism may have involved some form of molecular mimicry, supported by the observation that mice receiving the vaccine develop anti-ganglioside antibodies.[123]

While some studies have suggested a possible causal relationship between influenza vaccine and GBS,[124] most have not. One, for example, looked at two influenza seasons in the United States in the early 1990s and found an RR of 1.7 (95% CI 1.0, 2.8), corresponding to approximately one additional case of GBS per million people vaccinated.[125] It is important to keep a perspective here: in any given 6 week period of time, somewhere between 1 in 220,000 and 1 in 1.4 million people will develop GBS—*vaccine or no vaccine.*[126] Another study in the United Kingdom spanning the years 1992 to 2000 found 228 incident cases of GBS; seven cases occurred within 42 days of any immunization (three were after influenza immunization) and 221 were not associated with immunization, for a RR of 1.03 (95% CI 0.48, 2.18).[127] A study from Canada published in 2006 demonstrated no seasonality of GBS and no increase in hospital admissions for GBS after the introduction of a universal influenza immunization program.[128] Finally, as of early 2010, there were no reports linking 2009 H1N1 vaccine to GBS.

By September 2006, 17 cases of GBS associated with MCV4-D administration had been reported to VAERS (the vaccine was licensed in January 2005).[129] Most of the cases occurred within 2 weeks of vaccination, a time frame that would fit with a causal relationship. The rate of GBS among immunized teenagers, calculated based on doses distributed, was estimated to be about 0.20 per 100,000 person-months. This rate was similar to the background rate of GBS calculated from the VSD database, but it was slightly higher than that seen in the Healthcare Cost and Utilization Project, a multistate hospital discharge database. It was estimated that if GBS is truly caused by MCV4-D, there would be 1 extra case for every 800,000 teenagers vaccinated. Data are not available to evaluate the potential risk of GBS following administration of MCV4-CRM.

■ Do Vaccines Cause Multiple Sclerosis (MS)?

The hypothesis that vaccines might cause MS was fueled by anecdotal reports of MS following HepB administration and two case-control studies showing an increase in the incidence of MS in vaccinated persons that was not statistically significant. However, two large case-control studies evaluated whether HepB causes MS or whether HepB, tetanus, or influenza vaccines exacerbate symptoms of MS. The first study in a cohort of nurses identified 192 women with MS and 645 matched controls.[130] The RR of multiple sclerosis associated with exposure to HepB was 0.9 and the RR within 2 years before the onset of disease was 0.7. There also was no association between the number of doses of HepB and the risk of MS. The second study included 643 patients in Europe with MS relapse occurring between 1993 and 1997.[131] Exposure to vaccination in the 2-month period before relapse was compared with the four previous 2-month control periods. The RR of relapse associated with the use of any vaccine was 0.71, and with HepB, tetanus, and influenza vaccines it was 0.67, 0.75, and 1.08, respectively. In a case-control study in France, 143 cases of MS in children <16 years of age were matched to 1122 controls; 32% of cases and 32% of controls had received HepB in the 3 years before the index date.[132] A subsequent study by the same group looked at first ever episodes of acute inflammatory demyelination in children, irrespective of the subsequent course of the disease.[133] The rates of HepB vaccination in the 3 years before the index date were 24.4% for 349 cases and 27.3% for 2941 matched controls, for an adjusted OR of 0.74 (95% CI 0.54, 1.02), although a possible trend was seen for one vaccine type.

Other well-controlled studies also found that influenza vaccine did not exacerbate symptoms of MS. In a retrospective study of 180 patients with relapsing MS, *infection* with influenza virus was more likely than *immunization* with influenza vaccine to cause an exacerbation of symptoms, suggesting that influenza vaccine is actually likely to prevent exacerbations of MS.[134] In a multicenter, prospective, randomized, double-blind trial of influenza vaccine among 104 patients with MS, immunization was not associated with exacerbation of symptoms or change in disease course.[135]

■ Can Vaccines Transmit Mad Cow Disease (MCD)?

By July of 2000 approximately 175,000 cows in the United Kingdom had developed bovine spongiform encephalopathy, more commonly referred to as MCD, a progressive deterioration of the nervous system. At the same time, >70 people in the United Kingdom had developed a progressive neurologic condition termed *variant Creutzfeldt-Jakob disease* (vCJD) that likely resulted from eating meat prepared from cows with MCD. Both MCD and vCJD are caused by prions, which are proteinaceous, self-replicating infectious particles. In July 2000, the FDA convened a meeting to discuss the possibility that some vaccines were made using serum or gelatin derived from cows in countries that had MCD, including England. Although the risk of transmission of vCJD to humans from such vaccines was considered theoretic and remote, the recommendation was made that vaccines use bovine materials originating from countries without endogenous MCD.[136] Mathematical models suggest that the agent of MCD first entered cattle feed in the United Kingdom around 1980; since the vast majority of initial cases of vCJD were born well before then, childhood vaccines were not likely to be the cause.[137]

Prions are found in the brains of cows with MCD and in the brains of humans with vCJD. They can also be found in the spinal cord and retina. However, blood from infected animals and from infected people has never been shown to be a source of infection of humans. The likely source of prions for people in England was hamburger, not steak, and hamburger may be prepared in a manner that includes the spinal cord. Steak, on the other hand, represents only the muscles of cows and, therefore, does not contain prions.

Vaccines may contain trace amounts of animal products used during the manufacturing process. For example, vaccines are grown in laboratory cells that require growth factors for maintenance. An excellent source of these is fetal bovine serum, which is naturally filtered by the 6-layered bovine placenta. Many proteins are excluded from the bovine fetal circulation by these layers (for example, bovine fetal blood contains 1/500th of the antibodies found in bovine maternal blood). Maternal-fetal transmission of prions has never been documented in animals and fetal blood is not known to contain prions. Moreover, the fetal bovine serum used in vaccine manufacture is highly diluted and eventually removed from cells during purification of vaccine viruses. It should be pointed out as well that prions propagate in mammalian brain but not in cell culture.

Another product from cows and pigs that may be used in vaccines is gelatin, a protein formed by boiling skin or connective tissue such as hooves. Gelatin is used to stabilize vaccines so that they remain effective after distribution. Since prions are not detected in the skin or connective tissue of animals, gelatin does not represent a risk of transmission to patients.

Final reassurance comes from the fact that transmission of prions occurs from eating the brains of infected animals or from directly inoculating preparations of brains of infected animals into the brains of experimental animals. Transmission of prions has not been documented after inoculation into the muscles or under the skin, which are the routes used for vaccination. Taken together, the chances that currently licensed vaccines contain prions and represent a risk to humans is essentially zero.

■ Can Vaccines Cause Cancer?

The polio vaccine used in the late 1950s and early 1960s was contaminated with a monkey virus called simian virus 40 (SV40), present in the monkey kidney cells used to grow the vaccine.[138] Investigators found SV40 DNA in biopsy specimens obtained from patients with mesothelioma, osteosarcoma, and non-Hodgkin's lymphoma. Interestingly, SV40 DNA was present in the cancers of people who had received the polio vaccine that was contaminated with SV40, but it was also present in those who had not. SV40 DNA was even found in the cancers of people born after 1963, a time when the vaccine no longer contained SV40. A study published in 2004 shed some light on this.[139] Some of the primers that were being employed in the PCR reactions used to amplify DNA sequences of SV40 were directed at a region of the T antigen. As it turns out, these sequences are also present in common laboratory plasmids. How did they get there? They were engineered into the plasmids during the first attempts to create expression vectors for eukaryotic cells, but this happened so long ago that their presence was not well known. When alternative T-antigen primers were used, only a few cancers were positive. Moreover, this study found no evidence of T-antigen RNA transcript production and no T-antigen protein expression in the tumors. Finally, epidemiologic studies do not show an increased risk of cancers in those who received polio vaccine between 1955 and 1963.

■ Did the Polio Vaccine Cause the AIDS Pandemic?

In 1999, Edward Hooper published a book entitled *The River: A Journey to the Source of HIV and AIDS*. The central hypothesis was that the origin of AIDS could be traced to oral poliovirus vaccines that were administered in the Belgian Congo between 1957 and 1960. This assertion was based on the following assumptions: 1) all poliovirus vaccines were grown in monkey kidney cells; 2) those cells were contaminated with simian immunodeficiency virus (SIV), which is closely related to HIV; and 3) people were inadvertently infected with SIV that then mutated to HIV and caused the AIDS epidemic.

The following facts, however, exonerate polio vaccines as a cause of AIDS:

- SIV is found in chimpanzees, not monkeys, and chimpanzee cells were never used to grow polio vaccine.[140,141]
- SIV and HIV are not very close genetically and mutation from SIV to HIV would have required centuries, not years.[142,143]
- Both SIV and HIV are enveloped viruses that are easily disrupted by extremes of pH. If given by mouth (as was OPV), both of these viruses would likely be destroyed in the acid environment of the stomach.
- Original lots of the polio vaccine (including those used in Africa for the polio vaccine trials) did not contain HIV, SIV, or chimpanzee genetic sequences when analyzed by molecular amplification techniques.[144,145]

Unfortunately, fears of polio vaccine based on this unfounded theory adversely affected vaccine use where it is need most—in the developing world where the last vestiges of wild type poliovirus reside.[146]

■ Can Vaccines Cause SIDS?

In 1999, the ABC news program *20/20* aired a story claiming that HepB caused sudden infant death syndrome (SIDS). The story included a picture of a 1-month-old girl who died of SIDS only 16 hours after receiving the second dose of HepB. In 1991, before routine use of HepB was fully implemented for all infants, about 5000 children died every year from SIDS. Within 10 years of that recommendation, vaccine uptake had increased to about 90% and the incidence of SIDS had *decreased* dramatically to about 1600 cases per year. This decrease was due to the introduction of the "Back to Sleep" program, in which parents were encouraged to place their infants on their backs or sides when going to sleep. The lack of an ecologic correlation between SIDS and HepB was supported by VAERS data showing very few neonatal deaths following HepB after approximately 86 million doses were given.[147] Several studies actually show *lower* SIDS rates among infants who receive vaccines when compared with those who do not.[148,149] While this may reflect biases wherein healthier or better-cared-for infants are the ones who are immunized, the data clearly do not indicate vaccines as a risk factor for SIDS. Temporal associations arise because some vaccines happen to be given just at the time of the peak age incidence of SIDS.

A study published in 2004 looked at a cohort of 361,696 infants born between 1993 and 1998.[150] A total of 1363 infants in the cohort died in the first 29 days of life; only 5% of them had been vaccinated with HepB, whereas 66% of those who survived the first month of life had been immunized. Moreover, there was no difference in the proportion of vaccinated and unvaccinated infants who died of unexpected causes, and the SIDS death rate was the same (3.3 per 100,000) for vaccinated and unvaccinated infants.

■ Do Vaccines Trigger Kawasaki Disease (KD)?

KD is an acute, inflammatory, small-to-medium sized vessel vasculitis manifest by prolonged high fever and some combination of rash, conjunctival suffusion, changes in the oral mucosa or peripheral extremities, and cervical lymphadenopathy; desquamation occurs in the convalescent phase, and ectasia or aneurysms can develop in the coronary arteries. An infectious etiology is suspected based on clustering of cases, but a genetic predisposition is likely based on widely varying incidence in different racial and ethnic groups.

In June 2007 the label for RV5 was updated to include data regarding the occurrence of KD in Phase 3 clinical trials. The disease was reported within 42 days of vaccination in 5 of 36,150 vaccinees and 1 of 35,536 placebees, for an unadjusted RR of 4.9 (95% CI 0.6, 239.1). The wide confidence interval that includes 1.0 means that one cannot assume there is an association. Nevertheless this label change prompted renewed interest in the possibility that vaccine could trigger KD. Early reassurance came from the VSD, where there had been only one unconfirmed case of KD within 30 days of 65,000 RV5 doses.[151] A study published in 2009 provided further reassurance that RV5 was not a cause of KD.[152] VAERS reports from 1990 through mid-2007 were analyzed, yielding only 97 cases. No clustering of cases was seen after vaccination. The reporting rates for KD in the 30 days following vaccination were 0.65 per 100,000 person-years before the RV5 label change and 2.78 per 100,000 person-years after the change; both rates were lower than the expected background incidence of 9 to 19 per 100,000 person-years.

REFERENCES

1. Evans G, Bostrom A, Johnston RB, Fisher BL, Stoto MA. *Risk Communication and Vaccination: Summary of a Workshop.* Washington, DC: National Academy Press; 1997.
2. Bohlke K, et al. *Pediatrics.* 2003;112:815-820.
3. Salmon DA, et al. *JAMA.* 1999;282:47-53.
4. Freed GL, et al. *Pediatrics.* 2010;125:654-659.
5. Patja A, et al. *Pediatr Infect Dis J.* 2000;19:1127-1134.
6. Shermer M. *Sci Amer.* 2008;September:40.
7. Black S, et al. *Lancet.* 2009;374:2115-2122.
8. Shermer M. *Sci Amer.* 2009;June:36.
9. Opel DJ, et al. *Arch Pediatr Adolesc Med.* 2009;163:432-437.
10. LeBaron CW, et al. *Arch Pediatr Adolesc Med.* 1999;153:1154-1159.
11. Davis TC, et al. *Pediatrics.* 2001;107:e17.
12. Fredrickson DD, et al. *Pediatr Ann.* 2001;30:400-406.
13. Flanagan-Klygis EA, et al. *Arch Pediatr Adolesc Med.* 2005;159:929-934.
14. Freed GL, et al. *Am J Prev Med.* 2004;26:11-14.

15. Gust DA, et al. *Pediatrics.* 2004;114:e16-e22.

16. Smith PJ, et al. *Pediatrics.* 2004;114:187-195.

17. Gust DA, et al. *Pediatrics.* 2008;122:718-725.

18. Eisenberg D. The ethics of smallpox immunization. Aish.com Web site. http://www.aish.com/ci/sam/48943486.html. Accessed February 15, 2010.

19. Refusal to vaccinate. American Academy of Pediatrics Web site. http://www.aap.org/immunization/pediatricians/pdf/RefusaltoVaccinate.pdf. Accessed February 2, 2010.

20. Diekema DS, et al. *Pediatrics.* 2005;115:1428-1431.

21. AMA Code of Medical Ethics. American Medical Association Web site. http://www.ama-assn.org/ama/pub/category/2498.html. Accessed January 22, 2010.

22. Kata A. *Vaccine.* 2010;28:1709-1716.

23. Poland GA, et al. *Vaccine.* 2001 19:2440-2445.

24. Blume S. *Soc Sci Med.* 2006;62:628-642.

25. Colgrove J. *State of Immunity: The Politics of Vaccination in Twentieth-Century America.* Berkeley, CA: University of California Press; 2006.

26. Offit PA. *Autism's False Prophets: Bad Science, Risky Medicine, and the Search for a Cure.* New York, NY: Columbia University Press; 2008.

27. Offit PA. *Deadly Choices: How the Anti-Vaccine Movement Threatens Our Children.* New York, NY: Basic Books; 2011.

28. Wolfe RM, et al. *JAMA.* 2002;287:3245-3248.

29. Feikin DR, et al. *JAMA.* 2000;284:3145-3150.

30. Omer SB, et al. *Am J Epidemiol.* 2008;168:1389-1396.

31. Cherry JD. *Curr Prob Pediatr.* 1984;14:1-78.

32. Gangarosa EJ, et al. *Lancet.* 1998;351:356-361.

33. Measles once again endemic in the United Kingdom. Eurosurveillance Web site. http://www.eurosurveillance.org/viewarticle.aspx?articleid=18919. Accessed January 24, 2010.

34. Parker AA, et al. *N Engl J Med* 2006;355:447-455.

35. The National Vaccine Advisory Committee. *JAMA.* 1991;266:1547-1552.

36. Dayan GH, et al. *N Engl J Med.* 2008;358:1580-1589.

37. Black SB, et al. *Am J Dis Child.* 1991;145:746-749.

38. Otto S, et al. *J Infect.* 2000;41:172-175

39. Hviid A, et al. *JAMA.* 2005;294:699-705.

40. Storsaeter J, et al. *Pediatr Infect Dis J.* 1988;7:637-645.

41. Davidson M, et al. *Am J Dis Child.* 1991;145:750-754.

42. Offit PA, et al. *Pediatrics.* 2003;112:1394-1397.

43. Jefferson T, et al. *Lancet Infect Dis.* 2004;4:84-90.

44. Keith LS, et al. *Vaccine.* 2002;20:S13-S17.

45. Hot topics: aluminum. The Children's Hospital Vaccine Education Center Web site. http://www.chop.edu/service/vaccine-education-center/hot-topics/aluminum.html Accessed February 14, 2010.

237

46. Beutler B, et al. *Nat Rev Immunol.* 2003;3:169-176.

47. Verstraeten T, et al. *Vaccine.* 2008;26:6630-6638.

48. Integrated Risk Information System. Formaldehyde (CASRN 50-00-0). U.S. Environmental Protection Agency Web site. http://www.epa.gov/ncea/iris/subst/0419.htm#reforal. Accessed February 14, 2010.

49. Sears R. *The Vaccine Book: Making the Right Decision for Your Child.* New York, NY: Little, Brown and Co; 2007.

50. Offit PA, et al. *Pediatrics* 2009;123:e164-e169.

51. Hurie MB, et al. *Pediatrics.* 2001;107:755-758.

52. Smith MJ, Woods CR. On-time vaccine receipt in the first year does not adversely affect neurophysiological outcomes. *Pediatrics.* 2010. In press.

53. Schaub B, et al. *J Allergy Clin Immunol.* 2006;117:969-977.

54. Offit PA, et al. *Pediatrics.* 2003;111:653-659.

55. DeStefano F, et al. *Pediatr Infect Dis J.* 2002;21:498-504.

56. Spycher BD, et al. *Pediatrics.* 2009;123:944-950.

57. Spycher BD, et al. *J Allerg Clin Immunol.* 2008;37:656.

58. Anderson HR, et al. *Am J Public Health.* 2001;91:1126-1129.

59. Nilsson L, et al. *Arch Pediatr Adolesc Med.* 1998;152:734-738.

60. Nilsson L, et al. *Arch Pediatr Adolesc Med.* 2003;157:1184-1189.

61. Nakajima K, et al. *Thorax.* 2007;62:270-275.

62. Rosenlund H, et al. *Pediatrics.* 2009;123:771-778.

63. DeStefano F, et al. *Pediatrics.* 2001;108:e112.

64. Black SB, et al. *Pediatr Infect Dis J.* 2002;21:568-569.

65. Heijbel H, et al. *Diabetes Care.* 1997;20:173-175.

66. Graves PM, et al. *Diabetes Care.* 1999;22:1694-1697.

67. Hummel M, et al. *Diabetes Care.* 2000;23:969-974.

68. Hviid A, et al. *N Engl J Med.* 2004;350:1398-1404.

69. Hayflick L. *Exp Cell Res.* 1965;37:614-636.

70. Grabenstein JD. *Catholic Pharmacist.* 1996;29:2-4.

71. Zimmerman RK. *Vaccine.* 2004;22:4238-4244.

72. United States Conference of Catholic Bishops. Fact Sheet: Embryonic stem cell research and vaccines using fetal tissue. USCCB Web site. http://www.usccb.org/prolife/issues/bioethic/vaccfac2.shtml. Accessed January 29, 2010.

73. Wakefield AJ, et al. *Lancet.* 1998;351:637-641.

74. Murch SH, et al. *Lancet.* 2004;363:750.

75. Fitness to practise panel hearing: 28 January 2010. General Medical Council Web site. http://www.gmc-uk.org/static/documents/content/Wakefield__Smith_Murch.pdf. Accessed February 3, 2010.

76. Editors. *Lancet.* 2010;375:445.

77. Afzal MA, et al. *Lancet.* 1998;351:646-647.

78. D'Souza Y, et al. *Pediatrics.* 2006;118:1664-1675.

79. Hornig M, et al. *PLoS ONE.* 2008;9:e3140(1-8).

80. Davis RL, et al. *Arch Pediatr Adolesc Med.* 2001;155:354-359.

81. Shattuck PT. *Pediatrics*. 2006;117:1028-1037.

82. Kaye JA, et al. *BMJ*. 2001;322:460-463.

83. Dales L, et al. *JAMA*. 2001;285:1183-1185.

84. Fombonne E, et al. *Pediatrics*. 2006;118:139-150.

85. Taylor B, et al. *Lancet*. 1999;353:2026-2029.

86. Farrington CP, et al. *Vaccine*. 2001;19:3632-3635.

87. Taylor B, et al. *BMJ*. 2002;324:393-396.

88. Fombonne E, et al. *Pediatrics*. 2001;108:e58.

89. Smeeth L, et al. *Lancet*. 2004;364:963-969.

90. DeStefano F, et al. *Pediatrics*. 2004;113:259-266.

91. Madsen KM, et al. *N Engl J Med*. 2002;347:1477-1482.

92. CDC. *MMWR*. 1999;48:563-565.

93. Freed GL, et al. *Pediatrics*. 2002;109:1153-1159.

94. Luman ET, et al. *JAMA*. 2004;291:2351-2358.

95. Offit PA. *N Engl J Med*. 2008;358:2089-2091.

96. U.S. Court of Federal Claims. Autism decisions and background information. Available at: http://www.uscfc.uscourts.gov/node/5026. Accessed February 16, 2010.

97. Pichichero ME, et al. *Lancet*. 2002;360:1737-1741.

98. Pichichero ME, et al. *Pediatrics*. 2008;121:e208-e214.

99. Madsen KM, et al. *Pediatrics*. 2003;112:604-606.

100. Stehr-Green P, et al. *Am J Prev Med*. 2003;25:101-106.

101. Schechter R, et al. *Arch Gen Psychiatry*. 2008;65:19-24.

102. Andrews N, et al. *Pediatrics*. 2004;114:584-591.

103. Hviid A, et al. *JAMA*. 2003;290:1763-1766.

104. Heron J, et al. *Pediatrics*. 2004;114:577-583.

105. Verstraeten T, et al. *Pediatrics*. 2003;112:1039-1048.

106. Thompson WW, et al. *N Engl J Med*. 2007;357:1281-1292.

107. Autism Science Foundation Web site. http://www.autismscience foundation.org. Accessed February 16, 2010.

108. Eichler EE, et al. *N Engl J Med*. 2008;358:737-739.

109. Weiss LA, et al. *Nature*. 2009;461:802-808.

110. Kulenkampff M, et al. *Arch Dis Child*. 1974;49:46-49.

111. Miller DL, et al. *BMJ*. 1981;282:1595-1599.

112. Miller D, et al. *BMJ*. 1993;307:1171-1176.

113. Howson CP, Howe CJ, Fineberg HV, eds. *Adverse Effects of Vaccines: A Report of the Committee to Review the Adverse Consequences of Pertussis and Rubella Vaccines*. Washington, DC: National Academy Press; 1991.

114. Stratton KR, Howe CJ, Johnston RB, eds. *DPT Vaccine and Chronic Nervous System Dysfunction: A New Analysis*. Washington, DC: National Academy Press; 1994.

115. Pollock TM, et al. *Lancet*. 1983;1:753-757.

116. Shields WD, et al. *J Pediatr*. 1988;113:801-805.

117. Griffin MR, et al. *JAMA*. 1990;263 1641-1645.

118. Gale JL, et al. *JAMA*. 1994;271:37-41.

119. Ray P, et al. *Pediatr Infect Dis J*. 2006;25:768-773.

120. Berkovic SF, et al. *Lancet Neurol*. 2006;5:488-492.

121. Gaydos JC, et al. *Emerg Infect Dis*. 2006;12:23-28.

122. Haber P, et al. *Drug Safety*. 2009;32:309-323.

123. Nachamkin I, et al. *J Infect Dis*. 2008;198:226-233.

124. Haber P, et al. *JAMA*. 2004;292:2478-2481.

125. Lasky T, et al. *N Engl J Med*. 1998;339:1797-1802.

126. Evans D, et al. *J Infect Dis*. 2009;200:321-328.

127. Hughes RA, et al. *Arch Intern Med*. 2006;166:1301-1304.

128. Juurlink DN, et al. *Arch Intern Med*. 2006;166:2217-2221.

129. CDC. *MMWR*. 2006;55:1120-1124.

130. Ascherio A, et al. *N Engl J Med*. 2001;344:327-332.

131. Confavreux C, et al. *N Engl J Med*. 2001;344:319-326.

132. Mikaeloff Y, et al. *Arch Pediatr Adolesc Med* 2007;161:1176-1182.

133. Mikaeloff Y, et al. *Neurology*. 2009;72:873-880.

134. De Keyser J, et al. *J Neurol Sci*. 1998;159:51-53.

135. Miller AE, et al. *Neurology*. 1997;48:312-314.

136. CDC. *MMWR*. 2000;49:1137-1138.

137. Minor PD, et al. *Vaccine*. 2000;19:409-410.

138. Ferber D. *Science*. 2002;296:1012-1015.

139. López-Ríos F, et al. *Lancet*. 2004;364:1157-1166.

140. Plotkin SA. *Clin Infect Dis*. 2001;32:1068-1084.

141. Plotkin SA. *Vaccine*. 2004;22:1829-1830.

142. Korber B, et al. *Science*. 2000;288:1789-1796.

143. Worobey M, et al. *Nature*. 2004;428:820.

144. Berry N, et al. *Nature*. 2001;410:1046-1047.

145. Poinar H, et al. *Science*. 2001;292:743-744.

146. Butler D. *Nature*. 2004;428:109.

147. Niu MT, et al. *Arch Pediatr Adolesc Med*. 1999;153:1279-1282.

148. Griffin MR, et al. *N Engl J Med*. 1988;319:618-623.

149. Fleming PJ, et al. *BMJ*. 2001;322:822.

150. Eriksen EM, et al. *Pediatr Infect Dis J*. 2004;23:656-662.

151. Kawasaki syndrome. Centers for Disease Control and Prevention Web site. http://www.cdc.gov/vaccinesafety/Vaccines/Rotavirus .html. Accessed February 16, 2010.

152. Hua W, et al. *Pediatr Infect Dis J*. 2009;28:943-947.

8   Schedules

As discussed in *Chapter 2: Vaccine infrastructure in the United States—Policy and Recommendations*, the Advisory Committee on Immunization Practices (ACIP) has permanent working groups that make recommendations for changes to the routine childhood/adolescent and adult vaccination schedules.

Since 1995, the childhood schedule has been "harmonized" in its current graphic layout with the recommendations of the American Academy of Pediatrics (AAP) and the American Academy of Family Physicians (AAFP). The new schedule is released in January of each year. Beginning in 2007, the schedule was split into two—one giving the routinely recommended vaccines for children 0 to 6 years of age (**Tables 8.1** and **8.2**) and the other giving the recommendations for children and adolescents 7 to 18 years of age (**Table 8.3**). Two additional charts—the catch-up schedules (**Tables 8.4** and **8.5**)—are used to bring unimmunized and underimmunized children up-to-date as soon as possible. Catch-up can be accomplished by giving all vaccines for which a person is eligible at each visit, keeping in mind the minimum intervals between doses (**Table 5.1**). Remember, routine vaccine series do not need to be restarted, regardless of the time that has elapsed between doses.

The routine adult schedule, first published in its current form in 2002, is also updated each year. The recommendations are now developed in conjunction with the AAFP, the American College of Obstetricians and Gynecologists, and the American College of Physicians. The schedule is given in two different formats—by age group (**Table 8.6**) and by underlying medical condition (**Table 8.7**).

The routine schedules, given in simplified format in these tables, were derived from the published 2010 schedules with changes based on the ACIP meeting in February 2010.[1,2] The notes below are offered for clarification. Additional details, including vaccine composition, route of administration, contraindications, precautions, and high-risk groups are given in the individual vaccine chapters in *Section B*. Vaccination of special populations is discussed in more detail in *Chapter 6: Vaccination in Special Circumstances*.

Notes on the Routine Schedules (Tables 8.1 through 8.7)

■ **HepB**

Only monovalent HepB (Engerix-B or Recombivax HB) can be used under 6 weeks of age. A birth dose should be given to all newborns before hospital discharge. For infants of HBsAg-negative mothers, the birth dose should be delayed only by an order from the provider and a copy of the mother's negative hepatitis B serology laboratory report on the chart. Infants of HBsAg-positive mothers should receive both vaccine and hepatitis B immune globulin within 12 hours of birth and should be tested for HBsAg and HBsAb between 9 and 18 months of age (a few months after completion of the vaccine series). If the mother's status is unknown, vaccinate within 12 hours of birth and test the mother; hepatitis B immune globulin can still be given in the first week if the mother turns out to be HBsAg-positive.

The following pediatric combination vaccines containing HepB are available: HepB-Hib-OMP (Comvax) and DTaP-HepB-IPV (Pediarix). See **Table 8.2** for how these integrate into the schedule. Use of these combination vaccines may mean that children will get an unnecessary dose of HepB at 4 months of age. Such extraimmunization is permissible and safe.

The timing of the routine 3 doses of HepB is a little tricky. Dose 2 must be at least 4 weeks after Dose 1; Dose 3 must be at least 16 weeks after Dose 1 and 8 weeks after Dose 2; and the last dose (third or, in the case of HepB-containing combination vaccines, fourth) should not be given before 24 weeks of age.

A 2-dose series of Recombivax HB is licensed for adolescents 11 to 15 years of age. For patients on hemodialysis and for other immunocompromised adults, high-dose formulations are used—Recombivax HB 40 mcg/mL given at 0, 1, and 6 months, or 2 simultaneous doses of Engerix-B 20 mcg/mL given at 0, 1, 2, and 6 months. HepA-HepB (Twinrix) may be used for adults on a 0, 1, and 6 month schedule or a 0, 7, 21-to-30 day, and 12 month schedule.

■ RV

Either RV1 (Rotarix, 2 doses) or RV5 (RotaTeq, 3 doses) may be used. Dose 1 should be given between 6 weeks and 14 weeks 6 days of age. All doses should be administered by 8 months 0 days of age. Vaccination should not be deferred if the product used for the previous dose is unavailable or not known. If any of the doses in the series is RV5 or unknown, a total of 3 doses should be given.

■ DTaP

Dose 4 may be given as early as 12 months of age, provided at least 6 months have elapsed since Dose 3. Dose 5 is not necessary if Dose 4 was given at ≥4 years of age. DTaP is not indicated for children ≥7 years of age.

The following combination vaccines containing DTaP are available: DTaP-HepB-IPV (Pediarix), DTaP-IPV/Hib-T (Pentacel), DTaP/Hib-T (TriHIBit), and DTaP-IPV (Kinrix). See **Table 8.2** for how these integrate into the schedule.

TABLE 8.1 — Routine Schedule for Children 0 to 6 Years of Age, 2010

Vaccine	Birth	1	2	4	6	12	15	18	19-23	2-3	4-6
HepB	Dose 1	Dose 2		See notes	Dose 3						
RV			Dose 1	Dose 2	(Dose 3)						
DTaP			Dose 1	Dose 2	Dose 3		Dose 4				Dose 5
Hib			Dose 1	Dose 2	(Dose 3)	Dose 3 or Dose 4					
PCV			Dose 1	Dose 2	Dose 3	Dose 4					
IPV			Dose 1	Dose 2	Dose 3					See notes	Dose 4
Influenza					Annual (2 doses in first season)						
MMR						Dose 1					Dose 2
VAR						Dose 1					Dose 2
HepA						Dose 1			Dose 2	2 doses if high-risk	
MCV										1-2 doses if high-risk	

See notes for each vaccine in text. Doses in parentheses depend on which product is used.

Adapted from CDC. *MMWR.* 2010;58(51 & 52):1-4.

TABLE 8.2 — Use of Combination Vaccines in Children 0 to 6 Years of Age, 2010

Combination Vaccine	Months									Years	
	Birth	1	2	4	6	12	15	18	19-23	2-3	4-6
HepB-Hib	HepB		Dose 1	Dose 2			Dose 3				
DTaP-HepB-IPV	HepB		Dose 1	Dose 2	Dose 3			DTaP			DTaP IPV
DTaP-IPV/Hib	HepB		Dose 1	Dose 2	Dose 3			Dose 4			DTaP IPV
DTaP/Hib			DTaP Hib	DTaP Hib	DTaP (Hib)			Dose 1			DTaP
DTaP-IPV			DTaP IPV	DTaP IPV	DTaP		IPV	DTaP			Dose 1
MMRV							Dose 1				Dose 2

See notes for each vaccine in text. Only elements of the routine schedule relevant to each combination vaccine are shown. Doses in parentheses depend on which product is used.

Adapted from CDC. *MMWR*. 2010;58(51 & 52):1-4.

TABLE 8.3 — Routine Schedule for Children 7 to 18 Years of Age, 2010

Vaccine	7-10 Years	11-12 Years	13-18 Years
Tdap		Dose 1	Catch-up (1 dose)
HPV		Dose 1, Dose 2, Dose 3	Catch-up (3 doses)
MCV	1 dose if high-risk	Dose 1	Catch-up (1 dose)
Influenza	Annual (2 doses in first season if <9 years of age)		
PPSV	1 dose if high-risk, consider one-time revaccination in 5 years		
HepA		2 doses if high-risk	
HepB		Catch-up (3 doses)	
IPV		Catch-up (4 doses)	
MMR		Catch-up (2 doses)	
VAR		Catch-up (2 doses)	

See notes for each vaccine in text. Where vaccination is recommended, it is assumed the person has not previously been vaccinated, except in the case of influenza, where vaccination should occur every year. Thus, for example, MMR and VAR should be given to adolescents who have not previously been vaccinated and who do not meet the criteria for immunity. For Tdap, HPV, influenza, PPSV, and MCV, the vaccines should be given even if disease has been previously documented. Thus, for example, IIIV vaccine is given to girls known to have had cervical dysplasia or HPV infection, since the vaccine may prevent infection with serotypes that the person has not yet encountered.

Adapted from CDC. *MMWR.* 2010;58(51 & 52):1-4.

8

TABLE 8.4 — Catch-up Schedule for Children 4 Months to 6 Years of Age, 2010

Vaccine	Minimum Age for Dose 1	Minimum Interval to...			
		Dose 2	Dose 3	Dose 4	Dose 5
HepB	Birth	4 weeks	8 weeks and ≥16 weeks after Dose 1		
RV	6 weeks	4 weeks	(4 weeks)		
DTaP	6 weeks	4 weeks	4 weeks	6 months	6 months
Hib	6 weeks	Dose 1 at <12 months: 4 weeks Dose 1 at 12-14 months: 8 weeks (final dose) Dose 1 at ≥15 months: no further doses	Age <12 months: 4 weeks Age ≥12 months, Dose 1 at <12 months and Dose 2 at <15 months: 8 weeks (final dose) Any dose at ≥15 months: no further doses	Age 12-59 months and 3 doses at <12 months: 8 weeks (final dose)	
PCV	6 weeks	Dose 1 at <12 months: 4 weeks Dose 1 at ≥12 months: 8 weeks (final dose)	Age <12 months: 4 weeks Age ≥12 months: 8 weeks (final dose)	Age 12-59 months and 3 doses at <12 months: 8 weeks (final dose)	

		Age 24-59 months: 8 weeks (final dose) Dose 1 at ≥24 months: no further doses	Age ≥24 months: no further doses	
IPV	6 weeks	4 weeks	4 weeks	6 months
MMR	12 months	4 weeks		
VAR	12 months	3 months		
HepA	12 months	6 months		

See notes for each vaccine in text. This table should be used for children who start late or who are >1 month behind. No routine vaccine series needs to be restarted, regardless of how much time has elapsed. Some combination vaccines can be used for catch-up. A computer application that determines catch-up schedules for young children is available from the CDC at http://www.cdc.gov/vaccines/recs/scheduler/catchup.htm (accessed February 25, 2010).

Adapted from CDC. *MMWR.* 2010;58(51 & 52):1-4.

TABLE 8.5 — Catch-up Schedule for Children 7 to 18 Years of Age, 2010

Vaccine	Minimum Age for Dose 1	Minimum Interval to…			
		Dose 2	Dose 3	Dose 4	
Td, Tdap	7 years	4 weeks	Dose 1 at <12 months: 4 weeks Dose 1 at ≥12 months: 6 months	Dose 1 at <12 months: 6 months	
HPV	9 years		See notes		
HepA	12 months	6 months			
HepB	Birth	4 weeks	8 weeks and ≥16 weeks after Dose 1		
IPV	6 weeks	4 weeks	4 weeks	6 months	
MMR	12 months	4 weeks			
VAR	12 months	Age <13 years: 3 months Age ≥13 years: 4 weeks			

See notes for each vaccine in text. This table should be used for children who start late or who are >1 month behind. No routine vaccine series needs to be restarted, regardless of how much time has elapsed. Some combination vaccines can be used for catch-up.

Adapted from CDC. *MMWR*. 2010;58(51 & 52):1-4.

TABLE 8.6 — Adult Schedule by Age, 2010

Vaccine	19-26	27-49	50-59	60-64	>65
Td, Tdap	Substitute Tdap for Td one time, then Td every 10 years				Td every 10 years
HPV	3 doses for females				
VAR			2 doses		
ZOS				1 dose	
MMR	1 or 2 doses		1 dose if high-risk		
Influenza			Annual		
PPSV		1 or 2 doses if high-risk			1 dose
HepA			2 doses if high-risk		
HepB			3 doses if high-risk		
MCV, MPSV			≥1 dose if high-risk		

See notes for each vaccine in text. Where vaccination is recommended, it is assumed the person has not previously been vaccinated, except in the case of influenza, where vaccination should occur every year. Thus, for example, MMR and VAR should be given to adults who have not previously been vaccinated and who do not meet the criteria for immunity. For Tdap, HPV, ZOS, influenza, PPSV, and MCV or MPSV, the vaccines should be given even if disease has been previously documented. Thus, for example, HPV vaccine is given to women known to have had cervical dysplasia or HPV infection, since the vaccine may prevent infection with serotypes that the person has not yet encountered.

Adapted from CDC. *MMWR*. 2010;58(51 & 52):1-4. Updated with influenza recommendation from the February 2010 meeting of the ACIP.

TABLE 8.7 — Adult Schedule by Medical and Other Indications, 2010

Vaccine	Pregnancy	Immune compromised	HIV <200 CD4 per mcL	HIV ≥200 CD4 per mcL	Diabetes, heart disease, chronic lung disease, alcoholism	Asplenia, persistent complement deficiency	Chronic liver disease	Kidney failure, ESRD, hemodialysis	Health care personnel
Td, Tdap	Td	Substitute Tdap for Td one time if ≤64 years of age, then Td every 10 years							
HPV	See notes	3 doses for females ≤26 years of age							
VAR		Contraindicated		2 doses					
ZOS		Contraindicated		See notes	1 dose ≥60 years of age				
MMR		Contraindicated		1 or 2 doses					
Influenza			Annual IIV						Annual IIV or LAIV
PPSV	If otherwise indicated				1 or 2 doses				If otherwise indicated
HepA			If otherwise indicated				2 doses	If otherwise indicated	

HepB	If otherwise indicated	3 doses	If otherwise indicated	3 doses
MCV, MPSV	If otherwise indicated		≥1 dose	If otherwise indicated

See legend for **Table 8.6** and notes for each vaccine in text.

Adapted from CDC. *MMWR*. 2010;58(51 & 52):1-4.

8

■ Td and Tdap

Tdap has taken the place of the previously recommended Td booster at 11 to 12 years of age. In general, 5 years should elapse between the last tetanus or diphtheria toxoid-containing vaccine and Tdap, but shorter intervals are acceptable. As of 2010, only one lifetime dose of Tdap is recommended; Td boosters should continue every 10 years after a dose of Tdap.

Td should be used from 7 to 9 years of age if a booster is indicated (eg, wound management). One brand of Tdap (Boostrix) may be used starting at 10 years of age, the other (Adacel) starting at 11 years of age. Both products are licensed up to 64 years of age. If vaccination history is uncertain, a primary series consisting of 2 doses of Td separated by 4 weeks with a booster dose 6 to 12 months later should be given; Tdap can be substituted for any one of the Td doses. In general, 5 years should elapse between the last dose of Td and a dose of Tdap, but shorter intervals are recommended for postpartum women, close contacts of infants <12 months of age, and health care personnel (studies have demonstrated the safety of intervals as short as 2 years, but even shorter intervals are acceptable; in truth, there is no minimum interval between Td and Tdap). Td should be given to pregnant women in the second or third trimester if they have not been vaccinated in the past 10 years; however, in some circumstances Td can be deferred so that Tdap can be given postpartum, or, in certain circumstances, Tdap may be given during pregnancy. If a pregnant woman received Td in the past 10 years, Tdap should be given postpartum. Td or Tdap also may be used in wound management.

■ Hib

A dose at 6 months is not required if Dose 1 and Dose 2 were Hib-OMP (PedvaxHIB or Comvax). One brand of Hib-T (Hiberix) is only licensed for the final dose and should not be used as the only dose in a child who has received no previous doses (the labeled age range is 15 months to 4 years, but it may be used as early as 12 months). For catch-up, if Dose 1 was given at 7 to 11 months of age, give Dose 2 at least 4 weeks later and Dose 3 (final dose) at 12 to 15 months of age. If Dose 1 and Dose 2 were Hib-OMP and were both given at ≤11 months of age, Dose 3 (final dose) should be given at 12 to 15 months of age and ≥8 weeks after Dose 2.

The following combination vaccines containing Hib are available: HepB-Hib-OMP (Comvax), DTaP-IPV/Hib-T (Pentacel), and DTaP/Hib-T (TriHIBit). See **Table 8.2** for how these integrate into the schedule.

DTaP-IPV/Hib-T may be used for Dose 4 of Hib, even if the patient has already received Dose 4 of DTaP and Dose 3 of IPV. In this case, the doses of DTaP and IPV contained in Pentacel do not count as the final doses of DTaP and IPV, which must be given at 4 to 6 years of age. Since the doses of DTaP and IPV would be invalid, there is no minimum interval since the last DTaP and IPV doses. However, increased local reactions can be seen when multiple doses of diphtheria and tetanus toxoids are given too close together.

Hib is not routinely given ≥5 years of age, but it may be indicated for certain high-risk persons. One dose should be considered in unimmunized, high-risk persons, including those with sickle cell disease, leukemia, HIV infection, and those who have had a splenectomy.

■ PCV and PPSV

PCV7 (Prevnar) was routinely used from 2000 through 2009. PCV13 (Prevnar 13), which covers 6 additional pneumococcal serotypes, was licensed in February 2010 and replaced PCV7. Children who started the series with PCV7 should switch to PCV13 at any point in the schedule. Those who have already received 4 doses of PCV7 and are ≤59 months of age (≤71 months of age if high-risk) should receive a single supplemental dose of PCV13.

One dose of PCV should be given to all healthy children 24 to 59 months of age who are incompletely vaccinated, including those who have never received PCV. For children with high-risk conditions who have received <3 doses of PCV, give 2 doses at least 8 weeks apart. For children with high-risk conditions who have received 3 doses, give 1 dose. PPSV23 (Pneumovax 23) should be given to persons ≥2 years of age with high-risk conditions, and one-time revaccination in 5 years is recommended for the highest-risk patients. For adults, asthma and cigarette smoking are included as indicators of chronic pulmonary disease and reasons to give PPSV23.

■ IPV

The final dose of IPV (IPOL) should be given at ≥4 years of age, regardless of the number of previous doses. For example, if a child received 4 doses of IPV as DTaP-IPV/Hib-T by 18 months of age, a fifth dose should be given at 4 to 6 years of age. A fourth dose is not necessary if the third dose was given at ≥4 years of age and ≥6 months after the previous dose (if both IPV and OPV were used as part of the series, then a total of 4 doses is necessary, regardless of age). Minimum age and minimum intervals during the first 6 months of life should only be used if the child is at risk of imminent exposure to poliovirus. Catch-up immunization is recommended through 17 (not 18) years of age; this is why the box in **Table 8.3** is cut short.

The following combination vaccines containing IPV are available: DTaP-HepB-IPV (Pediarix), DTaP-IPV/Hib-T (Pentacel), and DTaP-IPV (Kinrix). See **Table 8**.2 for how these integrate into the schedule.

■ Influenza

In 2009, both 3-valent seasonal and monovalent 2009 H1N1 vaccines were recommended; each was available as IIV and LAIV. For the 2010-2011 season, the 2009 H1N1 strain will replace the previous H1N1 strain in the 3-valent vaccine.

Annual influenza immunization is recommended for everyone ≥6 months of age. IIV (multiple brands) may be used starting at 6 months of age and LAIV (FluMist) starting at 2 years of age. The dose of IIV between 6 and 35 months of age is 0.25 mL; beyond that it is 0.5 mL. LAIV may be used for healthy children; those who have underlying conditions that predispose to complications of influenza, as well as children 2 to 4 years of age with wheezing in the past 12 months, should not receive LAIV. Children <9 years of age who are receiving seasonal influenza vaccine for the first time, or who were vaccinated for the first time in the previous season and only received 1 dose, need 2 doses separated by 4 weeks (for the 2009 H1N1 vaccine, the age cut-off was <10 years).

High priority is given to persons with conditions that predispose to complications of influenza, as well as close contacts of those individuals.

■ MMR

Dose 2 may be given anytime ≥28 days after Dose 1. MMRV (ProQuad) may be used in place of MMR (M-M-R II) plus VAR (Varivax) in children 12 months to 12 years of age. If used, Dose 2 may be given anytime ≥3 months after Dose 1.

Criteria for immunity to measles, mumps, and rubella are given in **Table 17**.2.

■ VAR

For children <13 years of age, Dose 2 may be given any time ≥3 months after Dose 1. However, if the second dose is given ≥28 days after the first dose, this dose should be considered valid and should not be repeated. For adolescents ≥13 years of age, the minimum interval between doses is 4 weeks. MMRV may be used in place of MMR plus VAR in children 12 months to 12 years of age. If used, Dose 2 may be given anytime ≥3 months after Dose 1.

Special consideration should be given to those who have close contact with persons at high risk for varicella complications, exposure, or transmission. Pregnant women without evidence of immunity should receive a dose of VAR after delivery and before discharge from the hospital, with a second dose given 4 to 8 weeks later.

Criteria for immunity to varicella are given in **Table 25**.2.

HepA

HepA (Havrix or Vaqta) is recommended for universal use in young children and for older children and adults in certain high-risk groups. The usual timing of doses for Havrix is 0 and 6 to 12 months and for Vaqta 0 and 6 to 18 months. HepA-HepB (Twinrix) may be used for adults on a 0, 1, and 6 month schedule or a 0, 7, 21-to-30 day, and 12 month schedule. In some areas of the country, older children are routinely immunized. Vaccination should be offered to any person for whom immunity is desired.

In addition to persons with chronic liver disease, those who receive clotting factor concentrates should also be vaccinated.

MCV and MPSV

MCV (either MCV4-D [Menactra] or MCV4-CRM [Menveo]) is routinely recommended at 11 to 12 years of age. College freshmen living in dormitories should be vaccinated (but not routinely revaccinated). High-risk children 2 to 10 years of age should receive MCV4-D (as of February 2010, MCV4-CRM was not licensed for use in this age group). High-risk persons 11 to 55 years of age may receive either conjugate vaccine, but MPSV4 (Menomune—A/C/Y/W-135) should be used at ≥56 years of age. Persons who remain at high risk should be revaccinated on a regular basis.

HPV

HPV vaccine (either HPV2 [Cervarix] or HPV4 [Gardasil]) is routinely recommended for girls at 11 to 12 years of age to prevent cervical cancer. HPV4 may be used if prevention of genital warts is also desired. HPV4 may also be used in males to prevent genital warts. Either vaccine may be given as early as 9 years of age (although the Cervarix age indication starts at 10). Doses are given at 0, 1 to 2, and 6 months. At least 4 weeks should elapse between Dose 1 and Dose 2, 12 weeks between Dose 2 and Dose 3, and 24 weeks between Dose 1 and Dose 3.

HPV vaccine is not recommended for use in pregnancy, but testing is not needed before vaccination.

ZOS

Individuals should be vaccinated regardless of their personal history of chickenpox or shingles. While ZOS is contraindicated in immunocompromised persons, including those with HIV infection and CD4 counts <200 per mcL, consideration could be given to vaccinating HIV-infected persons who have no evidence of immunosuppression.

Combination Vaccines

Table 8.2 shows how various combination vaccines fit into the pediatric schedule. Use of combination vaccines is generally preferred over the separate component vaccines. There is one exception—no preference for MMRV over MMR plus VAR for the first dose, because of the increased risk of febrile seizures. The following factors should be considered in deciding whether or not to use combinations: patient preference, potential for adverse events, number of injections, vaccine availability, likelihood of improved coverage, likelihood of patient return, storage, and costs.

REFERENCES

1. CDC. *MMWR.* 2010;58(51 & 52):1-4.
2. CDC. *MMWR.* 2010;59(1):1-4.

9

Anthrax

Pathogen

Bacillus anthracis is a large, aerobic, spore-forming, toxin-producing gram-positive rod with a "jointed bamboo-rod" appearance and "Medusa's head" colony morphology. Pathogenicity is mediated by two secreted virulence factors: lethal toxin and edema toxin.

Clinical Features

Inhalational anthrax is characterized by a flu-like illness, dyspnea, and hemorrhagic thoracic lymphadenitis and mediastinitis.[1] *Cutaneous anthrax* is characterized by a painless ulcer with extensive surrounding edema, eschar formation, and regional adenopathy. Both of these forms of disease would be seen after a bioterrorism attack and either can lead to meningitis. The *gastrointestinal* (bloody diarrhea, hemorrhagic mesenteric adenitis) and *oropharyngeal* (oral or esophageal ulcers and regional adenopathy) forms of anthrax result from ingestion of large numbers of vegetative bacilli (usually in poorly cooked meat) and would therefore be unlikely to result from an attack. After the spores are ingested by phagocytes, they are transported to regional lymph nodes, where they germinate into vegetative cells after variable (and potentially extended) periods of time. Replicating cells then elaborate toxins that lead to massive hemorrhage, edema, necrosis, and cytokine release. Early antibiotic therapy for symptomatic disease is essential, but the effects of local tissue damage and systemic toxinosis may be irreversible.[2]

Epidemiology and Transmission

Anthrax spores are found in soil worldwide and may remain viable for years. Infection occurs in grazing animals that ingest the spores, and natural human infection occurs almost exclusively after contact with infected animals and animal products (one classic example is *woolsorter's disease*, inhalational anthrax linked to the processing of hides and wool in enclosed spaces). Up to 20,000 annual cases of anthrax are estimated to occur worldwide, but this disease in the United States was rare until October 2001. Only 18 cases of inhalational anthrax were reported between 1900 and 1976, and no cases of that particular form of the disease were reported after 1976. Between 1944 and 1994, only 224 cases of cutaneous anthrax were reported, with one case occurring in 2000.

Anthrax is an attractive agent of bioterrorism because the infection can be lethal, natural immunity does not exist, the organism can be engineered into antibiotic resistance, and the infectious dose of spores is very low.[3] It is easily grown in the laboratory, and the spores can be weaponized into a highly concentrated powder with uniform small particle size and low electrostatic charge, features that reduce clumping and facilitate aerosol dispersal. Such aerosols are odorless and invisible, can spread over large areas, and would probably not be detected until cases occurred. The lethality of aerosolized weapons-grade anthrax was demonstrated after the accidental release of anthrax spores (possibly as little as 1 g) on April 2, 1979, from a Soviet bioweapons facility in Sverdlovsk (now called Ekaterinburg). As many as 250 cases and 100 deaths occurred downwind (away from the city of over 1 million people) of the release, mostly from inhalational disease. Most cases occurred within 10 days, although some occurred 6 weeks later. While the majority of victims were exposed in a narrow 4-km band extending from the military facility to the southern city limit, cases did occur many miles away and livestock in several towns downwind of the release were affected.

In September and October 2001, at least five letters containing high-grade Ames strain anthrax spores were mailed through the United States postal service from Trenton, NJ, to sites in Florida, New York City, and Washington, DC. One letter was known to contain 2 g of powder and between 100 billion and 1 trillion spores. A total of 22 anthrax cases occurred in seven eastern states between September 22 and November 16; 11 were inhalational (five deaths) and 11 cutaneous (no deaths). Twelve victims were mail handlers, demonstrating the propensity for weaponized spores to disperse from relatively sealed containers. Cross-contamination was evidenced by the isolation of anthrax from over 100 environmental samples along the path of the letters.

In 1970, the WHO estimated that a release of 50 kg of spores over an urban population of 5 million would result in 250,000 cases and 100,000 deaths. The experience in the United States in 2001 indicates that this might have been an underestimate. Unlike smallpox, all cases occurring after an attack would result from primary exposure, because the infection is not transmitted from person to person. However, secondary aerosolization of particles that settle after a primary release could continue to cause disease for some time.

Immunization Program

The latest recommendations for civilian use of anthrax vaccine prior to the October 2001 attacks were published in 2000.[4] Following the attacks, occupational health guidelines for remediation workers[5] and vaccination recommendations in response to bioterrorism were released.[6] Updated provisional recommendations were posted in 2009.[7]

Antibiotic therapy after exposure can prevent inhaled spores from germinating and causing disease. In fact, there were no cases of anthrax among over 10,000 people who took antibiotics (primarily ciprofloxacin or doxycycline) for at least 60 days following the October 2001 attacks. In May 2002, the Working Group on Civilian Biodefense concluded that antibiotic therapy in conjunction with vaccination would be optimal for exposed persons, and current recommendations incorporate that concept.

Pre-exposure vaccination is based on a quantifiable risk for exposure and is not recommended for the general public. Although a vaccine has been licensed since 1970, it was in limited use until 1991 when the United States military immunized 150,000 service members deployed for the Gulf War. The Anthrax Vaccine Immunization Program was started in March 1998 with the routine immunization of personnel deployed to high-risk areas. In June 2002, the Department of Defense reintroduced the program (which had slowed because of dwindling vaccine supplies) because of intelligence assessments indicating possible risk of exposure to military personnel; the guidelines were updated as recently as 2009.[8]

Vaccines

Characteristics of the anthrax vaccine licensed in the United States are given in **Table 9.1**. This is an inactivated vaccine composed of proteins released by the bacterium into the medium during growth in culture. It contains no intact bacteria, live or dead.

Efficacy and/or Immunogenicity

Protection has been demonstrated in a macaque model of inhalational anthrax. One controlled trial of a similar vaccine among 1249 mill workers (379 were immunized) demonstrated 92.5% efficacy. No inhalational cases occurred among vaccinees, but three cutaneous cases occurred in incompletely vaccinated persons. Case surveillance data from 1962 to 1974 suggest that anthrax in mill workers or those living near mills occurred exclusively in unvaccinated or incompletely vaccinated persons. In a controlled trial conducted between 2002 and 2008 involving 1564 adults, the intramuscular route of administration was found to be noninferior to the subcutaneous route in terms of immunogenicity, and nearly all vaccinees demonstrated a $\geq$4-fold increase in antibody titer.

TABLE 9.1 — Anthrax Vaccine

Trade Name	BioThrax
Abbreviation	—
Manufacturer/distributor	Emergent BioDefense Operations Lansing[a]
Type of vaccine	Inactivated, purified subunits
Composition	Cell-free filtrate of microaerophilic cultures of an avirulent, noncapsulated *Bacillus anthracis* strain
	Includes 83kDa protective antigen
Adjuvant	Aluminum hydroxide (0.6 mg aluminum)
Preservative	Benzethonium chloride (12.5 mcg)
	Formaldehyde (50 mcg)
Excipients and contaminants	Sodium chloride (0.85%)
Latex	Vial stopper contains dry natural rubber
Labeled indications	Pre-exposure prophylaxis
Labeled ages	18 to 65 years
Dose	0.5 mL
Route of administration	Intramuscular (subcutaneous if patient has coagulopathy)
Labeled schedule	0, 4 weeks, 6, 12, 18 months (intramuscular)
	Booster doses every year (intramuscular)
Recommended schedule	Pre-event: same
	Postevent:[b] 0, 2 weeks, 4 weeks (subcutaneous)
How supplied (number in package)	10-dose vial (1)
Storage	Refrigerate
	Do not freeze
Cost per dose ($US, 2009):	
Public	—
Private	350.00
Reference package insert	December 2008

[a] Formerly manufactured by BioPort.

[b] For postevent prophylaxis, vaccine is given under Investigational New Drug or Emergency Use authorization. Antimicrobials may also be indicated (see **Table 9.2**).

In an open-label safety study, 15,907 doses of BioThrax were administered subcutaneously to 7000 at-risk persons. Mild local reactions (erythema only or induration <30 mm) occurred after 8.6% of doses administered, moderate reactions (edema or induration between 30 mm and 120 mm) after 0.9%, and severe reactions (edema or induration >120 mm accompanied by limitation of motion or axillary lymph node tenderness) in 0.15%. There were only four reports of systemic reactions such as fever, chills, nausea, and general body aches. In a study of 28 volunteers, injection-site tenderness was reported in 71% after Dose 1, 61% after Dose 2, and 58% after Dose 3. The respective rates of erythema were 43%, 32%, and 12%, occurrence of a subcutaneous nodule 36%, 39%, and 4%, and induration 21%, 18%, and 8%. Fewer than 10% of volunteers had notable systemic reactions, and all of these were transient.

In the 2002-2008 trial, intramuscular administration was found to cause less local reactogenicity than subcutaneous administration. Most local and systemic reactions were mild or moderate in severity; severe adverse reactions were reported in <1% of subjects. Interestingly, injection site reactions were more common in women, especially with subcutaneous administration. There were 44 pregnancies during the study; the majority of outcomes were good, although there was a spontaneous abortion and a clubbed foot abnormality among infants born to 15 women vaccinated in the first trimester. In an observational study of infants born to US military service women between 1998 and 2004, birth defects were slightly more common (odds ratio 1.18) among the 3465 infants born to women who were vaccinated during the first trimester when compared to the 33,675 infants whose mothers were vaccinated outside of the first trimester (most of these were vaccinated before pregnancy or after delivery).[9]

In a study involving >4300 service personnel in Korea, 2% of persons reported limitation in work performance after Dose 1 or Dose 2 but <1% lost ≥1 day of work. In 2002, an IOM study concluded that the anthrax vaccine is safe,[10] and epidemiologic studies provide no evidence linking the vaccine to Gulf War Syndrome.[11] Finally, from 1998 to 2007, approximately 6 million doses of anthrax vaccine were administered and slightly over 4700 adverse event reports were received by VAERS.[12] No unexpected risks were seen and there was no distinctive pattern of serious events or death.

- *Contraindications*
  - Allergic reaction to previous dose of vaccine or any vaccine component (risk of recurrent allergic reaction)

- *Precautions*
  - Moderate or severe acute illness (difficulty distinguishing illness from vaccine reaction)
  - Pregnancy (Pregnancy Category D—vaccine can cause fetal harm, so use only if the potential benefits outweigh the potential risks)
  - Previous anthrax disease (risk of more severe adverse events)

Recommendations

Recommendations for civilian use of anthrax vaccine are given in **Table 9.2**.

Use of anthrax vaccine in the military is summarized below:

- Vaccination is mandatory for Department of Defense service members, emergency-essential designated civilians, and contractor personnel performing mission-essential services assigned to Central Command area of responsibility for ≥15 consecutive days, Korean Peninsula for ≥15 consecutive days, special units with biowarfare or bioterrorism related missions, and specialty units with approved exception to policy
- Vaccination occurs up to 120 days prior to deployment or arrival in higher threat areas
- Vaccination is voluntary for Department of Defense service members and government civilian employees of the Department of Defense who are not in the mandatory groups and have received at least one dose of anthrax vaccine during or after 1998
- Vaccination is voluntary for Department of Defense civilians and adult family members, as well as contractors and their accompanying United States citizen family members
- Vaccine manufacturing and research personnel and others, as designated by the Assistant Secretary of Defense for Health Affairs, are vaccinated

REFERENCES

1. Dixon TC, et al. *N Engl J Med*. 1999;341:815-826.

2. Grabenstein JD. *Clin Infect Dis*. 2008;46:129-136.

3. Inglesby TV, et al. *JAMA*. 2002;287:2236-2252.

4. CDC. *MMWR*. 2000;49(RR-15):1-20.

5. CDC. *MMWR*. 2002;51:786-789.

6. CDC. *MMWR*. 2002;51:1024-1026.

7. ACIP provisional recommendations for use of anthrax vaccine adsorbed. Centers for Disease Control Web site. www.cdc.gov /vaccines/recs/provisional/default.htm. Accessed January 29, 2010.

8. Military Vaccine Agency, Office of the Army Surgeon General. Anthrax vaccine immunization program (AVIP): questions and answers. http://www.anthrax.osd.mil/documents/Anthrax_QA.pdf. Accessed February 4, 2010.

9. Ryan MAK, et al. *Am J Epidimiol*. 2008;168:434-442.

10. Joellenbeck LM, et al, editors. *The Anthrax Vaccine: Is It Safe? Does It Work?* Washington, DC: Institute of Medicine, National Academy Press; 2002.

11. Iowa Persian Gulf Study Group *JAMA*. 1997;277:238-245.

12. Niu MT, et al. *Vaccine*. 2009;27:290-297.

9

TABLE 9.2 — Recommendations for Civilian Use of Anthrax Vaccine

Group	Pre-event[a]	Postevent Prophylaxis[b]
General public	Not recommended	Recommended
Pregnant women	Not recommended	Recommended
Breastfeeding women	Not recommended	Recommended
Children 0 to 18 years of age	Not recommended	Determine on event-by-event basis
Medical professionals	Not recommended	Recommended
Persons engaged in handling animals or animal products	Not routinely recommended[c]	Recommended
Persons engaged in certain laboratory work[d]	Recommended	Based on pre-event vaccination status
Persons working in postal facilities	Not recommended	Recommended
Persons engaged in environmental investigations or remediation efforts	Recommended	Based on pre-event vaccination status
Emergency and other responders[e]	Not routinely recommended[f]	Recommended

[a] Pre-event vaccination is recommended for persons who are occupationally at risk for exposure to aerosolized *B anthracis* spores. See **Table 9.1** for vaccination schedule.

[b] Prophylaxis is recommended following natural, occupational, or intentional exposure to *B anthracis* spores in persons who have not completed pre-event vaccination. See **Table 9.1** for vaccination schedule. In addition to vaccination, appropriate antimicrobials are given for 60 days (see Anthrax: exposure management/prophylaxis. Centers for Disease Control and Prevention Web site. http://emergency.cdc.gov/agent/anthrax/exposure. Accessed March 25, 2010). Persons who already received 5 doses of the vaccine plus annual boosters before exposure do not need additional vaccination or antimicrobials unless there was a disruption in their personal protective equipment.

c Recommended if handling potentially infected animals in a research setting, animals with high incidence of enzootic anthrax, or if standards are insufficient to prevent exposure to spores. Potentially contaminated animal products include imported animal hides, furs, bone meal, wool, animal hair, or bristles.

d Includes persons handling high concentrations of spores, pure cultures, environmental samples associated with anthrax investigations, spore-contaminated areas or other settings with aerosol exposure. Does not include workers using standard Biosafety Level 2 practices in routine processing of clinical samples or environmental swabs.

e Includes police and fire departments, hazmat units, government responders, and National Guard who may perform site investigations, respond to "white powder incidents", perform evacuations or other activities critical to the maintenance of infrastructure.

f Vaccination may be offered on a voluntary basis under a comprehensive occupational health and safety program.

Adapted from CDC. *MMWR*. 2000;49(RR-15):1-20, CDC. *MMWR*. 2002;51:786-789, CDC. *MMWR*. 2002;51:1024-1026, and ACIP provisional recommendations for use of anthrax vaccine adsorbed. Centers for Disease Control Web site. www.cdc.gov/vaccines/recs/provisional/default.htm. Accessed January 29, 2010.

9

10
Diphtheria, Tetanus, Pertussis

The Pathogens

■ Diphtheria

Corynebacterium diphtheriae is an aerobic, nonencapsulated, nonspore-forming, pleomorphic gram-positive bacillus that has a club-like appearance on Gram stain. Infection occurs on mucous membranes of the upper respiratory tract or in the skin, where the organism elaborates a potent exotoxin that works by inactivating tRNA transferase, preventing amino acids from being added to nascent polypeptide chains during protein synthesis. On respiratory surfaces like the throat, necrotic cells, inflammatory exudate, bacteria, and fibrin coalesce into adherent *pseudomembranes*. Local effects of the toxin include paralysis of the palate and hypopharynx; distant effects can be seen in the kidneys, liver, heart, and nervous system.

■ Tetanus

Clostridium tetani is a nonencapsulated, gram-positive, obligately anaerobic bacillus that has a drumstick or tennis racket appearance on Gram stain because of terminally located spores. Initial infection usually takes place in a deep, penetrating wound, where the organism elaborates *tetanospasmin*, a potent neurotoxin. The toxin spreads via the bloodstream and lymphatics to distant sites, where it is taken up into nerves through the neuromuscular junction and transported to the CNS. There it prevents the release of neurotransmitters at inhibitory synapses, causing unopposed lower motor-neuron activity, with resultant spasms and rigidity.

■ Pertussis

Bordetella pertussis is a tiny, aerobic, gram-negative coccobacillus that is tropic for ciliated respiratory epithelium. Attachment is mediated by several proteins, including *filamentous hemagglutinin* (FHA), *fimbriae* (FIM), and *pertactin* (PRN). The major virulence factor is *pertussis toxin* (PT), a complex molecule that causes increased intracellular levels of cyclic adenosine monophosphate and disruption of cellular function. PT also facilitates adherence, promotes lymphocytosis, inhibits phagocytosis, increases insulin production (causing hypoglycemia) and increases sensitivity to histamine (causing vascular permeability and hypotension). PT and other toxins, including *tracheal cytotoxin* and *adenylate cyclase toxin*, are involved in the genesis of protracted cough.

Clinical Features

■ Diphtheria

The disease most often presents as *membranous nasopharyngitis* or *obstructive laryngotracheitis* associated with low-grade fever. Less commonly, cutaneous, vaginal, conjunctival, or otic infection can occur. Serious complications include upper airway obstruction caused by extensive membrane formation, myocarditis, and peripheral neuropathy. The case fatality rate is as high as 10% but is higher in young children and adults >40 years of age. Treatment includes antibiotics as well as equine antitoxin (available through the CDC), which neutralizes circulating toxin and prevents disease progression.

■ Tetanus

Most cases occur within 14 days of injury. Shorter incubation periods have been associated with more heavily contaminated wounds, more severe disease, and worse prognosis. *Generalized tetanus* (lockjaw) initially manifests with trismus, followed within a week by neck stiffness, dysphagia, rigidity of the abdominal muscles, and generalized muscle spasms. Severe spasms, often aggravated by external stimuli, persist for 3 to 4 weeks, and complete recovery may take months. *Neonatal tetanus* results from contamination of the umbilical stump. *Localized tetanus* manifests as muscle spasms in areas contiguous with an infected wound. *Cephalic tetanus* refers to cranial nerve dysfunction associated with infected wounds on the head and neck. Both localized and cephalic tetanus may precede generalized tetanus. Treatment includes tetanus immune globulin, which neutralizes unbound toxin. The case fatality rate is about 10%.

■ Pertussis

Classic *whooping cough* begins with mild upper respiratory tract symptoms (*catarrhal stage*) that last for 1 to 2 weeks. This progresses to severe paroxysms of cough (*paroxysmal stage*), often followed by a characteristic inspiratory whoop, that last for 4 to 6 weeks. Post-tussive emesis is common and the cough can be forceful enough to cause injury—rib fractures and even carotid artery dissections have been reported. Fever is minimal or absent and symptoms wane gradually (*convalescent stage*) over 6 to 10 weeks, giving rise to the colloquial term *the hundred-day cough*. Complications include seizures, pneumonia, and encephalopathy. Pertussis is most severe during the first year of life. During 2000 to 2004, approximately 2500 cases were reported each year in infants <12 months of age—63% were hospitalized for a median duration of 5 days.[1] Almost all deaths occur in young infants; of the 100 pertussis-related deaths reported from 2000 to 2004, 90 were among infants <4 months of age. Disease in infants <6 months of age may be atypical, with prominent apnea and absent whoop. Older children and adults may also have atypical disease, manifest solely as persistent cough, making recognition and treatment difficult. Infection in immunized children and older persons is often mild.

Epidemiology and Transmission

■ Diphtheria

Humans are the only known reservoir of *C diphtheriae*. Patients excrete the organism for 2 to 6 weeks in nasal discharge, from the throat, or from eye or skin lesions. Antibiotic treatment shortens the period of communicability. Transmission results from intimate contact, and illness is more common in crowded living situations. Although *infection* can still occur in immunized persons, *disease* generally does not because any elaborated toxin is neutralized by antibody. Respiratory diphtheria is seen in winter and spring; summer epidemics can occur in warm, moist climates where skin infections are prevalent. Despite dramatic declines in diphtheria in the United States since the 1940s (at the present time, an average of two to three annual cases are reported), toxigenic *C diphtheriae* can still be found in some populations. Diphtheria continues to be a significant cause of morbidity and mortality in developing countries.

■ Tetanus

Tetanus is not transmissible from person to person. Spores of *C tetani* are ubiquitous in the environment, especially where there is soil contaminated with excreta. Wounds, recognized or unrecognized, are where the organism multiplies and elaborates toxin. Contaminated wounds, those that result from deep puncture, and those with devitalized tissue are at greatest risk. Disease occurs worldwide but is more frequent in warmer climates and during warmer months, in part because contaminated wounds are more common. In 2003, the number of reported cases in the United States reached a low of 20. Neonatal tetanus is rare in the United States but common in developing countries, where pregnant women may not be fully immunized and nonsterile umbilical cord-care practices are followed.

■ Pertussis

Humans are the only known hosts for *B pertussis*. Transmission occurs through respiratory droplets and direct contact with respiratory secretions, and acquisition rates approach 80% in susceptible household contacts. Patients are most contagious during the catarrhal stage, before the onset of paroxysms; communicability then diminishes rapidly but may persist for ≥ 3 weeks after onset of cough. Antibiotic therapy decreases infectivity and may limit spread. Asymptomatic infection has been demonstrated but may not be a significant factor in transmission.

Pertussis is a common cause of prolonged-cough illness. For example, one study showed that 26% of university students with cough for ≥6 days had pertussis.[2] Many cases go unrecognized and untreated, and chemoprophylaxis of contacts does not take place, facilitating persistence and spread through communities. In fact, older people in the environment—parents, older siblings, non-household adults—are the most important source of transmission to young infants.[3] Nearly 26,000 cases of pertussis were reported in 2004, the highest number since 1959[4]; by 2007, the number of cases had fallen to around 10,000.[5] The actual annual disease burden probably exceeds 1 million[6]; in fact, about 1% of adolescents and young adults per year experience pertussis, although only 1 in 6 is symptomatic.[7] The *incidence* of disease—approximately 100 cases per 100,000—is highest among very young infants,[8] and hospitalization rates approach 240 per 100,000.[9] However, the greatest number of reported cases occurs among adolescents and young adults. School-based outbreaks are common.

Immunization Program

■ Diphtheria

Introduction of diphtheria toxoid vaccines in the United States in the 1940s led to a dramatic reduction in disease incidence. High levels of vaccination have made diphtheria rare in the United States, and most cases today occur in unvaccinated or inadequately vaccinated persons. However, immunization does not completely eliminate the potential for transmission because it does not prevent carriage of the organism in the nasopharynx or on the skin. The consequences of inadequate immunization at the population level were demonstrated in Russia and other former Soviet countries in the 1990s, when over 150,000 cases and 5000 deaths occurred.

■ Tetanus

Following the introduction of tetanus toxoid vaccines in the United States, the incidence of tetanus declined from 0.4 per 100,000 in 1947 to 0.05 per 100,000 since the mid 1970s. Currently, the majority of tetanus cases occur in persons who have not completed a 3-dose primary series or who have uncertain vaccination histories. From 1998 to 2000, only one death is known to have occurred in an individual who had completed a primary immunization series; in this case, however, the last dose of tetanus toxoid was 11 years before the onset of illness. In contrast, 19 deaths occurred in persons who had not completed a primary series or who had unknown vaccination histories. Because naturally acquired immunity to tetanus toxin does not occur, universal primary vaccination with appropriately timed boosters is the only way to protect persons in all age groups.

■ Pertussis

After the introduction of universal infant immunization in the 1940s, the number of cases dramatically declined; between 1980 and 2004, however, there was a dramatic *increase* in cases, making pertussis the only disease preventable by a routinely recommended vaccine that was on the rise. During this time, from 1991 to 1996, the whole-cell pertussis vaccine was gradually replaced by acellular vaccines, which were more effective and less reactogenic.[10] Some of the resurgence in reported pertussis cases was due to better diagnostic testing (eg, the use of PCR) and increased case-finding, but an important factor also was *waning immunity*. Protection from childhood immunization—and even from natural infection, for that matter—wanes after about 5 to 10 years. With the approval of Tdap vaccines for adolescents and adults in 2005, booster immunization became a possibility and, along with that, the opportunity to reduce disease in that age group as well as to impact a reservoir of pertussis in the community. The experience in Canada validated this approach— adolescent booster immunization was started there in 2000, and overall cases of pertussis steadily declined.[11] In 2006, Tdap was recommended for all adolescents and adults in the United States.[1,12] Recommendations for immunization of pregnant and postpartum women were published in 2008.[13]

Vaccines

Characteristics of the diphtheria, tetanus, and pertussis vaccines licensed in the United States are given in **Tables 10.1** and **10.2**. These vaccines contain diphtheria, tetanus, and pertussis toxins that are chemically treated to render them nontoxic (toxoids) but still immunogenic, as well as other physically purified bacterial subunits, such as PRN, FHA, and FIM, some of which are also chemically modified.

Efficacy and/or Immunogenicity

Essentially 100% of persons who receive a series of any of the available diphtheria or tetanus toxoid-containing vaccines achieve protective antibody levels. The acellular pertussis vaccines have not been compared directly in head-to-head clinical trials, but efficacy estimates overlap enough so as to consider the products equivalent in terms of protection.

Tripedia was studied in trials in Sweden and Germany. In the Swedish trial involving 1389 infants who received 2 doses, efficacy was estimated at 81% for culture-confirmed cases with coughing spasms ≥21 days. In a German case-control study involving 16,780 children, 75% of whom had received Tripedia,

TABLE 10.1 — Diphtheria, Tetanus, and Pertussis Vaccines

	Adacel	Boostrix	Daptacel[a]	Infanrix[b]	Tripedia[c]
Trade name					
Abbreviation	Tdap	Tdap	DTaP	DTaP	DTaP
Manufacturer/distributor	Sanofi Pasteur	GlaxoSmithKline	Sanofi Pasteur	GlaxoSmithKline	Sanofi Pasteur
Type of vaccine	Inactivated, purified subunits and toxoids	Inactivated, purified subunits and toxoids	Inactivated, purified subunits and toxoids	Inactivated, purified subunits and toxoids	Inactivated, purified subunits and toxoids
Composition:					
Diphtheria toxoid	2 Lf units	2.5 Lf units	15 Lf units	25 Lf units	6.7 Lf units
Tetanus toxoid	5 Lf units	5 Lf units	5 Lf units	10 Lf units	5 Lf units
Inactivated pertussis toxin	2.5 mcg	8 mcg	10 mcg	25 mcg	23.4 mcg
Filamentous hemagglutinin	5 mcg	8 mcg	5 mcg	25 mcg	23.4 mcg
Pertactin	3 mcg	2.5 mcg	3 mcg	8 mcg	—
Fimbriae types 2 and 3	5 mcg	—	5 mcg	—	—
Adjuvant	Aluminum phosphate (0.33 mg aluminum)	Aluminum hydroxide (≤0.39 mg aluminum)	Aluminum phosphate (0.33 mg aluminum)	Aluminum hydroxide (≤0.625 mg aluminum)	Aluminum potassium sulphate (≤0.17 mg aluminum)
Preservative	None	None	None	None	None

Excipients and contaminants:					
Formaldehyde	≤5 mcg	≤100 mcg	≤5 mcg	≤100 mcg	≤100 mcg
Glutaraldehyde	≤50 ng	—	≤50 ng	—	—
2-phenoxyethanol	3.3 mg	—	3.3 mg	—	—
Polysorbate 80	—	≤100 mcg	—	≤100 mcg	Unspecified amount
Thimerosal	—	—	—	—	≤0.3 mcg mercury
Gelatin	—	—	—	—	Unspecified amount
Latex	None	Tip cap and plunger of prefilled syringe contain dry natural rubber	Vial stopper contains dry natural rubber	Tip cap and plunger of prefilled syringe contain dry natural rubber	Vial stopper contains dry natural rubber
Labeled indications	Booster immunization against diphtheria, tetanus, and pertussis	Booster immunization against diphtheria, tetanus, and pertussis	Prevention of diphtheria, tetanus, and pertussis	Prevention of diphtheria, tetanus, and pertussis	Prevention of diphtheria, tetanus, and pertussis
Labeled ages	11 to 64 years	10 to 64 years	6 weeks to 6 years	6 weeks to 6 years	6 weeks to 6 years
Dose	0.5 mL	0.5 mL	0.5 mL	0.5 mL	0.5 mL
Route of administration	Intramuscular	Intramuscular	Intramuscular	Intramuscular	Intramuscular

Continued

10

273

TABLE 10.1 — *Continued*

	Adacel	Boostrix	Daptacel[a]	Infanrix[b]	Tripedia[c]
Trade name					
Abbreviation	Tdap	Tdap	DTaP	DTaP	DTaP
Labeled schedule	1 dose	1 dose	2, 4, 6, 15 to 20 months, 4 to 6 years of age	2, 4, 6, 15 to 20 months, 4 to 6 years of age	2, 4, 6, 15 to 18 months, 4 to 6 years of age
Recommended schedule	Same	Same	2, 4, 6, 15 to 18 months, 4 to 6 years of age	2, 4, 6, 15 to 18 months, 4 to 6 years of age	Same
How supplied (number in package):					
1-dose vial	(5, 10)	(10)	(1, 5, 10)	(10)	(10)
Prefilled syringe	(5)	(5)	—	(5)	—
Storage	Refrigerate Do not freeze	Refrigerate Do not freeze	Refrigerate Do not freeze	Refrigerate Do not freeze	Refrigerate Do not freeze
Cost per dose ($US, 2009):					
Public	27.52	28.54	13.75	13.75	13.25
Private	37.43	37.55	23.03	20.96	22.35
Reference package insert	January 2009	January 2009	March 2008	July 2009	December 2005

274

[a] A DTaP vaccine similar to Daptacel is also available in combination with Hib and IPV (Pentacel; Sanofi Pasteur); in this case, ActHIB is reconstituted with liquid DTaP-IPV that is packaged with the product.

[b] Infanrix is available in combination with HepB and IPV (Pediarix; GlaxoSmithKline). Pediarix is usually given at 2, 4, and 6 months of age. Infanrix is also available in combination with IPV (Kinrix; GlaxoSmithKline). Kinrix is indicated for the booster dose at 4 to 6 years of age.

[c] Tripedia is also available in combination with Hib (TriHIBit; Sanofi Pasteur); in this case, ActHIB is reconstituted with the liquid Tripedia that is packaged with the product. TriHIBit is indicated only for Dose 4 of DTaP.

TABLE 10.2 — Diphtheria and Tetanus Vaccines[a]

Trade name	Decavac	Diphtheria and Tetanus Toxoids (for Pediatric Use)	Tetanus and Diphtheria Toxoids Adsorbed	Tetanus Toxoid Adsorbed
Abbreviation	Td	DT	Td	TT
Manufacturer/distributor	Sanofi Pasteur	Sanofi Pasteur	MassBiologics[b]	Sanofi Pasteur
Type of vaccine	Inactivated, toxoids	Inactivated, toxoids	Inactivated, toxoids	Inactivated, toxoids
Composition:				
Diphtheria toxoid	2 Lf units	6.7 Lf units	2 Lf units	—
Tetanus toxoid	5 Lf units	5 Lf units	2 Lf units	5 Lf units
Adjuvant	Aluminum potassium sulfate (≤0.28 mg aluminum)	Aluminum potassium sulfate (≤0.17 mg aluminum)	Aluminum (≤0.53 mg aluminum)	Aluminum potassium sulfate (≤0.25 mg aluminum)
Preservative	None	None	None	Thimerosal (25 mcg mercury) or none
Excipients and contaminants:				
Formaldehyde	≤0.02%	≤0.02%	≤0.02%	≤0.02%
Thimerosal	≤0.3 mcg mercury	≤0.3 mcg mercury	≤0.3 mcg mercury	Preservative-free formulation: ≤0.3 mcg mercury

Latex	None	Vial stopper contains dry natural rubber	None	Multidose vial: vial stopper contains dry natural rubber
Labeled indications	Prevention of diphtheria and tetanus	Prevention of diphtheria and tetanus	Prevention of diphtheria and tetanus	Prevention of tetanus
Labeled ages	≥7 years	6 weeks to 6 years	≥7 years	≥7 years
Dose	0.5 mL	0.5 mL	0.5 mL	0.5 mL
Route of administration	Intramuscular	Intramuscular	Intramuscular	Intramuscular
Labeled schedule	2 doses 4 to 8 weeks apart; reinforcing dose 6 to 12 months after Dose 2; booster dose	3 doses 4 to 8 weeks apart; reinforcing dose 6 to 12 months after Dose 3; booster dose	2 doses 4 to 8 weeks apart; reinforcing dose 6 to 12 months after Dose 2; booster dose	2 doses 4 to 8 weeks apart; reinforcing dose 6 to 12 months after Dose 2; booster dose
Recommended schedule	Same	Same	Same	Same
How supplied (number in package)	1-dose vial (10) Prefilled syringe (10)	1-dose vial (10)	1-dose vial (10)	Preservative-free formulation: 1-dose vial (10) Thimerosal-containing formulation: 10-dose vial (1)
Storage	Refrigerate Do not freeze	Refrigerate Do not freeze	Refrigerate Do not freeze	Refrigerate Do not freeze

Continued

277

TABLE 10.2 — *Continued*

Trade name	Decavac	Diphtheria and Tetanus Toxoids (for Pediatric Use)	Tetanus and Diphtheria Toxoids Adsorbed	Tetanus Toxoid Adsorbed
Abbreviation	Td	DT	Td	TT
Cost per dose ($US, 2009):				
Public	18.17	—	15.00	—
Private	19.49	29.00	—	55.00
Reference package insert	December 2005	December 2005	April 2009	December 2005

[a] Tenivac, manufactured by Sanofi Pasteur, is licensed in the United States but not distributed.
[b] Formerly Massachusetts Public Health Biologic Laboratories.

efficacy of 3 doses was estimated at 80%; in this study, pertussis was defined as ≥21 days of cough plus a positive culture or a household contact with a positive culture.

In an Italian trial sponsored by the NIH that enrolled 15,601 infants, 4481 of whom received 3 doses of Infanrix, efficacy against typical pertussis (≥21 days of cough plus culture or serologic confirmation) was 84%. Efficacy against milder disease, defined as >7 days of cough, was 71%. Protection against typical pertussis was sustained to 6 years of age. In a German household contact study involving 22,000 children, Infanrix was 89% effective against typical pertussis and 81% effective against disease with ≥7 days of paroxysmal cough.

In a Swedish trial involving 9829 infants, 2587 of whom received 3 doses of Daptacel, efficacy against typical pertussis was 85%. Efficacy against milder disease, defined as ≥1 day of cough, was 78%. Protection was sustained during the 2-year follow-up period.

Both Tdap vaccines were licensed on the basis of immunogenicity rather than efficacy. In each case, the antibody response to pertussis antigens after a single dose was noninferior to the analogous infant DTaP vaccines, for which efficacy had been previously demonstrated. In a randomized, double blind trial among adolescents and adults, 1391 subjects received an acellular pertussis vaccine containing the same antigens as Boostrix and 1390 received HepA as a control.[6] Efficacy against pertussis was 92%, although there was no difference in the incidence of prolonged cough illness.

Safety

Local pain, swelling, and erythema are common after DTaP administration, reported in up to 40% of vaccinees during the primary series. The rate of local reactions is higher with Dose 4 and Dose 5, and swelling of the entire limb, sometimes accompanied by fever, has been reported. Such reactions are self-limited, resolve without sequelae, and are *not* contraindications to further doses.[14] Clinically significant fever is reported in <5% of DTaP recipients.

Tdap appears to be slightly more painful than Td, with local pain and/or tenderness in up to 75% of vaccinees (60% to 70% for Td); swelling and erythema occur in around 20% of recipients of either Tdap or Td. Fever occurs in <5%. In a large Vaccine Safety Datalink study, the risk of medically attended local reactions was 2.6 per 10,000 vaccinations.[15]

- *Contraindications for DTaP and Tdap*
  - Allergic reaction to previous dose of vaccine or any vaccine component (risk of recurrent allergic reaction)

- Encephalopathy within 7 days of receiving a pertussis-containing vaccine (risk of recurrent encephalopathy [causality not established] and difficulty distinguishing illness from vaccine reaction)
- *Contraindications for DT, Td, and TT*
  - Allergic reaction to previous dose of vaccine or any vaccine component (risk of recurrent allergic reaction)
- *Precautions for DTaP*
  - Moderate or severe acute illness (difficulty distinguishing illness from vaccine reaction)
  - Evolving neurologic disorder, uncontrolled epilepsy, infantile spasms, encephalopathy, seizures that have not been evaluated, and a neurological event between doses (risk of neurologic deterioration [causality not established] and difficulty distinguishing illness from vaccine reaction)
  - Any of these conditions after receiving a DTaP vaccine
    - Otherwise unexplained fever ≥105°F (40.5°C) within 48 hours (risk of recurrent fever)
    - Collapse or shock-like state (hypotonic hyporesponsive episode) within 48 hours (risk of recurrent reaction)
    - Persistent, inconsolable crying lasting ≥3 hours within 48 hours (risk of recurrent reaction)
    - Seizure with or without fever occurring within 72 hours (risk of recurrent seizure)
  - Personal history of Guillain-Barré syndrome within 6 weeks of receiving a tetanus toxoid-containing vaccine (risk of recurrent Guillain-Barré syndrome; family history not relevant)
  - Severe local (Arthus-type) reaction to previous dose of tetanus and/or diphtheria toxoid-containing vaccine in the last 10 years (risk of recurrent reaction)
- *Precautions for Tdap*
  - Moderate or severe acute illness (difficulty distinguishing illness from vaccine reaction)
  - Progressive neurologic disorder (including encephalopathy), uncontrolled epilepsy, or unstable neurological condition (including cerebrovascular events) (risk of neurologic deterioration [causality not established] and difficulty distinguishing illness from vaccine reaction)
  - Personal history of Guillain-Barré syndrome within 6 weeks of receiving a tetanus toxoid-containing vaccine (risk of recurrent Guillain-Barré syndrome; family history not relevant)
  - Severe local (Arthus-type) reaction to previous dose of tetanus and/or diphtheria toxoid-containing vaccine in the last 10 years (risk of recurrent reaction)

- *Precautions for DT, Td, and TT*
  - Moderate or severe acute il'
    illness from vaccine react'
  - Guillain-Barré syndron.
    a tetanus toxoid-containin
    Guillain-Barré syndrome; fam
  - Severe local (Arthus-type) react.
    tetanus and/or diphtheria toxoid-con.
    last 10 years (risk of recurrent reaction)

Recommendations

All persons should be vaccinated against diphtheria, tu
and pertussis, and immunity should be maintained through boo
immunization. The primary series of DTaP consists of doses a
2, 4, 6, and 15 to 18 months of age; Dose 4 may be given at 12
to 14 months of age if ≥6 months have elapsed since Dose 3 and
the child is unlikely to return at 15 to 18 months of age. A booster
dose of DTaP is given at 4 to 6 years of age (this is optional if
Dose 4 was given at ≥4 years of age), and while there is a preference to use the same brand of DTaP for all 5 doses, any brand may
be used if this is not feasible. An additional booster in the form
of Tdap is given at 11 to 12 years of age. If contraindications to
pertussis immunization exist, DT may be used for children and
Td may be used for adolescents. However, if pertussis vaccination
is deferred during the first year of life because of the possibility
of an evolving neurologic condition, DT should not be given
because the risk of diphtheria or tetanus is very low. By 1 year of
age, if the neurologic condition is deemed to be nonprogressive,
the DTaP series may be initiated; if the condition *is* progressive,
the series should be given as DT.

Children who have had well-documented pertussis (ie, laboratory confirmed or linked to a confirmed case) may not need
further pertussis immunization until they reach adolescence and
become eligible for the booster dose of Tdap. However, since the
duration of protection from natural disease is unknown and there
is no harm in continuing the vaccine series, it makes practical
sense to do so unless there are contraindications. Patients who
have had diphtheria or tetanus should still be immunized because
natural infection does not confer immunity (the amount of toxin
is too small to induce effective immune responses).

All persons 11 to 64 years of age who have never had a dose
of Tdap should have one. As a matter of routine, the dose should
be given at 11 to 12 years of age, in place of the historically
recommended dose of Td. Tdap may be given at the same time
as MCV4 and HPV vaccine. The AAP recommends a minimum
interval of 1 month between MCV4-D and Tdap if they are not

...e day; the ACIP does not recommend a minimum

...iven at 11 to 12 years of age, Tdap should be given at ...available opportunity, provided enough time has elapsed ...e last tetanus toxoid-containing vaccine (the risk of local ...ns increases when too many doses of tetanus toxoid are ...too close together). The manufacturers of Tdap recommend ...nimum interval of 5 years between the last dose of a tetanus ...oid-containing vaccine and a dose of Tdap. However, there are ...ta supporting the safety of intervals as short as 2 years, and in ...ruth there is no absolute minimum interval—Tdap may be given regardless of when the last tetanus toxoid-containing vaccine was received. Giving it earlier than 5 years should be considered when the risk of pertussis or its complications (in the individual or his or her contacts) is elevated (eg, outbreak situations, household exposure, chronic pulmonary and neurologic conditions, people who have close contact with infants <12 months of age, health care personnel, women who may become pregnant).

As a matter of routine, Tdap should replace the next scheduled 10-year Td booster for adults. For adolescents and adults who have not had a complete series (at least 3 doses) of tetanus or diphtheria toxoid vaccines, Tdap should be given followed by 2 doses of Td at least 4 weeks apart. Tdap should be used in place of Td for wound management for all persons who have not previously had a dose.

Postpartum women who have never received Tdap should receive a dose before discharge from the hospital. The recommended interval since the last dose of Td is 2 years, but shorter intervals may be used if there is no history of moderate-to-severe adverse reactions to previous doses of tetanus and diphtheria toxoid-containing vaccines. The dose of Tdap "resets the clock" for the next decennial dose of tetanus and diphtheria toxoid vaccines.

Pregnant women should have a tetanus and diphtheria booster if ≥10 years have elapsed since the previous Td. For those women who are likely to be tetanus immune, Td may be deferred during pregnancy and Tdap given postpartum (however, giving Tdap during pregnancy is also acceptable). Tetanus immunity is likely in the following situations:

- Women ≤30 years of age who received a complete childhood series of tetanus toxoid-containing vaccine and at least 1 booster as an adolescent or adult (the primary series in childhood consists of 4 or 5 doses, and in adolescents and adults, it consists of 3 doses)
- Women >30 years of age who received a complete childhood series and at least 2 boosters, or who received a primary series as an adolescent or adult
- Tetanus antibody level ≥0.10 IU/mL

The following should be taken into account when deciding whether or not a pregnant woman should receive Tdap during pregnancy:

- Tdap should be strongly considered if there is an increased risk of pertussis (the AAP favors giving Tdap to pregnant adolescents for this reason).
- There are no data on safety, immunogenicity, pregnancy outcomes, and protection of the infant against pertussis.
- There is the theoretic possibility that transplacental antibodies could interfere with infant immunization.
- If given, the second or third trimester is preferred.

The use of tetanus toxoid-containing vaccines and tetanus immune globulin for wound management is summarized in **Table 10.3**.

10

TABLE 10.3 — Tetanus Prophylaxis in Wound Management

Primary Series of Tetanus-Toxoid Vaccine	Age (Years)	Time Since Last Dose of Vaccine	Clean, Minor Wounds		Tetanus-Prone Wounds[a]	
			Vaccine	TIG[b]	Vaccine	TIG[b]
Complete[c]	≤6	<5 years	No	No	No	No
		≥5 years	DTaP[d,e]	No	DTaP[e]	No
	7 to 10	<5 years	No	No	No	No
		≥5 years	No	No	Td[f]	No
	≥11	<5 years	No	No	No	No
		≥5 years	Tdap[g]	No	Tdap[h]	No
Unimmunized, unknown, incomplete, or HIV-infected[i]	≤6	Not relevant	DTaP[d,e]	No	DTaP[e]	Yes
	7 to 10		Td[f]	No	Td[f]	Yes
	≥11		Tdap[g]	No	Tdap[h]	Yes

[a] Includes puncture, avulsion, crush, necrotic, and burn wounds; frostbite; and wounds contaminated with dirt, feces, soil, or saliva. Wounds should be cleaned, necrotic tissue debrided, and foreign material removed.

[b] The dose of TIG is 250 units given intramuscularly. Immune globulin intravenous can be used if TIG is not available. Equine tetanus antitoxin is not available in the United States. Vaccine and TIG should be given at separate sites.

[c] The primary series is considered complete if the patient has received ≥3 doses of an adsorbed (not fluid) tetanus toxoid. HIV-infected persons should be considered *unimmunized* even if they have received the vaccine series.

[d] A booster dose of DTaP is routinely indicated for all children at 4 to 6 years of age, so a dose should be given to children who have not received a routine booster, even for clean, minor wounds (vaccination here is for catch-up, not wound management).

[e] Use DT if pertussis immunization is contraindicated.

[f] Td is preferred but tetanus toxoid can be used; only adsorbed products are indicated. One brand of Tdap (Boostrix) is licensed down to 10 years of age and may be used instead of Td.

g One dose of Tdap is routinely indicated for all adolescents and adults, so a dose should be given (if not previously received) even for clean, minor wounds (vaccination here is for catch-up, not wound management). Use Td if pertussis immunization is contraindicated.

h If Tdap is not available or has been given previously, Td (or tetanus toxoid, if Td is not available) should be used. No Tdap is licensed for use in patients >64 years of age. Use Td if pertussis immunization is contraindicated.

i For infants <6 months of age who have not received the 3-dose primary series, decisions about the use of TIG should be based on the mother's vaccination history.

REFERENCES

1. Broder KR, et al. *MMWR*. 2006;55(RR-3):1-34.
2. Mink CM, et al. *Clin Infect Dis*. 1992;14:464-471.
3. Wendelboe AM, et al. *Pediatr Infect Dis J*. 2007;26:293-299.
4. Jajosky RA, et al. *MMWR*. 2006;53:1-79.
5. Hall-Baker PA, et al. *MMWR*. 2009;56:1-94.
6. Ward JI, et al. *N Engl J Med*. 2005;353:1555-1563.
7. Ward JI, et al. *Clin Infect Dis*. 2006;43:151-157.
8. Tanaka M, et al. *JAMA*. 2003;290:2968-2975.
9. Cortese MM, et al. *Pediatrics*. 2008;121:484-492.
10. CDC. *MMWR*. 1997;46(RR-7):1-25.
11. Greenberg DP, et al. *Pediatr Infect Dis J*. 2009;28:521-528.
12. Kretsinger K, et al. *MMWR*. 2006;55(RR-17):1-37.
13. Murphy TV, et al. *MMWR*. 2008;57(RR-4):1-51.
14. Rennels MB, et al. *Pediatr Infect Dis J*. 2008;27:464-465.
15. Jackson LA, et al. *Vaccine*. 2009;27:4912-4916.

11

Haemophilus influenzae Type b

The Pathogen

H influenzae type b is an aerobic gram-negative bacterium that appears as pleomorphic coccobacilli on Gram's stain. The organism produces a polysaccharide capsule that contributes to virulence by inhibiting complement-mediated lysis and phagocytosis by neutrophils. Colonization of the nasopharynx is facilitated by factors that mediate adherence to respiratory epithelium and interfere with ciliary clearance, as well as immune evasion mechanisms such as IgA1 protease. Disease results from bacteremia and spread to distant sites like the meninges.

Clinical Features

The most common forms of invasive *H influenzae* type b disease are *meningitis, bacteremia, epiglottitis, pneumonia, arthritis,* and *periorbital* and *buccal cellulitis*. Meningitis is the most common clinical manifestation, accounting for 50% to 65% of cases in the prevaccine era. Hallmark presenting features include fever, altered mental status, and stiff neck. The mortality rate is 2% to 5%, even with appropriate antimicrobial therapy, and neurologic sequelae occur in 15% to 30% of survivors. Osteomyelitis and pericarditis are less common. Otitis media and acute bronchitis due to *H influenzae* are generally caused by nontypeable (nonencapsulated) strains.

Epidemiology and Transmission

Humans are the only natural hosts and transmission occurs by direct person-to-person contact or via respiratory droplets. The organism does not survive on fomites. Asymptomatic nasopharyngeal colonization was seen in 2% to 5% of children in the prevaccine era, but widespread use of *H influenzae* conjugate vaccine (Hib) has resulted in much lower colonization rates. Invasive disease now is extremely rare. *H influenzae* type b disease was more frequent in boys, African-Americans, Alaska Eskimos, Apache and Navajo Indians, child care center attendees, children living in overcrowded conditions, and children who were not breast-fed. Unimmunized children, particularly those <4 years of age who were in prolonged close (eg, household) contact with an infected child, were at high risk. Other factors predisposing to invasive infection included sickle cell disease, asplenia, HIV infection, certain immunodeficiency syndromes, and malignant neoplasms.

Many laboratories are now relatively inexperienced in identifying *H influenzae* type b, and many isolates that are labeled as such turn out to be other serotypes or nontypeable strains when subjected to molecular analysis.

Immunization Program

Prior to the introduction of routine childhood immunization, *H influenzae* type b was a major cause of invasive bacterial infection in the United States, with an estimated 12,000 cases of meningitis and 8000 other invasive syndromes annually. A striking one out of every 200 children in the first 5 years of life developed invasive *H influenzae* type b infection, with peak incidence in 6- to 12-month-olds. In high-risk populations, disease rates were even higher.

After 1991, when Hib was recommended for all infants,[1] the incidence of invasive disease in infants and young children declined by >99% (see **Table 1.5**). This remarkable reduction in disease burden was partly due to the ability of conjugate vaccines to reduce nasopharyngeal carriage, leading to reduced rates of exposure and infection even in those not immunized (this is an example of herd immunity; see *Chapter 1: Introduction to Vaccinology—Herd Immunity*). The standing recommendations for Hib were first published in 1993[2]; the only recent changes have been updates on available products[3] and use of the vaccine for high-risk persons >5 years of age. Today, invasive *H influenzae* type b disease is seen primarily in underimmunized children and infants too young to have completed the primary series; in 2008, attention focused on a resurgence of cases in infants and children who were intentionally not immunized because of parental concerns about vaccine safety.[4]

Vaccines

Characteristics of the Hib vaccines licensed in the United States are given in **Table 11.1**. Each of these is a protein-polysaccharide conjugate, and two are available in combination with other antigens.

Efficacy and/or Immunogenicity

Efficacy of Hib-OMP (PedvaxHIB) was first demonstrated in Navajo infants who had very high rates of invasive infection. After a primary regimen given at 2 and 4 months of age, 91% of infants had anti-PRP antibody levels >0.15 mcg/mL (the so-called *short term* correlate of protection) and 60% had levels >1 mcg/mL (the so-called *long-term* correlate of protection), and efficacy at 15 to 18 months of age was 93%. In infants drawn from the general US population who received the 2-dose primary series, 97% achieved anti-PRP antibody levels >0.15 mcg/mL and 80%, >1 mcg/mL; the proportions after a booster at 12 to 15 months were 99% and 95%, respectively. Hib-OMP is the only vaccine that induces significant antibody levels after a single injection in infants <6 months of age.

Licensure of ActHIB (Hib-T) was based on immunogenicity that was comparable to that of the other licensed products. Overall, about 90% of infants achieve anti-PRP antibody levels of ≥1 mcg/mL after the primary series of 3 doses, and 98% achieve this level after a booster dose.

Hiberix (Hib-T) has been used outside the United States for both primary series and booster dose since 1996. Immunogenicity studies conducted in Germany and Canada involving slightly over 200 subjects led to licensure for the booster dose only in the United States in 2009. In these studies, the proportion of subjects with anti-PRP antibody levels ≥0.15 mcg/mL went from 71.4%-77.8% to 100% one month after a booster dose, and the proportion with anti-PRP antibody levels ≥1.0 mcg/mL went from 12.7%-35.7% to 97.6%-100%.

Children ≥15 months of age respond well to a single dose of any of the vaccines.

Safety

Local reactions such as redness, swelling and pain occur in 5% to 30% of recipients, but typically are mild and last <24 hours. Systemic reactions, such as high fever and irritability, are infrequent. Serious adverse events such as anaphylaxis are rare.

• *Contraindications*
  – Allergic reaction to previous dose of vaccine or any vaccine component (risk of recurrent allergic reaction)
  – Age <6 weeks (risk of induction of immune tolerance)
• *Precautions*
  – Moderate or severe acute illness (difficulty distinguishing illness from vaccine reaction)

Recommendations

All infants should be vaccinated against *H influenzae*. The primary series for Hib-T consists of doses at 2, 4, and 6 months of age; the primary series for Hib-OMP consists of doses at 2 and 4 months of age. For both of these vaccines, booster doses are given at 12 to 15 months of age. Hiberix may be used for the booster

TABLE 11.1 — *H influenzae* Type b Vaccines[a]

	ActHIB[b,c]	PedvaxHIB[b,d]	Hiberix[b]
Trade name	ActHIB[b,c]	PedvaxHIB[b,d]	Hiberix[b]
Abbreviation	Hib-T	Hib-OMP	Hib-T
Manufacturer/distributor	Sanofi Pasteur	Merck	GlaxoSmithKline
Type of vaccine	Inactivated, engineered subunit	Inactivated, engineered subunit	Inactivated, engineered subunit
Composition	Polyribosylribitol phosphate (10 mcg) conjugated to tetanus toxoid (24 mcg)	Polyribosylribitol phosphate (7.5 mcg) conjugated to *N meningitidis* serogroup B (strain B11) outer membrane protein (125 mcg)	Polyribosylribitol phosphate (10 mcg) conjugated to tetanus toxoid (25 mcg)
Adjuvant	None	Aluminum hydroxide (0.225 mg aluminum)	None
Preservative	None	None	None
Excipients and contaminants	Sucrose (8.5%)	Sodium chloride (0.9%)	Lactose (12.6 mg) Residual formaldehyde (≤0.5 mcg)
Latex	Vial stopper contains dry natural rubber	None	None
Labeled indications	Prevention of invasive *H influenzae* type b disease	Prevention of invasive *H influenzae* type b disease	Booster immunization against invasive *H influenzae* type b disease
Labeled ages	2 to 18 months	2 to 71 months	15 months to 4 years

Dose	0.5 mL	0.5 mL	0.5 mL
Route of administration	Intramuscular	Intramuscular	Intramuscular
Labeled schedule	2, 4, 6, 12 to 15 months of age	2, 4, 12 to 15 months of age[e]	15 months of age
Recommended schedule	Same	Same	12 to 15 months of age
How supplied (number in package)	1-dose vial (5), lyophilized, with diluent	1-dose vial (10)	1-dose vial (10), lyophilized, with diluent in prefilled syringes
Storage	Vaccine: Refrigerate Do not freeze Diluent: Refrigerate Do not freeze Reconstituted vaccine: Use within 24 hours	Refrigerate Do not freeze	Vaccine: Refrigerate Do not freeze Protect from light Diluent: Refrigerate or controlled room temperature Do not freeze Reconstituted vaccine: Refrigerate Do not freeze Use within 24 hours
Cost per dose ($US, 2009):			
Public	8.66	11.29	8.66
Private	22.83	22.77	22.83
Reference package insert	December 2005	January 2001	August 2009

11

Continued

TABLE 11.1 — *Continued*

---

[a] ProHIBit (Hib-D; Connaught) and HibTITER (Hib-CRM; Pfizer [formerly Wyeth]) are no longer available.

[b] Hib-T and Hib-OMP are considered interchangeable in the primary series. However, if either the 2-month or 4-month dose is given as Hib-T, a dose of either product must be given at 6 months. If the first 2 doses are Hib-OMP, the 6-month dose is omitted. Hib-OMP and Hib-T are considered interchangeable for the booster dose.

[c] ActHIB is also available in combination with DTaP (TriHIBit; Sanofi Pasteur); in this case, ActHIB is reconstituted with liquid DTaP (Tripedia) that is packaged with the product. TriHIBit is indicated only for the fourth dose of DTaP at 15 to 18 months of age. ActHIB is also available in combination with DTaP and IPV (Pentacel; Sanofi Pasteur); in this case, ActHIB is reconstituted with liquid DTaP-IPV that is packaged with the product. Pentacel is usually given at 2, 4, 6, and 15 to 18 months of age.

[d] Hib-OMP is also available in combination with HepB (Comvax; Merck). Comvax is usually given at 2, 4, and 12 to 15 months of age.

[e] The primary series for Hib-OMP consists of only 2 doses.

---

dose at 12 to 15 months of age (be aware that the package insert gives a minimum age of 15 months). Previously unimmunized children 15 to 59 months should receive a single dose of ActHIB or PedvaxHIB (Hiberix should not be given as the only Hib dose in a child with no prior Hib doses).

REFERENCES

1. CDC. *MMWR*. 1991;40(RR-1):1-7.
2. CDC. *MMWR*. 1993;42(RR-13):1-15.
3. CDC. *MMWR*. 2009;58:1008-1009.
4. CDC. *MMWR*. 2009;58(3):58-60.

11

12
Hepatitis A

The Pathogen

Hepatitis A virus (HAV) is a small, nonenveloped, single-stranded RNA virus in the Picornaviridae family. There is only one known serotype. Initial infection occurs in the pharynx and lower gastrointestinal tract, with hematogenous spread to the liver, where the virus replicates in hepatocytes and Kupffer cells (resident macrophages). It is believed that most of the injury to the liver is immune mediated rather than the direct result of viral replication. Virus is excreted in the bile and ultimately shed in the stool. Unlike HBV, HAV does not establish chronic infection and does not cause chronic liver disease.

Clinical Features

Ninety percent of children <5 years of age with HAV infection are asymptomatic, whereas 90% of adults experience symptoms such as jaundice. The incubation period ranges from 15 to 50 days. Onset is usually abrupt, with low-grade fever, myalgia, poor appetite, nausea, vomiting, malaise, and fatigue, followed by dark-colored urine, scleral icterus, pale stools, jaundice, and weight loss. Diarrhea is more common in children. Hepatomegaly, right upper quadrant tenderness, and occasionally splenomegaly or rash may be present. Symptoms generally subside within 3 to 4 weeks, although 10% to 15% of patients experience prolonged or relapsing disease for up to 6 months. Fulminant hepatitis is rare. Extrahepatic manifestations include arthralgias, pruritus, cutaneous vasculitis, cryoglobulinemia, hemophagocytic syndrome, and Guillain-Barré syndrome.

Epidemiology and Transmission

Humans are the only natural hosts and transmission occurs by the fecal-oral route. Peak infectivity occurs during the 2-week period before the onset of jaundice, and infants and children can shed the virus for several months. Since infants and young children often have clinically silent infection and exposure to their feces may unavoidable, they are often the source of infection for adults in households or day care centers. Contaminated water and undercooked food (especially shellfish) are also common sources of transmission—often a food handler somewhere up the line is infected.[1] Transient viremia in a blood donor occasionally leads to transmission through transfusion of blood products.

Hepatitis A is most prevalent in Southeast Asia, Africa, and Latin America. In countries with high endemicity, the infection is usually acquired in childhood, whereas in developed countries many adults have not yet been exposed. Childhood disease often correlates with overcrowding, poor sanitation, limited access to clean water, and inadequate sewage systems. Prior to the institution of a universal immunization program in the United States, the incidence of *disease* was highest among children 5 to 14 years of age, but the incidence of *infection* was highest in those <4 years of age. Infection was more common among American Indians, Alaska Natives, and Hispanics. Disease rates were substantially higher in the western United States; between 1987 and 1997, half of all cases occurred in 11 states west of the Mississippi. The majority of patients in the United States in 2007 (67.7%) had no known risk factor for hepatitis A.[2] The most important *known* risk factor was international travel (17.5% of cases)[3]; other risk factors were sexual or household contact with a case (7.8%), male homosexual activity (5.9%), food- or waterborne outbreaks (6.5%), employment or attendance at a day care center (3.8%), contact with a day care employee or attendee (4.6%), injection drug use (1.2%), and other known contact with a case (9.0%).

Immunization Program

In the prevaccine era, there were 22,000 to 36,000 annual reported cases of hepatitis A and an estimated 271,000 annual HAV infections in the United States. Up to 22% of patients were hospitalized, and the average work lost for these patients was 33 days. Annual direct and indirect costs were as high as $488 million (1997 dollars).

In 1996, HepA was recommended for high-risk groups and children living in communities with the highest rates of infection.[4] In 1999, universal vaccination of all children ≥ 2 years of age was recommended in states, counties, and communities whose average annual reported incidence of hepatitis A was ≥ 20 cases per 100,000 population (at least twice the national average between 1987 and 1997).[5] At the time, those states were Arizona, Alaska, Oregon, New Mexico, Utah, Washington, Oklahoma, South Dakota, Idaho, Nevada, and California. Routine immunization was also considered for children living in areas where the average annual reported incidence was ≥ 10 but <20 cases per 100,000 population; those states were Missouri, Texas, Colorado, Arkansas, Montana, and Wyoming. For areas with high rates of disease, routine vaccination of children beginning at 2 years of age, catch-up vaccination of preschool children, and vaccination of older children (10 to 15 years of age) was recommended.

After these recommendations were instituted, hepatitis A declined dramatically in the United States, a demonstration of the remarkable ability of childhood immunization to prevent disease in an entire population (see *Chapter 1: Introduction to Vaccinology—Herd Immunity* and **Figure 1.6**). In fact, HepA is a model for the benefits of herd immunity effects in immunization programs, more than doubling the expected cost savings compared to direct effects alone.[6] By 2007, there were only 2979 symptomatic cases reported, for an incidence of 1.0 per 100,000, the lowest ever recorded (the estimated number of infections was 25,000).[7] As might have been expected, the disease burden decreased overall and shifted from the West to other regions of the country. In 2006, new age indications for both available vaccines (down to 12 months) made it easier to consider incorporation of HepA into the routine childhood schedule, and the final step in the incremental national strategy to control hepatitis A was taken—the recommendation to immunize all young children.[8] This was seen as creating the foundation for eventual elimination of indigenous transmission.

Recommendations for control of hepatitis A in correctional facilities were issued in 2003,[9] updates on post-exposure prophylaxis and international travel in 2007,[10] and vaccination of contacts of international adoptees in 2009.[11] In 2010, the recommendations for HepA were broadened to include vaccination of anyone who desires protection from the disease.

Vaccines

Characteristics of the hepatitis A vaccines licensed in the United States are given in **Table 12.1**. These are inactivated, whole-virus vaccines made much the same way as was the Salk polio vaccine.

Efficacy and/or Immunogenicity

Nearly 100% of persons who receive 2 doses of either vaccine achieve protective levels of antibody to HAV. Seroconversion rates within 1 month of the first dose exceed 95%. Based on kinetic models of antibody decay, protective antibody may persist for up to 20 years in children and ≥25 years in adults.

The efficacy of Havrix was evaluated in a study of 40,119 school children in Thailand aged 1 to 16 years. Two doses of vaccine (360 ELISA units each) or placebo were administered 1 month apart. Two children in the vaccine group and 32 in the control group developed hepatitis A, indicating an efficacy of approximately 94%. In children 2 to 19 years of age ($N=314$), 1 dose (720 ELISA units) resulted in seroconversion rates of 96.8% to 100%, and 2 doses given 6 months apart resulted in seroconversion rates of 100%. In studies involving over 400 adults, 1 dose (1440 ELISA units) resulted in seroconversion

TABLE 12.1 — Hepatitis A Vaccines

	Havrix[a,b]	Vaqta[b]
Trade name	Havrix[a,b]	Vaqta[b]
Abbreviation	HepA	HepA
Manufacturer/distributor	GlaxoSmithKline	Merck
Type of vaccine	Inactivated, whole agent	Inactivated, whole agent
Composition:[c]		
Virus strain	HM175	CR326F
Propagation	Human diploid (MRC-5) cells	Human diploid (MRC-5) cells
Inactivation	Formalin	Formalin
Antigen content:		
Pediatric/adolescent formulation	720 ELISA units/0.5 mL	25 U/0.5 mL
Adult formulation	1440 ELISA units/mL	50 U/mL
Adjuvant	Aluminum hydroxide (0.25 mg/0.5 mL aluminum)	Aluminum hydroxide (0.225 mg/0.5 mL aluminum)
Preservative	None	None
Excipients and contaminants	Amino acid supplement (0.3%) Phosphate-buffered saline Polysorbate 20 (0.05 mg/mL) Residual MRC-5 cellular proteins ($\leq$5 mcg/mL) Formalin ($\leq$0.1 mg/mL) Neomycin ($\leq$40 ng/mL)	Formaldehyde ($\leq$0.8 mcg/mL) Nonviral protein (<0.1 mcg/mL) DNA ($<4 \times 10^{-6}$ mcg/mL) Bovine albumin ($\leq$0.0001 mcg/mL) Sodium borate (70 mcg/mL) Sodium chloride (0.9%)

Latex	Tip cap and plunger of prefilled syringe contain dry natural rubber	Vial stopper and plunger of prefilled syringe contain dry natural rubber
Labeled indications	Prevention of hepatitis A	Prevention of hepatitis A
Labeled ages	≥12 months	≥12 months
Dose:[d]		
Pediatric (1 to 18 years)	0.5 mL	0.5 mL
Adult (≥19 years)	1.0 mL	1.0 mL
Route of administration	Intramuscular	Intramuscular
Labeled schedule	0, 6 to 12 months	0, 6 to 18 months
Recommended schedule	Same	Same
How supplied (number in package):		
Pediatric/adolescent formulation	1-dose vial (10)	1-dose vial (1, 10)
	Prefilled syringe (5, 10)	Prefilled syringe (6)
Adult formulation	1-dose vial (10)	1-dose vial (1, 10)
	Prefilled syringe (5)	Prefilled syringe (1, 6)
Storage	Refrigerate	Refrigerate
	Do not freeze	Do not freeze

12

Continued

TABLE 12.1 — *Continued*

Trade name	Havrix[a,b]	Vaqta[b]
Abbreviation	HepA	HepA
Cost per dose, pediatric ($US, 2009):		
Public	12.75	13.00
Private	28.74	30.37
Cost per dose, adult ($US, 2009):		
Public	20.59	—
Private	63.10	—
Reference package insert	October 2009	December 2007

[a] Havrix is also available in combination with HepB (Twinrix; GlaxoSmithKline).
[b] Havrix and Vaqta are considered interchangeable.
[c] The units used to measure antigen content for these vaccines are different and cannot be directly compared.
[d] The patient's age at the time of the dose determines which formulation is used.

rates of >96%; 100% of adults ($N=269$) were seropositive 1 month after a booster dose. In children immunized with 2 doses 6 months apart beginning at 11 to 13 months of age ($N=218$), the vaccine response rate was 99%. Persistence of antibody was evaluated in a study of 1016 subjects who had received a 3-dose schedule as adults; 10 years out, 98.3% still had protective levels of antibody.[12]

The efficacy of Vaqta was evaluated in a study of 1037 healthy seronegative children 2 to 16 years of age in Monroe County, New York, a small community with a historically high infection rate.[13] A single dose of vaccine (25 units) or placebo was administered. Beyond the immediate postvaccination period, there were no cases of hepatitis A in the vaccine group and 21 confirmed cases in the placebo group, for an efficacy of 100%. After this study, a subset of vaccinees received a booster dose of vaccine. No cases of hepatitis A occurred among these individuals in the 9 years they were monitored.[14] In Butte County, CA, a mass immunization campaign in children 2 to 12 years of age between 1995 and 2000 resulted in a 93.5% decline in cases in the entire county population (see **Figure 1.6**).[15]

In studies of children 12 to 23 months of age, seroconversion rates were 96% of 471 and 100% of 343, respectively, for 1 or 2 doses of Vaqta (25 units). In studies of children 2 to 18 years of age, seroconversion rates were 97% in 1230 and 100% in 1057, respectively, for 1 or 2 doses (25 units). In studies of adults, seroconversion rates were 95% in 1411 and 99.9% in 1244, respectively, for 1 or 2 doses (50 units).

Safety

Reactions are usually mild and subside within 24 hours. Mild injection-site reactions, including erythema, swelling, pain, or tenderness, occur in 20% to 50% of patients. Systemic reactions, including low-grade fever, malaise, and fatigue, are reported in <10% of vaccinees. No serious adverse events have been reported.

- *Contraindications*
  - Allergic reaction to previous dose of vaccine or any vaccine component (risk of recurrent allergic reaction)
- *Precautions*
  - Moderate or severe acute illness (difficulty distinguishing illness from vaccine reaction)
  - Pregnancy (theoretic risk to the fetus or attribution of birth defects to vaccination, although no deleterious effects from HepA administered during pregnancy have been demonstrated and the risk of adverse fetal effects from an inactivated vaccine is extremely low; it is not clear why pregnancy is listed as a precaution for some inactivated vaccines but not others)

■ **Pre-exposure Prophylaxis**

All children should be vaccinated against hepatitis A during the second year of life. The first dose of HepA is usually given at 12 months of age and the second at 18 to 23 months of age. Vaccination for children 2 to 18 years of age should continue in areas that had catch-up programs in place based on the 1999 recommendations; catch-up vaccination for children 2 to 18 years of age in other communities is optional. Anyone who wants protection from hepatitis A should be vaccinated.

The following persons are at increased risk for hepatitis A and *should be routinely vaccinated*:

- Persons traveling to or working in countries with high or intermediate endemicity
- Persons (eg, household members) who will be in close contact with an adoptee from an endemic country during the first 60 days after arrival (the first dose should be given at least 2 weeks before arrival)
- Men who have sex with men (the risk is thought to relate to fecal-oral contact)
- Injection and noninjection illegal drugs users (transmission probably occurs through percutaneous and fecal-oral routes)
- Persons who work with HAV-infected primates or with HAV in a research laboratory
- Persons who have clotting-factor disorders (outbreaks presumably due to blood from donors who were viremic at the time of donation were reported in the early 1990s)
- Persons who have chronic liver disease, including those who are waiting for or have received liver transplants (these persons are particularly susceptible to severe disease)

Vaccination *should be considered* for juveniles in correctional facilities. For most travelers to endemic areas, vaccination is now preferred to the use of immune globulin (see *Chapter 6: Vaccination in Special Circumstances—Travel*).

Routine vaccination is *not* considered necessary for the following based on occupation:

- Health care workers
- Persons attending or working in child care centers
- Caretakers in institutions for the developmentally challenged
- Persons working in correctional facilities
- Persons working in waste management
- Food service workers, unless recommended by state or local authorities

■ **Postexposure Prophylaxis**

In the past, prophylaxis with immune globulin was recommended for susceptible persons after exposure to hepatitis A.

However, immune globulin is expensive, relatively painful, difficult to obtain, and only offers transient protection. A randomized, double-blind trial results published in 2007, as well as experience from other countries, suggest that postexposure vaccination also is effective.[16] The recommendations below are for *unimmunized persons* exposed to hepatitis A (persons who received at least 1 dose of vaccine at least 1 month before exposure are considered immune). Prophylaxis should be initiated as soon as possible after exposure, but preferably within 2 weeks (efficacy beyond 2 weeks is questionable). Only monovalent HepA should be used in the following situations:

- *12 months to 40 years of age*: Vaccination is preferred.
- *>40 years of age*: Immune globulin (0.02 mL/kg intramuscularly) is preferred but vaccine can be given if immune globulin is not available. If the person has other reasons to be vaccinated with HepA, he or she should receive a dose of the vaccine simultaneously (at a separate site) and receive the second dose at the appropriate interval.
- *<12 months of age, immunocompromised individuals, those with chronic liver disease, and those in whom vaccination is contraindicated*: Immune globulin (0.02 mL/kg intramuscularly) should be given. Immunocompromised individuals and those with chronic liver disease should receive a dose of the vaccine simultaneously (at a separate site) and receive the second dose at the appropriate interval.

12

The following situations constitute a high risk of exposure to hepatitis A and warrant postexposure prophylaxis (if the persons were not previously immunized):

- Household and sexual contacts of a case (consider also for persons with ongoing close personal contact such as occurs with regular babysitting)
- Persons who have shared illicit drugs with a case
- Staff members and attendees at day care centers and day care homes if there has been one or more case in employees or attendees, or if two or more cases occur in the households of attendees. If the center does not have children who are in diapers, prophylaxis should be given only to classroom contacts of the index case. If three or more families are affected, prophylaxis should be considered for members of households that have children in diapers who attend the center.
- Other food handlers at an establishment where there is an index case in a food handler. Prophylaxis of patrons should be considered if the index case could have contaminated food because of diarrhea and poor hygienic practices, and only if the patrons can be identified and treated within 2 weeks of exposure. Institutional cafeterias might represent a higher risk to patrons than other establishments. In a common-source

outbreak, prophylaxis should not be given once cases begin to occur since by then, the 2-week window for effective prophylaxis will have been exceeded.
• Prophylaxis is indicated in the school or hospital setting only if transmission from an index case has been demonstrated.

REFERENCES

1. Fiore AE. *Clin Infect Dis*. 2004;38:705-715.
2. Daniels D, et al. *MMWR*. 2009;58(SS-3):1-27.
3. Mutsch M, et al. *Clin Infect Dis*. 2006;42:490-497.
4. CDC. *MMWR*. 1996;45(RR-15):1-30.
5. CDC. *MMWR*. 1999;48(RR-12):1-37.
6. Armstrong GL, et al. *Pediatrics*. 2007;119:e22-e29.
7. Wasley A, et al. *MMWR*. 2008;57(SS-2):1-24.
8. CDC. *MMWR*. 2006;55(RR-7):1-23.
9. Weinbaum C, et al. *MMWR*. 2003;52(RR-1):1-36.
10. CDC. *MMWR*. 2007;56:1080-1084.
11. CDC. *MMWR*. 2009;58:1006-1007.
12. Rendi-Wagner P, et al. *Vaccine*. 2007;25:927-931.
13. Werzberger A, et al. *N Engl J Med*. 1992;327:453-457.
14. Werzberger A, et al. *Vaccine*. 2002;20:1699-1701.
15. Averhoff F, et al. *JAMA*. 2001;286:2968-2973.
16. Victor JC, et al. *N Engl J Med*. 2007;357:1685-1694.

13 Hepatitis B

The Pathogen

Hepatitis B virus (HBV) is a nonenveloped, partially double-stranded DNA virus in the Hepadnaviridae family. The virus infects hepatocytes but is not directly cytopathic; instead, damage occurs through the action of cytotoxic T-cells directed against virus-infected hepatocytes.[1] Immune tolerance leads to persistent infection in some individuals; hallmark features include low-grade chronic hepatitis and HBsAg (a surface protein of the virion that is overproduced) in the serum, as well as an increased lifetime risk of hepatocellular carcinoma. One factor that contributes to carcinogenesis is chronic inflammation, with attendant regeneration, fibrosis, and the accumulation of cellular mutations.[2] Another factor is the random integration of HBV DNA into the host chromosome, resulting in mutations that either inactivate tumor suppressor genes or activate oncogenes. Finally, much attention has focused on the viral X protein, which can upregulate the expression of host cell oncogenes.

13

Clinical Features

The incubation period ranges from 6 weeks to 6 months and averages 120 days.[3] The clinical course of acute infection is indistinguishable from that of other types of viral hepatitis. While infants and children are usually asymptomatic, clinical signs and symptoms occur in about 50% of adults. The prodromal phase usually lasts 3 to 10 days and is characterized by the insidious onset of malaise, anorexia, nausea, vomiting, right upper-quadrant abdominal pain, fever, headache, myalgia, rash, arthralgia, arthritis, and dark urine. The icteric phase, which usually lasts from 1 to 3 weeks, is characterized by jaundice, elevated hepatic transaminases, light or gray-colored stools, liver tenderness, and hepatomegaly (splenomegaly is less common). During convalescence, malaise and fatigue may persist for weeks to months, while jaundice, anorexia, and other symptoms disappear.

Most acute HBV infections in adults result in complete recovery, with disappearance of HBsAg from the blood and the production of HBsAb (antibody directed against HBsAg), which provides for lasting immunity. However, 90% of infants, 30% of young children, and <5% of adults with acute infection become persistently infected (so-called *chronic carriers*). Premature death from cirrhosis, liver failure, or hepatocellular carcinoma occurs in

25% of those who become persistently infected in childhood and in 15% of those who become persistently infected after childhood.

Epidemiology and Transmission

Humans are the only natural hosts and transmission occurs by contact with contaminated secretions, including semen, vaginal secretions, blood, and saliva; through percutaneous inoculation (eg, accidental needlesticks or sharing of needles with infected people); or by maternal-neonatal transmission (the risk is about 10% if the mother is a chronic carrier). Almost half of the world's population lives in areas where ≥8% of the population is persistently infected; in China, southeast Asia, most of Africa, most of the Pacific Islands, parts of the Middle East, and the Amazon basin, 8% to 15% of the population are chronic carriers, and most persons are infected at birth or in early childhood. The lifetime risk of infection in these areas exceeds 60%. An estimated 2 billion people worldwide have been infected with HBV and 350 million are chronic hepatitis B carriers.

In the United States as of 2007, 58% of patients with acute hepatitis B have no known risk factor for infection; 38% have had multiple sex partners, 15% have engaged in injection-drug use, 12% have had recent surgery, and 11% are men who have sex with men.[4]

Immunization Program

While acute hepatitis B can cause significant morbidity and even death, a major rationale for immunization is to prevent chronic carriage. This is because chronic carriers are often asymptomatic, can infect others over long periods of time, and are at increased risk for developing cirrhosis and primary hepatocellular carcinoma. Data from Hawaii[5] and China[6] show that universal childhood immunization, including a birth dose, can dramatically decrease the prevalence of chronic carriage, and data from Taiwan demonstrate that universal HepB immunization can decrease the incidence of hepatocellular carcinoma.[7] This makes HepB vaccine the first vaccine that prevents a human cancer.

Selective vaccination of high-risk populations in the 1980s failed to impact disease burden. In fact, from 1988 to 1994, the age-adjusted prevalence of HBV infection in the United States population remained about 5%; approximately 1 million people, or 0.4%, were chronically infected.[8] Universal infant vaccination, which was first recommended in 1991,[9] aims to prevent perinatal transmission; arguably, transmission cannot occur if the mother is HBsAg-negative, but many pregnant women are not tested and those who test negative early in pregnancy may develop infection close to delivery (it is even possible that the mother's HBsAg status may be inaccurately reported). HepB is known to be immunogenic in infants and protection persists at least into young adulthood. Other advantages of the birth dose include potentially reducing the number of concurrent injections that must be given at the 2-month visit, increasing the likelihood that the entire 3-dose series (and other vaccine series) will be completed,[10] and emphasizing the importance of immunization for new parents, laying the groundwork for the routine schedule in infancy.

In 2007, there were 4519 reported cases of acute hepatitis B, for an overall incidence of 1.5 per 100,000 population (the actual number of cases is estimated at 43,000).[4] This was the lowest rate ever recorded and represents an 82% decline since 1990, a direct result of the universal immunization program. The decline in incidence occurred in all age groups but was greatest among children <15 years of age. Recommendations for prevention of hepatitis B in children were updated in 2005[11] and in adults in 2006.[12] Recommendations for immunization of health care personnel were published in 2001[13] and for control of hepatitis B in correctional facilities in 2003.[14]

In situations where exposure has occurred, the long incubation period allows for postexposure prophylaxis through vaccination. However, even an accelerated vaccine series requires a minimum of 4 months to complete, and the series cannot be completed in neonates until 24 weeks of age. Therefore, passive immunization with hepatitis B immune globulin (HBIG) is a necessary adjunct to active vaccination for immediate protection after exposure.

Vaccines

Characteristics of the hepatitis B vaccines licensed in the United States are given in **Table 13.1**. Both are inactivated subunit vaccines consisting of HBsAg expressed in yeast using recombinant DNA technology.

HBIG is a hyperimmune globulin preparation made from the plasma of donors who have high levels of HBsAb. The donors are screened for antibodies to HIV and hepatitis C virus, as well as for hepatitis C virus RNA. In addition, the manufacturing process inactivates known bloodborne viruses. HBIG is administered intramuscularly at the same time as HepB but at a different site (the deltoid or gluteal regions are preferred). Available products in the United States include Nabi-HB (North American Biologicals), HepaGam B (Cangene), and HyperHEP B S/D (Talecris). The only contraindication is a history of anaphylaxis to a previous dose of human immune globulin. Certain safety issues are common to all immune globulin products, including the possibility of allergic reaction to residual IgA in the product

TABLE 13.1 — Hepatitis B Vaccines

	Engerix-B[a]	Recombivax HB[b]
Trade name	Engerix-B[a]	Recombivax HB[b]
Abbreviation	HepB	HepB
Manufacturer/distributor	GlaxoSmithKline	Merck
Type of vaccine	Inactivated, engineered subunit	Inactivated, engineered subunit
Composition:		
Antigen content:	HBsAg	HBsAg
Expression system	Yeast (S cerevisiae)	Yeast (S cerevisiae)
Pediatric/adolescent formulation	10 mcg/0.5 mL	5 mcg/0.5 mL
Adult formulation	20 mcg/mL	10 mcg/mL
Dialysis formulation	—	40 mcg/mL
Adjuvant	Aluminum hydroxide (0.25 mg/0.5 mL aluminum)	Aluminum hydroxide (0.25 mg/0.5 mL aluminum)
Preservative	None	None
Excipients and contaminants	Yeast protein (≤5%) Sodium chloride (9 mg/mL) Disodium phosphate dihydrate (0.98 mg/mL) Sodium dihydrogen phosphate dihydrate (0.71 mg/mL)	Yeast protein (≤1%)
Latex	Tip cap and plunger of prefilled syringe contain dry natural rubber	None

	Prevention of hepatitis B	Prevention of hepatitis B
Labeled indications		
Labeled ages	All ages	All ages
Dose:		
Pediatric/adolescent formulation (≤19 years)	0.5 mL[c]	0.5 mL
Adult formulation (≥20 years)	1 mL[c]	1 mL[d]
Hemodialysis formulation	2 simultaneous adult doses of 1 mL each[e,f]	1 mL[f]
Route of administration	Intramuscular[g]	Intramuscular[g]
Labeled schedule:		
Hemodialysis patients	0, 1, 6 months of age[h]	0, 1, 6 months of age[h]
	0, 1, 2, and 6 months; periodic boosters[i]	0, 1, 6 months; periodic boosters[i]
Alternate dosing for 11 to 15 years of age	—	Adult formulation at 1 and 4 to 6 months[d]
Recommended schedule	Same	Same
How supplied (number in package):		
Pediatric/adolescent formulation	1-dose vial (10); Prefilled syringe (5, 10)	1-dose vial (1, 10); Prefilled syringe (6)
Adult formulation	1-dose vial (10); Prefilled syringe (5)	1-dose vial (1, 10); Prefilled syringe (1, 6)
Hemodialysis formulation	—	1-dose vial (1)
Storage	Refrigerate; Do not freeze	Refrigerate; Do not freeze

13

Continued

TABLE 13.1 — Continued

Trade name	Engerix-B[a]	Recombivax HB[b]
Abbreviation	HepB	HepB
Cost per dose, pediatric ($US, 2009):		
Public	9.75	10.00
Private	21.37	23.20
Cost per dose, adult ($US, 2009):		
Public	26.70	—
Private	52.50	—
Reference package insert	August 2009	December 2007

[a] Engerix-B is also available in combination with DTaP and IPV (Pediarix; GlaxoSmithKline) and with HepA (Twinrix; GlaxoSmithKline).

[b] Recombivax HB is also available in combination with Hib (Comvax; Merck).

[c] Adolescents 11 to 19 years of age may receive the adult formulation.

[d] An adult dose (10 mcg/mL) may be constituted by 2 separate injections of the pediatric (5 mcg/0.5 mL) formulation at the same site or by combining 2 pediatric doses in the same syringe.

[e] There is no specific hemodialysis formulation. The 40-mcg/2 mL dose can be constituted by 2 separate injections of the adult (20-mcg/mL) formulation at the same site or by combining 2 adult doses in the same syringe.

[f] Hemodialysis patients need higher doses to respond.

[g] May be administered subcutaneously in patients who are at risk of hemorrhage with intramuscular injections (eg, hemophiliacs). However, reactogenicity may be increased and immunogenicity decreased.

[h] Other dosing regimens are contained in the package insert.

[i] Booster doses are given when annual testing shows that HBsAb levels have fallen below 10 mIU/mL. Annual testing with periodic booster doses may be indicated for other immunocompromised persons, such as those with HIV infection, hematopoietic stem-cell transplant recipients, and those receiving chemotherapy.

in IgA-deficient individuals and the possibility of transmission of bloodborne pathogens that are not killed in the manufacturing process.

Efficacy and/or Immunogenicity

Engerix-B was found to be 95% effective in preventing peri-natal infection when given without immunoglubulin to newborns ($N=58$; 0, 1, 2 month schedule) of mothers who were chronic carriers. Of neonates ($N=52$) given the vaccine at 0, 1, and 6 months of age, 97% achieved a protective level of antibody (≥ 10 mIU/mL). Seroprotection rates of 98% were seen in children 6 months to 10 years of age ($N=242$) and 97% in adolescents ($N=119$) after a 3-dose schedule. Studies in adolescents and adults demonstrate seroprotection rates of >95% after 3 doses, although responses are somewhat lower in those >40 years of age.

Recombivax HB was found to be 95% effective in preventing perinatal transmission among 130 high-risk infants who were given concomitant HBIG. With 3 doses of vaccine, protective levels of antibody were achieved in 100% of infants ($N=92$), 99% of children ($N=129$), and 99% of adolescents ($N=112$). Response rates in adults were 98% in those 20 to 29 years of age ($N=787$), 94% in those 30 to 39 years of age ($N=249$), and 89% in those ≥ 40 years of age ($N=177$). Seroprotection rates in adolescents who received the 2-dose regimen ($N=255$) were 99%.

Although antibody levels after HepB vaccination in infancy wane with time, immune memory remains intact at least into adolescence, when it may be needed the most.[15] Protection lasts as well. A study from The Gambia, for example, showed that 50% of persons followed for ≥ 15 years had antibody levels that fell below 10 mIU/mL. Despite this, efficacy was 83% against infection and 97% against chronic carriage.[16] In a 2010 meta-analysis that looked at 34 cohorts with a total of 9356 vaccinated subjects, the cumulative incidence of breakthrough hepatitis B 5 to 20 years after vaccination was <1%.[17]

Safety

The most common adverse reaction following HepB vaccination is pain at the site of injection, reported in 13% to 29% of adults and 3% to 9% of children. Mild systemic complaints, such as fatigue, headache, and irritability, have been reported in 11% to 17% of adults and up to 20% of children. Low-grade fever is seen in 1% of adults and in up to 6% of children. It should be noted that well over 1 billion doses of HepB have been given worldwide since the 1980s, and serious systemic adverse events and allergic reactions have rarely been reported. There is no

13

evidence that HepB causes or exacerbates multiple sclerosis (see *Chapter 7: Addressing Concerns About Vaccines—Do Vaccines Cause Multiple Sclerosis [MS]?*)

- *Contraindications*
  - Allergic reaction to previous dose of vaccine or any vaccine component (risk of recurrent allergic reaction; this includes reactions to baker's yeast)
- *Precautions*
  - Moderate or severe acute illness (difficulty distinguishing illness from vaccine reaction)
  - Infant weight <2000 g, unless the mother is HBsAg-positive (risk of poor response to vaccination)

Recommendations

■ Universal Infant, Child, and Adolescent Immunization

All infants should be vaccinated against hepatitis B. The usual schedule for HepB is a dose at birth (before hospital discharge), 1 to 2 months of age, and 6 to 18 months of age (6 to 12 months of age for high-risk groups such as Alaska Natives, Pacific Islanders, and immigrants from areas like Asia and Africa). Only monovalent vaccine may be used for the birth dose. Infants who receive subsequent doses as DTaP-HepB-IPV or HepB-Hib-OMP may receive an extra dose at 4 months of age; this does not increase reactogenicity or impair the immune response. The birth dose should be implemented by *standing order* and should be deferred only by a physician's order, with a copy of the mother's *recent* negative HBsAg test result on the infant's chart. If the birth dose is deferred, the first dose of HepB should be administered before 2 months of age. The birth dose *should not be deferred* if the mother is HBsAg-positive (see below), had any behavioral risk factors for HBV infection during pregnancy, or if the infant is unlikely to return for follow-up. However, the birth dose *should be deferred* for preterm infants weighing <2000 g whose mothers are HBsAg-negative. These infants should be vaccinated at 1 month of age or at hospital discharge, whichever comes first (babies are assumed to be medically stable and gaining weight consistently if discharged before 1 month of age).

All children and adolescents ≤18 years of age who were not vaccinated as infants should receive the HepB series. Routine postvaccination testing for HBsAb is not recommended. Engerix-B and Recombivax HB are considered interchangeable except for the 2-dose schedule in adolescents, for which only Recombivax HB is approved.

■ Adult Vaccination

Vaccination is recommended for the following:
- Sex partners of persons who are HBsAg-positive
- Persons with more than one sex partner in the past 6 months

- Persons seeking evaluation or treatment for a sexually transmitted disease
- Men who have sex with men
- Injection drug users
- Household contacts of HBsAg-positive persons
- Residents and staff of facilities for developmentally disabled persons
- Health care and public safety workers at risk for infection through exposure to blood or blood-contaminated body fluids, including hospital, institutional, and laboratory employees, students, contractors, physicians, emergency medical technicians, paramedics, and volunteers
- Patients with end-stage renal disease, including those on hemodialysis and peritoneal dialysis (vaccination of patients with renal failure is encouraged before they require hemodialysis)
- Patients with chronic liver disease
- Persons with HIV infection
- Travelers to regions where the prevalence of chronic infection is ≥2%
- Inmates undergoing medical evaluation at a correctional facility, as well as staff who may have contact with blood or body fluids
- Anyone who wants protection from hepatitis B

Standing orders for HepB administration should be implemented in settings where high-risk individuals are seen, including sexually transmitted disease and HIV clinics, drug abuse treatment centers, correctional facilities, facilities that care for men who have sex with men, kidney disease programs, and facilities for the developmentally disabled. Prevaccination testing might reduce costs by avoiding vaccination of persons who are already immune, and is recommended for the following groups: persons born in areas where the prevalence of chronic infection is ≥8%; household, sex, and needle-sharing contacts of HBsAg-positive persons; HIV-infected persons; and other populations in whom the prevalence of chronic infection exceeds 20%. The preferred test is for antibody to hepatitis B core antigen, since this identifies all people with previous infection. Testing for HBsAb can be used, but must be done along with testing for HBsAg, since chronic carriers may have negative tests for HBsAb.

Testing for HBsAb 1 to 2 months after vaccination is recommended for the following groups: health care and public safety workers at high risk for exposure to blood or body fluids; chronic hemodialysis patients; HIV-infected and other immunocompromised persons; and sex partners of HBsAg-positive persons. Levels ≥10 mIU/mL are considered protective. Patients with antibody levels <10 mIU/mL should receive a second 3-dose series of HepB, followed by repeat testing. If the result is still <10 mIU/mL, the person should be tested for HBsAg, since chronic carriage is a reason for nonresponse to vaccination. If they are negative for HBsAg, they are considered primary nonresponders; these persons may respond to intradermal vaccination, although neither HepB product is labeled for this route of administration. Periodic (eg, annual) testing for HBsAb after vaccination is only recommended for dialysis patients and other immunocompromised persons, including those with HIV infection, hematopoietic stem-cell transplant recipients, and persons receiving chemotherapy.

The recommendation to test HIV-infected and immunocompromised persons after vaccination makes the most sense if the individual is at high risk of being exposed to hepatitis B. This might be the case for a person who acquired HIV from injecting drug use, for example, but not for an otherwise healthy congenitally infected individual who is at low risk of exposure to hepatitis B.

■ Postexposure Prophylaxis for Infants of HBsAg-Positive and HBsAg-Unknown Mothers

All pregnant women should be tested for HBsAg early on in each pregnancy. Women who were not screened prenatally, those who are at high risk for infection, and those with clinical hepatitis should be tested at the time of delivery. A physical copy of the test results should be provided to the birthing hospital and the newborn's health care provider.

Infants born to mothers who are HBsAg-positive should receive HepB and HBIG (0.5 mL intramuscularly) at separate sites within 12 hours of birth. The vaccine series should be completed with Dose 2 at 1 to 2 months of age and Dose 3 at 6 months of age. For preterm infants weighing <2000 g, both vaccine and HBIG should be given as well, but the vaccine dose should not count toward the complete series, since responses are not reliable; the first valid dose is given at 1 month of age, the second at 2 to 3 months, and the third at 6 months. Both term and preterm infants of HBsAg-positive mothers should be tested for HBsAg and HBsAb at 9 to 18 months of age (not earlier than 4 weeks after the last dose). Those with protective levels of antibody and a negative HBsAg test need no further medical management. Those without protective levels of antibody who are HBsAg-negative should receive a second 3-dose vaccine series and should be tested again 1 to 2 months after completion. Those who are HBsAg-positive should receive appropriate medical management.

Infants born to mothers whose HBsAg status is unknown or not documented at the time of delivery should be vaccinated within 12 hours of birth, and the mother should be tested. If she is HBsAg-positive, the baby should receive HBIG before 7 days of age and should complete the HepB series at 6 months of age. If she is HBsAg-negative, the HepB series should be completed by

6 to 18 months of age. If the mother is not tested, the baby should complete the HepB series by 6 months of age, but HBIG should not be given—unless the baby is preterm and weighs <2000 g. In this situation, if the mother's status will not be known within 12 hours of birth, both vaccine and HBIG should be given and the infant should be followed as if born to an HBsAg-positive mother.

■ Postexposure Prophylaxis in Other Settings

Recommendations for the management of potential occupational and nonoccupational exposures to HBV are given in **Tables 13.2** and **13.3**, respectively.

REFERENCES

1. Liaw Y-F, et al. *Lancet*. 2009;373:582-592.
2. Azam F, et al. *Ann Hepatol*. 2008;7:125-129.
3. Ganem D, et al. *N Engl J Med*. 2004;350:1118-1129.
4. Daniels D, et al. *MMWR*. 2009;58(SS-3):1-27.
5. Perz JF, et al. *Pediatrics*. 2006;118:1403-1408.
6. Liang X, et al. *J Infect Dis*. 2009;200:39-47.
7. Chang MH, et al. *N Engl J Med*. 1997;336:1855-1859.
8. Shepard CW, et al. *Pediatr Infect Dis J*. 2005;24:755-760.
9. CDC. *MMWR*. 1991;40(RR-13):1-20.
10. Yusuf HR, et al. *JAMA*. 2000;284:978-983.
11. Mast EE, et al. *MMWR*. 2005;54(RR-16):1-31.
12. Mast EE, et al. *MMWR*. 2006;55(RR-16):1-33.
13. CDC. *MMWR*. 2001;50(RR-11):1-52.
14. Weinbaum C, et al. *MMWR*. 2003;52(RR-1):1-36.
15. Boxall EH, et al. *J Infect Dis*. 2004;190:1264-1269.
16. van der Sande MA, et al. *J Infect Dis*. 2006;193:1528-1535.
17. Poorolajal J, et al. *Vaccine*. 2010;28:623-631.

13

TABLE 13.2 — Management of Potential Occupational Exposures to HBV[a]

Vaccination Status of Exposed Person	Response to Vaccination[b]	HBsAg Status of Source Individual		
		Positive	Negative	Unknown[c]
Not vaccinated or incompletely vaccinated (<3 doses)	—	Give HBIG[d] and initiate or complete HepB series[e]	Initiate or complete HepB series[e]	Initiate or complete HepB series[e]
Vaccinated	Responder[f]	No treatment	No treatment	No treatment
	Nonresponder[f]	Patients who *have not* received a second complete 3-dose HepB series: 1 dose of HBIG[d] and initiate second 3-dose HepB series[e]	No treatment	If high-risk, assume HBsAg-positive and treat accordingly[g]
		Patients who *have* received a second complete 3-dose HepB series: 2 doses of HBIG[d] separated by 1 month	No treatment	If high-risk, assume HBsAg-positive and treat accordingly[g]
	Antibody level unknown—test exposed person for HBsAb:			
	Adequate response[f]	No treatment	No treatment	No treatment
	Inadequate response[f]	Give HBIG[d] and a booster dose of HepB[e,h]	No treatment	Give booster dose of HepB[e,i]

a Percutaneous exposures include needle sticks, lacerations, and bites. Permucosal exposures include splashes of blood, any fluid containing visible blood, other potentially infectious fluid (including semen; vaginal secretions; CSF; synovial, pleural, peritoneal, pericardial, or amniotic fluids; tracheal secretions; and saliva), or tissue onto any mucosal surface, including the conjunctival, oral, and buccal mucosa.

b Testing for HBsAb 1 to 2 months after vaccination is recommended for health care and public safety workers at high risk for exposure to blood or body fluids.

c Efforts should be made to test the source individual for HBsAg.

d The dose is 0.06 mL/kg given intramuscularly. HBIG should be given as soon as possible after exposure, preferrably within 24 hours. Intervals exceeding 7 days are unlikely to be of benefit after percutaneous exposure.

e In cases where the source is HBsAg-positive or -unknown, the first dose should be given as soon as possible, preferably within 24 hours. In cases where the source is HBsAg-negative, the HepB series should be initiated or completed because of occupational risk of exposure in the future.

f An adequate response is ≥10 mIU/mL of HBsAb 1 to 2 months postvaccination.

g HBIG is given in this situation because the exposed person, for whatever reason, did not respond to previous doses of the vaccine, and therefore might remain vulnerable if only vaccine were given (as is recommended for previously unvaccinated persons exposed to an unknown, but presumed high-risk, source it is assumed they will respond to vaccination).

h Test for HBsAb in 4 to 6 months. If the level is inadequate, give 2 more doses to complete a second 3-dose series.

i Test for HBsAb in 1 to 2 months. If the level is inadequate, give 2 more doses to complete a second 3-dose series.

Adapted from Centers for Disease Control and Prevention. *Epidemiology and Prevention of Vaccine-Preventable Diseases*. 11th ed. Atkinson W, et al, eds. Washington, DC: Public Health Foundation, 2009:99-122.

13

TABLE 13.3 — Management of Potential Nonoccupational Exposures to HBV[a]

Status of Exposed Individual	Source HBsAg Status[b]	Management
Not vaccinated or incompletely vaccinated (<3 doses)	Negative	Catch-up vaccination
	Positive	Initiate or complete HepB series[c] Give HBIG[d]
	Unknown	Initiate or complete HepB series[c]
Vaccinated[e]	Negative	No treatment
	Positive	Give a booster dose of HepB[c]
	Unknown	No treatment

[a] Percutaneous exposures include needle sticks (needle sharing), lacerations, and bites. Permucosal exposures include splashes of blood, any fluid containing visible blood, other potentially infectious fluid (including semen; vaginal secretions; CSF; synovial, pleural, peritoneal, pericardial, or amniotic fluids; tracheal secretions; and saliva), or tissue onto any mucosal surface, including the conjunctival, oral and buccal mucosa.

[b] Efforts should be made to test the source individual for HBsAg. Needles and syringes discarded in public places, presumably by injection drug users, pose a risk of transmission since HBV can survive on environmental surfaces for up to 7 days. However, the risk depends on the prevalence of hepatitis B in the drug-abusing population and the amount of blood in the needle. There is no consensus opinion regarding the use of HBIG in these situations.

[c] The first dose should be given as soon as possible, preferably within 24 hours.

[d] The dose is 0.06 mL/kg given intramuscularly. HBIG should be given as soon as possible after exposure, preferably within 24 hours. Intervals exceeding 7 days after percutaneous exposure and 14 days after sexual exposure are unlikely to be of benefit.

[e] Written documentation of a complete 3-dose series of HepB should be provided.

Adapted from CDC. *MMWR.* 2006;55(RR-16):1-33.

14
Human Papillomavirus

The Pathogen

Human papillomavirus (HPV) is a small, nonenveloped, double-stranded DNA virus in the family Papillomaviridae that is tropic for epithelial surfaces. The virion capsid is composed of major and minor late proteins, L1 and L2. The oncogenic HPV types—most notably 16 and 18, but including types 33, 45, 31, 58, 52, as well as others—are a *necessary* but not *sufficient* cause of cervical cancer.[1] In other words, the virus *must* be present for cervical cancer to develop, but the majority of women who acquire the virus do not develop cancer. Approximately 90% of new infections clear within 2 years, and it is only the remaining 10% of persistent infections that can lead to cancer. It is important to note that certain biologic factors put young women at particularly high risk for infection, persistence, and neoplasia. The most important of these is the *cervical transformation zone*, an area of immature metaplasia between the prepubertal squamocolumnar junction (where the squamous cells of the vagina meet the columnar epithelial cells of the endocervix, originally found peripheral to the cervical opening) and the postpubertal junction, found inside the cervical opening. The cells in this region are particularly susceptible to malignant transformation.

HPV initially reaches dividing cells in the basal layer of the cervical epithelium through minute fissures and abrasions. DNA replication and early cell differentiation occur together, but expression of the viral proteins E6 and E7 prevents further cell differentiation and causes delayed cell-cycle arrest. This, along with the virus' clever mechanisms for evading host immune surveillance,[2] results in vertical expansion of the dividing cell population. Integration of viral DNA into the host genome causes overexpression of E6 and E7, leading to further unchecked cell proliferation and the accumulation of germ-line mutations, which ultimately lead to invasive cancer.

Some HPV types—most notably 6 and 11—cause genital warts rather than cancer, although they may cause low-grade cervical dysplasia that eventually regresses.

Clinical Features

HPV is one of the few human viruses unequivocally linked to cancer (others include HBV and Epstein-Barr virus). *Squamous cell carcinoma of the cervix* comprises 75% of cervical cancers in the United States; the remainder are *adenocarcinomas*. HPV

16 and 18 cause approximately 70% of squamous cell carcinomas and 80% of adenocarcinomas. Most HPV infections are asymptomatic and self-limited. In a minority of women, persistent infection leads to progressive dysplasia, referred to as *cervical intraepithelial neoplasia* grades 1 (CIN 1) through 3 (CIN 3). Approximately 60% of CIN 1 cases spontaneously regress and <1% lead to cancer. On the other hand, only 30% to 40% of CIN 2 or 3 lesions regress, and >12% develop into cancer. The Pap test is used to detect dysplasia early so treatment can be initiated. The duration of time from the first intraepithelial lesion to invasive cancer is 15 to 20 years.

HPV also causes *vaginal and vulvar intraepithelial neoplasia* (VaIN and VIN) that can progress to cancer; up to 50% of vulvar and vaginal cancers are caused by HPV. Up to 90% of *anal cancers*, 50% of *penile cancers*, and 20% of *oropharyngeal cancers* are also caused by HPV. For most of these tumors, types 16 and 18 predominate.

Approximately 90% of *anogenital warts* are caused by types 6 and 11. These are typically small, soft flesh-colored growths that are raised to varying degrees; some develop into large, cauliflower-like clusters called *condyloma acuminata*. In women, warts can be seen anywhere from the cervix to the vagina, urethra, inguinal region or upper thighs. In males, the most common site is the shaft of the penis. Most individuals are asymptomatic, but some experience itching, burning, pain, bleeding, and tenderness. *Recurrent respiratory papillomatosis*, defined by wart-like lesions that develop on the larynx, nasopharynx, oropharynx, trachea and/or esophagus, is also caused by types 6 and 11. This is seen most commonly in infants and children <5 years of age and is acquired from the mother during vaginal delivery. Infants may present with hoarseness, weak cry, stridor, feeding difficulties, and failure to thrive. Airway obstruction can result from enlarged lesions, and multiple surgical laser procedures are often necessary. Malignancy can develop, albeit rarely.

Epidemiology and Transmission

Whereas papillomaviruses are widely distributed in nature, HPV is only transmitted among humans. Direct *skin-to-skin* or *skin-to-mucosa* contact is required; generally, this means sexual activity where there is direct contact between the genitalia, anus, and/or mouth. Direct transfer of virus from the hands can occur. Not surprisingly, the risk of HPV infection correlates directly with sexual activity. Studies in female college students demonstrate that over half acquire HPV infection within 4 years of their first sexual intercourse,[3] and the prevalence of HPV infection among women 20 to 24 years of age in the United States approaches 50%.[4] Estimates of the prevalence of infection in men vary widely, but some are as high as 70%,[5] and the dominant risk factor for HPV acquisition in men is clearly the lifetime number of sexual partners.[6] The prevalence of antibody to the 4 HPV types contained in HPV4 is as high as 42% among women 30 to 39 years of age and 18% among men 50 to 59 years of age.[7]

Worldwide there are 500,000 new cases of cervical cancer and 250,000 cervical cancer deaths each year—virtually all of these caused by HPV. In the United States, an estimated 6.2 million new HPV infections occur every year among teenagers and young adults. The annual disease burden includes approximately 5000 deaths, 17,000 cancers, 300,000 high-grade cervical dysplasias, 1,250,000 low-grade cervical dysplasias, and 1,400,000 cases of genital warts. The estimated direct medical costs are at least $4 billion (2004 dollars).

Immunization Program

HPV4, which provides protection against cervical cancer caused by types 16 and 18 as well as genital warts caused by types 6 and 11, was licensed in 2006 and recommended for universal use in girls and young women.[8] The major reason for a universal recommendation was prevention of cervical cancer due to types 16 and 18. Other anticipated benefits included prevention of anogenital warts due to types 6 and 11, reductions in the direct and indirect costs associated with cervical cancer screening and follow-up of abnormal Pap tests, fewer cases of recurrent respiratory papillomatosis, and reductions in the incidence of anal, penile, and oral cancers. HPV2, which provides protection against cervical cancer caused by types 16 and 18, was licensed in October 2009. At the same time, HPV4 was granted an indication for prevention of genital warts in males 9 to 26 years of age. Provisional recommendations incorporating these changes were released in December 2009.[9]

In 2003, the Youth Risk Behavior Survey showed that 62% of high school seniors in the United States were sexually active.[10] Seven percent of high school students had sexual intercourse before 13 years of age, and 14% had ≥4 lifetime partners. Since the benefits of vaccination can best be realized before sexual debut, adding HPV vaccine to the routine adolescent health care visit for girls at 11 to 12 years of age makes sense. For those girls who will abstain from sex and ultimately enter a monogamous relationship, vaccination still makes sense because exposure through involuntary sexual contact is a possibility and the sexual history of the eventual partner may not be known.

Studies suggest that protection lasts at least 5 years without waning, and antibody levels achieved by young adolescents are actually higher than those achieved by older women. Vaccination does not lead to clearance of persistent HPV infection nor does it prevent neoplasia in women who are already infected with a particular serotype of HPV. However, sexually active women or those known to be infected with HPV can still benefit from vaccination due to protection against serotypes with which they are not infected.

At the beginning of the HPV vaccination program, it was estimated that vaccination of an entire cohort of girls at 12 years of age would reduce the lifetime risk of cervical cancer by 20% to 66%. Models that included only direct effects placed the cost per QALY saved at slightly more than $20,000 (2001 dollars)[11]; models that incorporated herd immunity effects yielded estimates as low as $3000 (2005 dollars) per QALY saved.[12] Subsequent estimates have been as high as $43,600 per QALY saved for routine vaccination of all girls at 12 years of age (2006 dollars).[13] Catch-up programs are estimated to be more expensive—from $97,300 per QALY saved for vaccination of all girls through 18 years of age to $152,700 for all females through 26 years of age. Routine inclusion of boys in a universal vaccination program would not likely be cost-effective, even when transmission dynamics and other HPV related conditions in both males and females are considered.[14]

Vaccines

Characteristics of the HPV vaccines licensed in the United States are given in **Table 14**.**1**. Both are produced by recombinant DNA techniques and consist exclusively of the L1 major capsid protein of the virus, which self-assembles into virus-like particles that do not contain genetic material and are incapable of replicating or causing infection or disease. HPV2 contains a novel adjuvant (see *Chapter 1: Introduction to Vaccinology—The Germinal Center Reaction*).

Efficacy and/or Immunogenicity

Prelicensure efficacy studies of HPV4 involved >20,000 women between 16 and 26 years of age. These studies necessarily used CIN 2 or 3 and adenocarcinoma in situ as outcomes, since invasive cervical cancer was not a feasible or ethical end point. Two large Phase 3 studies were conducted: FUTURE (**F**emales **U**nited **T**o **U**nilaterally **R**educe **E**ndo/Ectocervical Disease) I,[15] which enrolled 5442 women, and FUTURE II,[16] which enrolled 12,167. Licensure was based on pooled efficacy data from these trials as well as from two smaller Phase 2 studies. Ninety-four percent of the women were sexually active at enrollment, 73% were HPV-naïve, and the median follow-up period ranged from 2.3 to 4 years.

The primary efficacy analyses included women who received all 3 doses of vaccine, had no major protocol deviations, and remained HPV-negative through 1 month after Dose 3 (so-called *per protocol* analyses). Efficacy against types 16- or 18-related CIN 2 or 3 or adenocarcinoma in situ (AIS) was 98%—2 cases occurred among 8493 vaccinees and 112 occurred among 8464 placebees. Efficacy was 100% against types 16- or 18-related VIN 2 or 3 and VaIN 2 or 3. Efficacy against any grade of CIN or AIS caused by any of the 4 types was 96% and efficacy against genital warts was 99%. Among women who were already infected with one of the HPV types in the vaccine, efficacy against the remaining types was excellent.

In the real world, not all women will complete the full series of shots, some women will already be infected with one or more HPV type at the time they start vaccination, and some will become infected right after the first shot. Additional analyses were therefore performed to estimate the impact that a vaccine program would have in practice, where none of these things is controlled. Among women who received at least 1 vaccine dose (a so-called *intention-to-treat* population) and were HPV-naïve at baseline, efficacy against CIN 2 or 3 or AIS caused by any HPV type was 43% and against CIN of any grade or AIS was 30%; considering all women regardless of baseline HPV status, the respective efficacies were 18% and 19%. The majority of cases in these analyses occurred in women who were HPV-infected at the time of first vaccination and thus represent *prevalent*, not *incident*, disease.

Cross-protection is a component of the overall impact of HPV4 on disease rates. In an intention-to-treat analysis of HPV-naïve women, HPV4 demonstrated 25% efficacy against infection with types 31, 33, 45, 52, or 58 (considered as a group) and 29% against CIN of any grade or AIS caused by those types.[17] Among all women regardless of baseline HPV status, the respective efficacies were 18% and 19%.[18] Efficacy against infection with type 31 among HPV-naïve women was 46%.

Nearly 100% of vaccinated persons develop antibodies to all four types after 3 doses of HPV4, and antibody levels are higher than those seen after natural infection. Licensure for use in girls 9 to 15 years of age was based on immunogenicity bridging studies that demonstrated noninferiority of antibody responses compared with those in women 16 to 26 years of age. In fact, the antibody levels in young adolescents a year and a half postvaccination were 2- to 3-fold higher than those in the older women.[19,20]

HPV4 was tested in a Phase 3 study involving 4055 boys and men. Among those who were HPV-naïve at baseline, per-protocol efficacy against external genital lesions caused by vaccine types was 90%. In intention-to-treat analyses, efficacy among HPV-naïve subjects was 76% and among all subjects regardless of baseline status was 66%.

Efficacy of HPV2 in preventing high-grade cervical lesions (CIN 2 or 3) or AIS was assessed in 2 studies that enrolled nearly

TABLE 14.1 — Human Papillomavirus Vaccines

	Gardasil	Cervarix
Trade name	Gardasil	Cervarix
Abbreviation	HPV4	HPV2
Manufacturer/distributor	Merck	GlaxoSmithKline
Type of vaccine	Inactivated, engineered subunit	Inactivated, engineered subunit
Composition:	Virus-like particles composed of self-assembled L1 major capsid protein molecules	Virus-like particles composed of self-assembled L1 major capsid protein molecules
Expression system	Yeast (*Saccharomyces cerevisiae*)	Insect (*Trichoplusia ni*) cells using a Baculovirus vector
Antigen content:		
HPV 6 L1	20 mcg	—
HPV 11 L1	40 mcg	—
HPV 16 L1	40 mcg	20 mcg
HPV 18 L1	20 mcg	20 mcg
Adjuvant	Aluminum hydrophosphate sulfate (0.225 mg aluminum)	AS04 (3-*O*-desacyl-4'-monophosphoryl lipid A (a derivative of bacterial lipopolysaccharide, 50 mcg) adsorbed to aluminum hydroxide (0.5 mg)
Preservative	None	None
Excipients and contaminants	Sodium chloride (9.56 mg) L-histidine (0.78 mg) Polysorbate 80 (50 mcg) Sodium borate (35 mcg) Yeast protein (<7 mcg)	Sodium chloride (4.4 mg) Sodium dihydrogen phosphate dihydrate (0.624 mg) Residual insect cell and viral protein (<40 ng) Residual bacterial cell protein (<150 ng)

Latex	None	Tip cap and plunger of prefilled syringe contain dry natural rubber
Labeled indications:		
Females: prevention of diseases caused by HPV types 6, 11, 16, and 18	Cervical cancer Vulvar cancer Vaginal cancer Cervical intraepithelial neoplasia grades 1, 2, and 3 Cervical adenocarcinoma in situ Vulvar intraepithelial neoplasia grades 2 and 3 Vaginal intraepithelial neoplasia grades 2 and 3 Prevention of genital warts caused by HPV types 6 and 11	
Females: prevention of diseases caused by HPV types 16 and 18		Cervical cancer Cervical intraepithelial neoplasia grades 1, 2, and 3 Adenocarcinoma in situ
Females and males		
Labeled ages	9 to 26 years (females and males)	10 to 25 years (females)[a]
Dose	0.5 mL	0.5 mL
Route of administration	Intramuscular	Intramuscular
Labeled schedule	0, 2, 6 months	0, 1, 6 months
Recommended schedule[b]	0, 1-2, 6 months	0, 1-2, 6 months
How supplied (number in package)	1-dose vial (1, 10) Prefilled syringe (6)	1-dose vial (10) Prefilled syringe (1, 5)
Storage	Refrigerate or room temperature for up to 72 hours Do not freeze Protect from light	Refrigerate Do not freeze

Continued

14

325

TABLE 14.1 — *Continued*

Trade name	Gardasil	Cervarix
Abbreviation	HPV4	HPV2
Cost per dose ($US, 2009):		
Public	105.58	—
Private	130.27	—
Reference package insert	October 2009	October 2009

[a] ACIP recommendations allow use of Cervarix from 9 to 26 years of age.
[b] The series should be completed with the same product, but vaccination should not be deferred if the same product is unknown or not available.

20,000 females 15 to 25 years of age. The first study enrolled 1113 women who were naïve for HPV infection; follow-up at a mean of 5.9 years was available for 776 subjects.[21-23] Efficacy against HPV 16- or 18-related CIN 2 or 3 or AIS was 100%, as was efficacy against 12-month persistent infection with HPV 16 or 18. In the second study, referred to as PATRICIA (PApilloma TRIal against Cancer In young Adults), 18,665 women were enrolled regardless of baseline HPV status and were randomized to receive HPV2 or HepA at 0, 1, and 6 months.[24,25] Prior to vaccination, 73.6% of subjects were naïve to HPV 16 and/or 18, and the mean follow-up period after the first dose was 39 months. Among women who were HPV-naïve at baseline and were vaccinated according to protocol, efficacy against HPV 16- or 18-related CIN 2 or 3 or AIS was approximately 93%. Among all women who received at least 1 dose of vaccine, regardless of current infection with or prior exposure to HPV 16 or 18 and including all cases starting on Day 1, efficacy against HPV 16- or 18-related CIN 2 or 3 or AIS was 52.8%; the majority of cases that occurred were due to prevalent infection at the time of vaccination rather than incident infection after vaccination. Among all women who received at least 1 dose of vaccine, regardless of current infection with or prior exposure to any HPV type and including all cases starting on Day 1, efficacy against CIN 2 or 3 or AIS related to any HPV type was 30.4%. This approximates what might be expected in the general population.

Among women who were vaccinated according to protocol, efficacy against CIN 2 or 3 or AIS caused by 12 non-vaccine types (considered as a group) was 54.0%. When lesions that contained HPV 16 and/or 18 DNA were excluded in the outcomes analysis, efficacy against CIN 2 or 3 or AIS caused by these types was 37.4%; arguably, if the vaccine did not protect against any of these other types, this number should have been 0%. Among women who were vaccinated according to protocol and were HPV 31 DNA negative through month 6, efficacy against CIN 2 or 3 or AIS caused by HPV 31 was 89.4% when lesions also containing 16 and 18 were excluded.

Virtually all subjects develop antibodies to HPV 16 and 18 after 3 doses of HPV2 as measured by ELISA as well as a pseudovirion-based neutralization assay. Persistent responses were seen in 98% when measured 76 months post-vaccination. The immune response in girls 10 to 14 years of age was noninferior to older women, allowing the assumption that similar disease protection will ensue. In a head-to-head trial involving 1106 women 18 to 45 years of age, geometric mean titers of neutralizing antibody to type 16 were 2.3 to 4.8-fold higher in HPV2 recipients than in HPV4 recipients; for type 18, they were 6.8 to 9.1-fold higher.[26] It is not known whether higher antibody titers predict better or longer-lasting protection.

Before licensure, safety data were collected from approximately 12,000 HPV4 recipients, about 5100 of whom kept detailed diaries for 2 weeks after each dose. Pain at the injection site occurred in 84%, compared with 75% of controls who received an aluminum-containing placebo and 49% who received a saline placebo (despite anecdotal accounts and media hype regarding pain, a survey study showed that HPV4 vaccination was less painful than other adolescent vaccinations[27]). Swelling and erythema were reported in about 25% of vaccinees, and fewer than 3% of local reactions were believed to be severe. Approximately 5% of female vaccinees reported a temperature of $\geq100°F$ ($\geq38°C$) after any dose, and temperatures $\geq102°F$ ($\geq38.9°C$) occurred in <1%. The rates of fever, other systemic adverse events, serious adverse events, and new medical conditions arising within 4 years were similar in vaccinees and placebees. There were 10 deaths among vaccinees and 7 among placebees, none of which were considered to be vaccine related (causes of death included motor vehicle accidents, intentional drug overdose or suicide, thromboembolic disease, sepsis, cancer, arrhythmia, and asphyxia).

In a postlicensure review of safety data from clinical trials, there were 6 serious adverse events (vaginal hemorrhage, bronchospasm, gastroenteritis, ulcerative colitis, hypertension and headache, and injection site reaction) thought to be possibly, probably, or definitely related to vaccine among vaccinees ($N=11,778$) and 2 (hypersensitivity and chills/headache/fever) among placebees ($N=9686$).[28] There were 11 deaths among vaccinees and 7 among placebees, none of which were related to the study vaccine. New autoimmune phenomena were reported in 2.4% of both groups. Between licensure and the close of 2008, >23 million doses of HPV4 had been distributed; 12,424 VAERS reports had been received, only 6% of which were considered serious (21% of these were headache, 16% nausea, 15% dizziness, 13% vomiting, 13% fever, 13% fatigue, and 13% syncope).[29] There were 32 deaths, with a mean time from the last vaccination to event onset of 39 days (range 2 to 288) and no common pattern. Causes of death included diabetes, viral illness, illicit drug use, and heart failure. Reporting rates for GBS (0.2 per 100,000 doses distributed), transverse myelitis (0.04 per 100,000), and motor neuron disease (0.009 per 100,000) were extremely low; this was reassuring given the well-publicized case of a 14-year-old girl who developed a peripheral motor neuropathy 4 months after Dose 3 of HPV4. The reporting rate for syncope was 8.2 per 100,000; 90% of cases occurred on the day of vaccination, and >50% of these occurred within 15 minutes. There were 56 reports of venous thromboembolic events; in 90% of the 31 that could be reviewed, known risk factors for such events were present.

In prelicensure trials, local reactions (pain, 91.8%; redness, 48.0%; swelling, 44.1%) occurred more frequently among HPV2 recipients than placebees; the majority of reactions were mild or moderate in intensity. Approximately half of vaccinees experienced fatigue, headache, and myalgia. In a pooled safety analysis, serious adverse events were reported in 5.3% of 16,142 vaccinees and 5.9% of 13,811 placebees during a follow-up period of 7.4 years. In a database of studies including 57,323 females, there were 20 deaths among HPV2 recipients and 17 among control recipients. The causes of death were as expected for the patient population under study. In the largest randomized controlled trial in women 15 to 25 years of age, new-onset autoimmune disease was seen in 78 (0.8%) of 9,319 vaccinees as compared to 77 (0.8%) of 9,325 HepA controls.

- *Contraindications*
  - Allergic reaction to previous dose of vaccine or any vaccine component (risk of recurrent allergic reaction; for HPV4, this includes reactions to baker's yeast)
- *Precautions*
  - Moderate or severe acute illness (difficulty distinguishing illness from vaccine reaction)
  - Pregnancy (theoretic risk to the fetus or attribution of birth defects to vaccination, although no deleterious effects from HPV vaccine administered during pregnancy have been demonstrated and the risk of adverse fetal effects from an inactivated vaccine is extremely low; it is not clear why pregnancy is listed as a precaution for some inactivated vaccines but not others)

Recommendations

All adolescent girls and young women should be vaccinated against cervical cancer caused by HPV. The usual schedule is 3 doses of HPV vaccine (given at 0, 1 to 2, and 6 months) at 11 to 12 years of age. The series may be started as early as 9 years of age. There is no preference for HPV2 or HPV4 for prevention of cervical cancer, but if prevention of genital warts is also desired, HPV4 should be used (HPV4 also protects against vulvar and vaginal precancers and cancers). All females 13 to 26 years of age also should be vaccinated, whether or not they are sexually active. Screening for HPV infection before vaccination is not needed, and vaccine should be given regardless of personal history of HPV infection, cervical, vaginal, or vulvar dysplasia, genital warts, and Pap test results. Vaccination of women >26 years of age is not recommended, but if a woman turns 27 after initiation of the vaccine series, the series may be completed.

HPV4 may be given to males 9 to 26 years of age for prevention of genital warts (this is a "permissive" statement; see

Chapter 2: Vaccine Infrastructure in the United States—Policy and Recommendations).

Routine cytologic screening of women for cervical cancer should continue even if they are vaccinated. New guidelines from the American College of Obstetricians and Gynecologists, issued in November 2009,[30] include the following: 1) no screening <21 years of age, regardless of sexual history; 2) screening every 2 years from 21 to 29 years of age; 3) screening every 3 years from 30 to 65 or 70 years of age, provided there have been 3 consecutive negative tests (exceptions include women with HIV infection, compromised immunity, history of CIN 2 or CIN 3, or in utero exposure to diethylstilbestrol; and 4) discontinuation of screening in women 65 to 70 years of age who have had ≥3 consecutive negative tests and no abnormal tests in the preceding 10 years (exceptions include women with multiple sexual partners).

REFERENCES

1. Schiffman M, et al. *Lancet.* 2007;370:890-907.
2. Einstein MH, et al. *Lancet Infect Dis.* 2009;9:347-356.
3. Winer RL, et al. *Am J Epidemiol.* 2003;157:218-226.
4. Dunne EF, et al. *JAMA.* 2007:297:813-819.
5. Dunne EF, et al. *J Infect Dis.* 2006;194:1044-1057.
6. Lu B, et al. *J Infect Dis.* 2009;199:362-371.
7. Markowitz LE, et al. *J Infect Dis.* 2009;200:1059-1067.
8. Markowitz LE, et al. *MMWR.* 2007;56(RR-2):1-24.
9. Centers for Disease Control and Prevention Web site. ACIP provisional recommendations for HPV vaccine. http://www.cdc.gov/vaccines/recs/provisional/downloads/hpv-vac-dec2009-508.pdf. Accessed February 4, 2010.
10. Grunbaum JA, et al. *MMWR.* 2004;53(SS-2):1-96.
11. Sanders GD, et al. *Emerg Infect Dis.* 2003;9:37-48.
12. Elbasha E, et al. *Emerg Infect Dis.* 2007;13:29-41.
13. Kim JJ, et al. *N Engl J Med.* 2008;359:821-832.
14. Kim JJ, et al. *BMJ.* 2009;339:b3884.
15. Garland SM, et al. *N Engl J Med.* 2007;356:1928-1943.
16. The FUTURE II Study Group. *N Engl J Med.* 2007;356:1915-1927.
17. Brown DR, et al. *J Infect Dis.* 2009;199:926-935.
18. Wheeler CM, et al. *J Infect Dis.* 2009,199:936-944.
19. Block SL, et al. *Pediatrics.* 2006;118:2135-2145.
20. Reisinger KS, et al. *Pediatr Infect Dis J.* 2007;26:201-209.
21. Harper DM, et al. *Lancet.* 2004;364:1757-1765.
22. Harper DM, et al. *Lancet.* 2006;367:1247-1255.
23. The GlaxoSmithKline HPV-007 Study Group. *Lancet.* 2009;374:1975-1985.
24. Paavonen J, et al. *Lancet.* 2007;369:2161-2170.
25. Paavonen J, et al. *Lancet.* 2009;374:301-314.
26. Einstein MH, et al. *Human Vaccines.* 2009;5:705-719.
27. Reiter PL, et al. *Vaccine.* 2009;27:6840-6844.
28. Block SL, et al. *Pediatr Infect Dis J.* 2010;29:95-101.
29. Slade BA, et al. *JAMA.* 2009;302:750-757.
30. American College of Obstetricians and Gynecologists. *Obstet Gynecol.* 2009;114:1409-1420

14

15

Influenza

The Pathogen

Influenza viruses are enveloped and have a segmented, single-stranded RNA genome. Two major surface proteins are involved in infectivity and generation of protective immune responses: hemagglutinin (H), which mediates attachment, and neuraminidase (N), which mediates release from cells. Proteolytic cleavage of the H molecule is required for infectivity. H and N types for influenza A viruses are designated by numbers—since 1977, the predominant circulating strains have been A(H1N1) and A(H3N2). The H and N molecules undergo minor changes from year to year that result in slight variation in antigenicity, termed *antigenic drift*. This accounts for the fact that a person's experience with influenza in the prior year does not prevent infection with the current year's strain, although severity of illness might be mitigated (depending on how much drift has occurred). Occasionally, a major change occurs, resulting in strains that express novel H or N molecules to which few people have immunity—this is termed *antigenic shift*. Influenza B viruses do not change as much from year to year because they have a limited host range (humans and seals) and they mutate at a slower rate.

Antigenic shift can occur when an animal (usually a pig) is simultaneously infected with an animal strain of influenza A (usually an avian strain) and a human strain (pigs are in a position to be exposed to both). Through *ressortment*, the human strain may package the RNA segment encoding the avian H or N molecule, creating a human virus with the avian H or N type. If this reassortant is capable of spreading from person to person, a pandemic may ensue. A global reservoir of influenza viruses (and gene segments) exists in aquatic birds.[1] These viruses are adapted to the avian enteric tract and do not cause disease. However, when they enter the pig along with human influenza strains, new strains can emerge that spread from person to person and cause disease. Pigs are good "mixing vessels" because their respiratory epithelial cells express both alpha 2,3-linked sialic acid residues, to which avian influenza viruses bind (via the H molecule), as well as alpha 2,6-linked sialic acid residues, to which human influenza viruses bind.

Pandemic strains can also emerge if animal influenza viruses adapt directly to humans. This is what happened in 1918, leading to the "mother of all influenza pandemics."[2] The A(H1N1) Spanish flu that appeared that year killed 50 million people worldwide; more Americans died from influenza in 1918 than were killed during World Wars I and II and the Korean, Vietnam,

Gulf, Afghanistan, and Iraq wars—*combined*.[3] The adaptation of this virus to human-to-human transmission was facilitated by a single amino acid change in the H molecule; the exceptional virulence was due to its ability to cause dysregulation of the host inflammatory response.[4] All interpandemic influenza A *epidemics* since 1918 have been caused by descendants of the 1918 strain that underwent antigenic drift; all influenza A *pandemics* since 1918, including those caused by the 1957 H2N2 "Asian" flu and the 1968 H3N2 "Hong Kong" flu, were caused by descendants of the 1918 virus that underwent antigenic shift.

2009 A(H1N1) is a reassortant, but it appears to have derived from a number of exchange events between circulating viruses.[5] In particular, the H gene is most closely related to classic swine influenza and the N gene is closely related to Eurasian swine influenza (both of which are descendants of the 1918 virus); and other genes apparently came from a human H3N2 strain and an avian strain. Antibodies recognizing the 2009 virus have been found in very few children and in only 6% to 9% of adults under 65 years of age, suggesting that the virus has not circulated among humans for several generations.[6] Antibody *has* been detected in about a third of adults over 60 years of age, suggesting that something similar may have circulated years ago, or that a previous version of the seasonal vaccine may have had shared antigenic determinants. The H of 2009 A(H1N1) is only 72% to 73% homologous at the amino acid level with seasonal H1 viruses; it is not surprising, therefore, that vaccination with recent seasonal vaccines does not induce protective responses. Transmissibility appears to be less than previous pandemic influenza viruses.[7]

The influenza A(H5N1) strain that emerged in humans in Southeast Asia in 2005 (bird flu) is entirely of avian origin (ie, not the product of reassortment).[8] Its ability to spread to humans also appears to have resulted from a change in its H molecule, allowing binding to alpha 2,6-linked sialic acid residues. Its increased virulence compared with human strains (which are virulent enough) may be explained by the presence of multiple basic amino acids in the region of the connecting peptide that links the two H subunits—this allows for cleavage by ubiquitous intracellular proteases—thus enhancing infectivity and expanding tissue tropism. Other virulence factors also may be involved.

Influenza virus infects columnar epithelial cells of the respiratory tract, causing necrosis, edema, and inflammation. Systemic symptoms are probably caused by circulating interleukin-6 and interferon-alpha induced by the infection. Influenza A virus infects all age groups and causes the most severe disease. Influenza B is milder and occurs more often in children.

Clinical Features

The incubation period is 1 to 4 days. Classic symptoms include abrupt onset of fever, myalgia, headache, sore throat, photophobia, tearing, rhinitis, and nonproductive cough. Older children may experience nausea and vomiting, and infants may present with a sepsis-like syndrome. Fever is usually 101° to 102°F (38.3° to 38.9°C) and may be accompanied by prostration. Uncomplicated illness lasts from 3 to 7 days, and while recovery is usually rapid, some patients may have lingering cough and fatigue for several weeks.

Secondary bacterial infection (eg, pneumonia, sinusitis, and otitis media) is the most common complication of influenza. The risk of complications and hospitalization with influenza is highest among persons ≥65 years of age, the very young, and in persons with certain underlying medical conditions. The virus itself may cause pneumonia, encephalitis, myocarditis, myositis, and exacerbation of underlying chronic medical conditions such as cardiopulmonary disease.

The clinical features of 2009 H1N1 are similar to the seasonal flu, although gastrointestinal symptoms are more common. Complications are similar as well. Pregnant women are at particular risk for complications.[9] So are young children. For example, the pediatric hospitalization rate in Argentina during the initial wave of illness was twice that for the seasonal flu and the death rate was 10 times higher.[10] Most of the admitted children were <2 years of age, and most of the deaths were due to refractory hypoxemia in infants <1 year of age. Most children who died had underlying chronic conditions, particularly neurological and pulmonary.

Bird flu typically manifests as febrile pneumonia that progresses rapidly to respiratory failure. Additional clinical and laboratory features include dyspnea, sore throat, headache, elevated transaminases, leukopenia, and thrombocytopenia. Mortality rates are extremely high, ranging from 39% to 88% in various studies, and young adults are disproportionately affected. Death usually occurs during the second week of illness.

Epidemiology and Transmission

Influenza virus is transmitted from person to person through large-particle respiratory droplets that are expelled during coughing or sneezing. Maximum communicability occurs from 1 day before the onset of illness to 5 days thereafter. Disease activity peaks between December and March in temperate climates. During 1976 to 2006, peak influenza activity in the United States occurred most frequently in January (19% of seasons) and February (45% of seasons).[11] However, peak activity occurred in March, April, or May in 19% of seasons. During average interpandemic years, anywhere from 5% to 15% of the population may become infected, and up to half of these infections will result in medical attention. Illness rates are highest among school-aged children, sometimes as high as 30%. Among adults, influenza illness results in an average of 2 lost workdays per episode.

School-aged children are at low risk for complications, but they play a key role in spreading the virus throughout the community. This was demonstrated in a classic study in Houston showing that school absenteeism during the influenza season preceded workplace absenteeism by several weeks.[12] Moreover, routine vaccination of school children in Japan between the 1960s and early 1980s resulted in dramatic reductions in excess (influenza-related) mortality among the elderly and other high-risk groups.[13]

Annual hospitalization rates for laboratory-confirmed influenza are around 20 per 100,000 for children 2 to 5 years of age, but as high as 240 to 720 per 100,000 for infants <6 months of age.[14] The rate of hospitalization for infants is similar to the rate for children with high-risk conditions and is comparable to that for adults ≥65 years of age. The annual outpatient burden of influenza may be as high as 100 clinic visits and 30 emergency department visits per 1000 children.

During the 1980s and 1990s in the United States, influenza resulted in an average of 226,000 hospitalizations and 36,000 deaths.[15,16] In fact, the number of deaths increased over that period of time, due in large part to the aging of the population (90% of deaths occur in persons ≥65 years of age). Although the number of deaths in children is small (153 in the 2003-2004 season), it is notable that nearly two thirds occur in children without underlying medical conditions.

Influenza peaks between April and September in temperate regions of the Southern Hemisphere and occurs throughout the year in tropical areas. Traveling with large tourist groups (eg, on cruise ships) that include persons from these areas increases the risk of infection during the summer.

On April 17, 2009, CDC determined that 2 children in southern California had respiratory infections caused by a strain of influenza A(H1N1) that had never been seen before (the first cases probably occurred in Mexico).[17] The words in the initial report proved to be prophetic: "...concern exists that this new strain of swine influenza A(H1N1) is substantially different from human influenza A(H1N1) viruses, that a large proportion of the population might be susceptible to infection, and that the seasonal influenza vaccine H1N1 strain might not provide protection. The lack of known exposure to pigs in the two cases increases the possibility that human-to-human transmission of this new influenza virus has occurred." On June 11, 2009, the WHO announced that the criteria for an influenza pandemic had been met.[18] At that point in time, infection with 2009 H1N1 had been reported in approximately 30,000 people from 74 countries across the globe. By December 2009 in the United States alone there had been an estimated 55 million cases, 246,000 hospitalizations, and 11,160 deaths.[19] Most cases (32 million), hospitalizations (145,000), and deaths (8620) had occurred among persons 18 to 64 years of age.

Between May 2005 and December 2007, bird flu was reported in 340 humans, most of whom lived in Southeast Asia, Eurasia, and Africa. The median age of affected persons was around 18 years, and the vast majority of patients were <40; this is strikingly different from seasonal influenza, which disproportionately affects the young and the old, but it is reminiscent of the 1918 pandemic. Humans are infected directly from birds; risk factors include handling of sick or dead poultry; slaughtering, defeathering, or preparing sick poultry for consumption; eating undercooked poultry products; and other close contact with birds, such as ducks. Some cases may have been acquired through contaminated fomites, and whereas there is no evidence of sustained human-to-human transmission, limited transmission might have occurred from very close contact with severely affected persons.

Immunization Program

The first influenza vaccines became commercially available in 1945. Between then and 2008, the focus was on protecting individuals from complications, hospitalization, and death related to influenza. High-risk groups were identified and recommended for annual immunization, and increasing emphasis was placed on immunizing close contacts of those individuals. Immunization of all adults ≥65 years of age was recommended until 2000, when the recommendation was broadened to include all adults ≥50 years of age. In 2002, immunization of all children 6 to 23 months of age was "encouraged"[20]; in 2004, this was changed to a strong recommendation.[21] In 2006, all children 24 to 59 months of age were added to the routine vaccination list.[22]

In 2008, an unprecedented step was taken—going beyond protecting individuals to protecting the general community. The recommendation was made to extend routine childhood immunization to include all children 6 months to 18 years of age.[23] As noted earlier, there is good reason to believe that preventing influenza in school-aged children will change the epidemiology of influenza transmission in the community. In 2009, there was a subtle but important change in the language surrounding universal childhood immunization, from "if feasible" to, essentially, "just do it."[24] Finally, at the February 2010 ACIP meeting, it was decided to recommend yearly influenza immunization for all persons ≥6 months of age.[25]

Recommendations for seasonal influenza are updated in the summer of each year. In 2009, separate recommendations for use of 2009 H1N1 vaccine were issued.[26] Recognizing that initial supplies would be limited, a risk-based tiered approach to vaccination was adopted. By 2010, vaccine supply was replete and in essence, the recommendations for 2009 H1N1 were the same as those for seasonal vaccine. In February 2010, it was decided that the 2009 H1N1 strain would be incorporated into the 3-valent seasonal vaccine for 2010-2011, in place of the previous H1N1 strain.

Studies among working adults suggest that influenza immunization reduces health care provider visits and lost workdays by nearly half.[27] A study in 2001 looked at the direct and indirect costs of both vaccination and disease, assuming that vaccination occurred in a low-cost setting, such as the workplace.[28] This analysis demonstrated that routine vaccination of healthy working adults would result in an average cost saving of $13.66 per person vaccinated (1998 dollars). The cost of immunization per QALY saved (2000 dollars) is estimated to be $980 for persons ≥65 years of age and $28,000 for persons 50-64 years of age.[29] The cost per quality-adjusted life year saved in healthy children 6 to 23 months of age is estimated to be around $12,000 (2003 dollars), and for adolescents around $119,000.[30] The additional benefits that would accrue from the herd-immunity effects of immunizing all school-aged children are difficult to assess.

Recommendations for influenza vaccination of health care personnel were updated in 2006.[31]

Vaccines

Characteristics of the influenza vaccines licensed in the United States are given in **Table 15.1a** and **15.1b**, and differences between LAIV and IIV are summarized in **Table 15.2**.

Influenza vaccines are made using the very same reassortment process that leads to pandemic strains.[32] In the case of IIV, the circulating wild-type viruses are reassorted with a strain that is well adapted to growth in embryonated hen's eggs (allantoic fluid provides the protease necessary for cleavage of the H molecule that is in turn necessary for infectivity). The reassortants have the backbone of the adapted strain and therefore grow efficiently to bulk levels; however, they express the H and N of the wild-type strain and therefore yield useful vaccine antigens. Reassortants can also be made using *reverse genetics*, whereby the relevant genes are harvested and introduced into cells to produce viruses. Vaccine viruses are inoculated into large numbers of hen's eggs; progeny virions are concentrated from allantoic fluids, chemically inactivated, and disrupted ("split"); the H and N proteins are then purified and formulated into a final product.

In the case of LAIV, the wild-type strains are reassorted with a master donor virus (MDV) that is *attenuated*, *cold adapted* (replication is efficient at 25°C), and *temperature sensitive* (replication is restricted at 37°C to 39°C). The reassortants have the backbone of MDV and can therefore be produced in bulk (MDV also grows well in embryonated eggs); because they carry the H and N of the wild-type viruses, they can engender protective immune responses to the circulating strains. The vaccine viruses are grown in hen's eggs; progeny viruses are concentrated from allantoic fluids, suspended in stabilizing buffer, and packaged for IN administration. LAIV replicates in the nasopharynx but is incapable of replicating lower in the respiratory tract.

Traditional seasonal influenza vaccines immunize against 3 strains: A(H1N1), A(H3N2), and influenza B. The specific strains used to manufacture the vaccines are chosen early each year based on the predominant circulating strains and how similar—or different—they are from the previous years' strains. The 2009 H1N1 strain emerged too late for inclusion in the seasonal vaccine; this necessitated 2 separate immunizations for full protection during that year. It is important to point out that the 2009 H1N1 vaccines were made in exactly the same way that the seasonal vaccines were made. In that sense, they were not "new" or "experimental".

There is an influenza A (H5N1) vaccine licensed in the United States. Manufactured by Sanofi Pasteur and approved in 2007, the vaccine is based on a laboratory strain of influenza A that was modified to carry the genes encoding the H and N of the human isolate A/Vietnam/1203/2004 (H5N1, clade 1). The H gene was mutated to prevent cleavage of the mature protein, reducing pathogenicity and allowing the vaccine to grow efficiently in embryonated eggs. The vaccine virus is inactivated with formaldehyde, chemically disrupted, and purified, in much the same way as is IIV-seasonal. Licensure was based on immunogenicity. Among 99 subjects receiving 2 doses of the 90-mcg formulation of the vaccine, 43% achieved a 4-fold or greater rise in hemagglutination inhibition antibody titer and a minimum titer of 1:40. The vaccine is not commercially available but will be purchased by the federal government for inclusion in the National Stockpile for distribution by public health officials, if necessary.

Efficacy and/or Immunogenicity

Each years' influenza vaccines are licensed based on immunogenicity, not efficacy. The accepted correlate of protection is a hemagglutination inhibition titer of $\geq 1:40$ (this test measures the ability of serum to compete with the binding of influenza virus to red blood cells); 50% of individuals who achieve this level of antibody are presumed to be protected.[33] Practically speaking, vaccine-induced immunity to influenza is good for only 1 year because antibody wanes. In addition, the vaccine strains chosen for a given year may not be a good antigenic match with the prevailing strains. For example, during the 2007 to

TABLE 15.1a — Influenza Vaccines[a]

	Agriflu	Afluria	Fluarix	Flulaval
Trade name				
2009 H1N1 version available[b]	No	Yes	No	Yes
Abbreviation[c]	IIV	IIV	IIV	IIV
Manufacturer/distributor	Novartis	CSL Biotherapies/Merck	GlaxoSmithKline	ID Biomedical/GlaxoSmithKline
Type of vaccine	Inactivated, purified subunits (split virus)	Inactivated, purified subunits (split virus)	Inactivated, purified subunits (split virus)	Inactivated, purified subunits (split virus)
Composition[d]:				
Inactivation (IIV)	Formaldehyde	Beta-propiolactone	Formaldehyde	Ultraviolet light and formaldehyde
Hemagglutinin (IIV)	15 mcg from each strain	15 mcg from each strain	15 mcg from each strain	15 mcg from each strain
Adjuvant	None	None	None	None
Preservative	None	Thimerosal (24.5 mcg mercury) or none	None	Thimerosal (25 mcg mercury)
Excipients and contaminants	Egg protein (<0.4 mcg) Formaldehyde (≤10 mcg) Polysorbate 80 (≤50 mcg) Cetyltrimethylammonium bromide (≤12 mcg) Neomycin (≤0.02 mcg) Kanamycin (≤0.03 mcg)	Sodium chloride (4.1 mg) Monobasic sodium phosphate (80 mcg) Dibasic sodium phosphate (300 mcg) Monobasic potassium phosphate (20 mcg)	Octoxynol-10 (≤0.085 mg) Alpha-tocopherol hydrogen succinate (≤0.1 mg) Polysorbate 80 (≤0.415 mg) Hydrocortisone (≤0.0016 mg) Gentamicin sulfate (≤0.15 mcg) Ovalbumin (≤1 mcg)	Ovalbumin (≤1 mcg) Formaldehyde (≤25 mcg) Sodium deoxycholate (≤50 mcg)

		None	Potassium chloride (20 mcg) Calcium chloride (1.5 mcg) Sodium taurodeoxycholate (≤10 ppm) Ovalbumin (≤1 mcg) Neomycin sulfate (≤0.2 pg) Polymyxin B (≤0.03 pg) Beta-propiolactone (<25 ng)	Formaldehyde (≤50 mcg) Sodium deoxycholate (≤50 mcg)
Latex	None	None	Tip cap and plunger of pre-filled syringe contain dry natural rubber	None
Labeled indications	Protection against influenza	Protection against influenza	Protection against influenza	Protection against influenza
Labeled ages[e]	≥18 years	≥6 months	≥3 years	≥18 years
Dose	0.5 mL	0.25 mL or 0.5 mL	0.5 mL	0.5 uL
Route of administration	Intramuscular	Intramuscular	Intramuscular	Intramuscular
Labeled schedule	1 dose annually	1 dose annually	1 dose annually	1 dose annually
Recommended schedule	Same	Same	Same	Same

Continued

15

TABLE 15.1a — *Continued*

Trade name	Agriflu	Afluria	Fluarix	Flulaval
How supplied (number in package)	Prefilled syringe (10)	10-dose vial (1), with preservative Prefilled syringe (10), 0.25 mL or 0.5 mL, without preservative	Prefilled syringe (5)	10-dose vial (1)
Storage	Refrigerate Do not freeze Protect from light	Refrigerate Do not freeze Protect from light Multidose vial should be discarded 28 days after first use	Refrigerate Do not freeze Protect from light	Refrigerate Do not freeze Protect from light Multidose vial should be discarded 28 days after carded 28 days after use
Cost per dose, pediatric ($US, 2009):				
Public	—	—	—	—
Private	—	—	—	—
Cost per dose, adult ($US, 2009):				
Public	—	6.00	8.90	6.70
Private	—	7.00	13.25	10.50
Reference package insert	November 2009	November 2009	October 2009	July 2009

342

TABLE 15.1b — Influenza Vaccines[a]

	FluMist	Fluvirin	Fluzone	Fluzone-High Dose
Trade name				
2009 H1N1 version available[b]	Yes	Yes	Yes	No
Abbreviation[c]	LAIV	IIV	IIV	IIV
Manufacturer/distributor	MedImmune (AstraZeneca)	Novartis	Sanofi Pasteur	Sanofi Pasteur
Type of vaccine	Live-attenuated, engineered	Inactivated, purified subunits (split virus)	Inactivated, purified subunits (split virus)	Inactivated, purified subunits (split virus)
Composition[d]:				
Inactivation (IIV)	Contains cold-adapted temperature-sensitive, attenuated reassortants	Beta-propiolactone	Formaldehyde	Formaldehyde
Hemagglutinin (IIV)	$10^{6.5\text{-}7.5}$ fluorescent focus units of each reassortant strain	15 mcg from each strain	15 mcg from each strain	60 mcg from each strain
Adjuvant	None	None	None	None
Preservative	None	Thimerosal (24.5 mcg mercury) or none	Thimerosal (25 mcg mercury) or none	None

Continued

15

TABLE 15.1b — *Continued*

Trade name	FluMist	Fluvirin	Fluzone	Fluzone-High Dose
Excipients and contaminants	Monosodium glutamate (0.188 mg) Hydrolyzed porcine gelatin (2 mg) Arginine (2.42 mg) Sucrose (13.68 mg) Dibasic potassium phosphate (2.26 mg) Monosodium phosphate (0.96 mg) Gentamicin sulfate (<0.015 mcg/mL)	Preservative-free formulation: thimerosal (≤1 mcg mercury) Ovalbumin (≤1 mcg) Polymyxin (≤3.75 mcg) Neomycin (≤2.5 mcg) Betapropiolactone (≤0.5 mcg) Nonylphenol ethoxylate (≤0.015%)	Sodium phosphate-buffered isotonic sodium chloride Gelatin (0.05%) Formaldehyde (≤100 mcg) Polyethylene glycol p-iso-octylphenyl ether (≤0.02%) Sucrose (≤2.0%)	Sodium phosphate-buffered isotonic sodium chloride Formaldehyde (≤100 mcg) Octylphenol ethoxylate (≤250 mcg)
Latex	None	None	None	None
Labeled indications	Protection against influenza	Protection against influenza	Protection against influenza	Protection against influenza
Labeled ages	2 to 49 years	≥4 years	≥6 months	≥65 years
Dose[e]	0.2 mL (0.1 mL per nostril)	0.5 mL	0.25 mL or 0.5mL	0.5 mL
Route of administration	Intranasal[f]	Intramuscular	Intramuscular	Intramuscular
Labeled schedule	1 dose annually	1 dose annually	1 dose annually	1 dose annually
Recommended schedule	Same	Same	Same	Same

	Prefilled sprayer (10)	10-dose vial (1), with preservative Prefilled syringe (10), without preservative	10-dose vial (1), with preservative 1-dose vial (10), without preservative Prefilled syringe (10), 0.25 mL or 0.5 mL, without preservative	Prefilled syringe (10)
How supplied (number in package)				
Storage	Refrigerate[v] Do not freeze[h]	Refrigerate Do not freeze Protect from light	Refrigerate Do not freeze	Refrigerate Do not freeze
Cost per dose, pediatric ($US, 2009):				
Public	15.25	7.75	9.09	—
Private	19.70	9.75	9.72	—
Cost per dose, adult ($US, 2009):				
Public	15.25	4.90	8.15	—
Private	19.70	9.75	9.72	—
Reference package insert	June 2009	April 2009	May 2009	December 2009

15

Continued

TABLE 15.1b — *Continued*

a Influenza vaccines are interchangeable in the sense that one product (any inactivated influenza vaccine or live influenza vaccine) can be used one year and another product the next year. Although no data are available regarding 2 consecutive doses of different products in the same year, it is assumed that this is acceptable. Other inactivated or live vaccines may be given at any time in relation to IIV; other inactivated vaccines may be given at any time in relation to LAIV, but LAIV and other live vaccines should not be given within 4 weeks of each other. Also, LAIV-seasonal and LAIV-2009 H1N1 should not be given at the same time.

b The monovalent 2009 H1N1 vaccines had no trade names and were distributed by the government free of charge. The presentation, preservative, and approved ages were the same as the analogous seasonal vaccines. For the 2010-2011 season, the 2009 H1N1 strain will be incorporated into the 3-valent seasonal vaccine, replacing the previous H1N1 strain.

c "IIV" stands for "inactivated influenza vaccine" (other publications may refer to this as "TIV", for "trivalent [inactivated] influenza vaccine). "LAIV" stands for "live-attenuated influenza vaccine". The (trivalent) seasonal versions are "IIV-seasonal" and "LAIV-seasonal", and the analogous monovalent 2009 H1N1 vaccines are "IIV-2009 H1N1" and "LAIV-2009 H1N1".

d The table shows the composition of the seasonal vaccines. The strains used vary from year to year depending on the strains that are anticipated to circulate during the influenza season. Each vaccine contains a strain of influenza A(H1N1), A(H3N2), and B. The vaccine viruses are propagated in embryonated eggs; for IIV, they are inactivated by the method listed.

e The dose of IIV for children 6 months through 35 months of age is 0.25 mL; for persons ≥36 months of age, it is 0.5 mL.

f If the patient sneezes after administration, the dose should not be repeated. Influenza antiviral medications should be avoided in the 48 hours before and 2 weeks after vaccination. No data exist regarding concomitant use of intranasal medications, including nasal steroids. Individuals who are too old to receive LAIV themselves or who have medical contraindications other than severe immunosuppression may administer the vaccine.

g Ideally, live influenza vaccine should be administered shortly after removal from the refrigerator. However, the vaccine may be used if left at room temperature for up to 12 hours. Unused vaccine kept at room temperature for less than 12 hours can be returned to the refrigerator and subsequently used.

h If inadvertently frozen, live influenza vaccine can be thawed in the refrigerator and subsequently used.

2008 influenza season, the circulating A(H3N2) and B viruses (A/Brisbane/10/2007-like and B/Florida/04/2006-like, respectively) were substantially different from the strains in the vaccine (A/Wisconsin/67/2005-like and B/Malaysia/2506/2004-like, respectively). Effectiveness against medically attended influenza A infection was 58% but no effectiveness against influenza B was seen.[34]

Efficacy (reduction in laboratory-confirmed cases) and effectiveness (reduction in symptomatic cases) may differ markedly. For example, a systematic review in 2005 found that efficacy of LAIV in children >2 years of age was 79% but effectiveness was 38%; for IIV, the respective numbers were 65% and 28%.[35] One reason for this is the large proportion of cases of influenza-like illness that are caused by other viruses.

■ IIV

Most vaccinees develop serum hemagglutination inhibition and neutralizing antibodies. Children 6 months to 8 years of age require 2 doses in the same season to ensure protective responses. In a study among children conducted between 1985 and 1990, annual vaccination with IIV-seasonal reduced laboratory-confirmed influenza A by 77% to 91%.[36] A 1-year placebo-controlled study yielded efficacy estimates of 56% among healthy children 3 to 9 years of age and 100% among adolescents,[37] and a retrospective study of 30,000 young children showed approximately 50% effectiveness against medically-attended, clinically diagnosed pneumonia or influenza.[38] IIV-seasonal may also reduce episodes of otitis media in children by as much as 30%.

Randomized controlled trials demonstrate efficacy against laboratory-confirmed influenza illness of 70% to 90% among healthy adults <65 years of age.[24] Whereas estimates of efficacy drop to 50% to 77% when the vaccine and circulating strains are not well matched, protection against hospitalization appears to be preserved. Efficacy against illness is lower among adults >65 years of age, but protection against influenza-related death may be as high as 80%.

Immunogenicity may be lower among immunocompromised individuals and those with chronic medical conditions. A 2009 study compared the immunogenicity of high-dose IIV containing 60 mcg of H from each strain to that of the standard vaccine (containing 15 mcg of H from each strain) among 2575 adults ≥65 years of age.[39] The geometric mean titer of antibody against influenza A strains was almost twice as high for the high-dose vaccine, and the seroprotection rate for A(H1N1) was 13% higher.

Efficacy data for 2009 H1N1 vaccines are not available. In an Australian study involving infants and children 6 months to 8 years of age, 2 doses of IIV-2009 H1N1 containing 15 mcg of H were administered 21 days apart.[40] Antibody titers ≥1:40 were seen in 93% of children after one dose and 100% after 2 doses,

347

TABLE 15.2 — Differences Between Live and Inactivated Influenza Vaccines

Characteristic	Live	Inactivated
Route of administration	Intranasal spray	Intramuscular injection
Type of vaccine	Live attenuated, engineered	Inactivated, purified subunits
Labeled age indication	2-49 years of age	≥6 months of age[a]
Minimal interval between doses	4 weeks (for LAIV-2009 H1N1, the official interval is "approximately" 4 weeks)	4 weeks (for IIV-2009 H1N1, ≥21 days is acceptable)
Simultaneous administration with other vaccines	Yes, except that LAIV-seasonal and LAIV-2009 H1N1 should not be given at the same time[b]	Yes
Minimum interval for any inactivated vaccine not given on the same day	None	None
Minimum interval for any live vaccine not given on the same day	4 weeks	None
Can the vaccine be used in the following situations?		
Persons with medical conditions that place them at increased risk for complications of influenza	No	Yes

Persons with asthma or children 2 to 4 years of age with wheezing in the past year	No	Yes
Close contacts of immunosuppressed persons who *do not* require a protected environment	Yes	Yes
Close contacts of immunosuppressed persons who *do* require a protected environment	No	Yes
Close contacts of persons at high risk but who are not severely immunosuppressed	Yes	Yes

[a] Approved ages vary by product (see **Tables 15.1a** and **15.1b**).

[b] The concern here is the potential for interference between the vaccine viruses.

Adapted from CDC. *MMWR.* 2009;58(RR-8):1-52, and CDC. *MMWR.* 2009;58(RR-10):1-8.

15

regardless of age, baseline serostatus, and history of seasonal influenza vaccination. In a similar study in adults, 97% of 120 subjects who received a single injection achieved protective antibody levels.[41]

■ LAIV

Immunologic correlates of protection after administration of live influenza vaccine have not been established but probably include antibodies in nasal secretions. LAIV was evaluated in a placebo-controlled study between 1996 and 1998 involving 1602 healthy children 15 to 71 months of age. Efficacy against culture-confirmed influenza was 89% for those who received 1 dose and 94% for those who received 2 doses. In the second year, despite a poor match with the circulating A(H3N2) strain, efficacy was 86%.[42] Efficacy against pneumonia, other lower respiratory tract disease, and influenza-associated otitis media was also demonstrated. In a multinational trial conducted during the 2004-2005 influenza season, 3916 children <5 years of age were randomized to receive LAIV and 3936 to receive IIV.[43] Culture-confirmed influenza illness caused by any strain was reduced by 55% in recipients of LAIV compared with recipients of IIV; for matched strains, the reduction was 45% and for mismatched strains it was 58%, suggesting that LAIV provides broader cross-protection. Additional prelicensure, placebo-controlled trials involving >4000 children demonstrated efficacy of 73% to 93% for culture-confirmed influenza due to any strain. A meta-analysis published in 2009 suggested that LAIV was 46% more effective than IIV in preventing influenza illness due to matched strains among young children receiving 2 doses in one season[44]; the relative efficacy among older children receiving one dose was 35%. The efficacy of LAIV and IIV are more comparable in adults.[45]

A multicenter placebo-controlled trial among 4561 healthy, working adults was conducted during 1997-1998, a season when the A(H3N2) strain in the vaccine was not well matched with the circulating strain.[46] Febrile illnesses were not reduced among vaccinees, but severe febrile illnesses (19% reduction) and febrile upper respiratory tract illnesses (24% reduction) were. There were also reductions in days of illness (23% for febrile illnesses, 27% for severe febrile illnesses), days of work lost (18% for severe febrile illnesses, 28% for febrile respiratory tract illnesses), and days with health care provider visits (25% for severe febrile illnesses, 41% for febrile upper respiratory tract illnesses). Use of prescription antibiotics and over-the-counter medications was reduced.

In experiments using LAIV as a challenge, subjects previously immunized with LAIV shed less virus than those previously immunized with inactivated vaccine. These results suggest that LAIV-seasonal may reduce carriage of natural influenza virus and help to control spread of infection in the community.

IIV

Inactivated influenza vaccine cannot cause influenza. Less than one third of vaccinees have been reported to develop local redness or induration for 1 to 2 days at the site of injection. Fever, chills, headache, and malaise, although infrequent, most often affect children who have had no previous exposure to the antigens contained in the vaccine. These reactions generally begin 6 to 12 hours after vaccination and persist for only 1 to 2 days. Immediate reactions, presumably allergic, may consist of hives, angioedema, allergic asthma, or systemic anaphylaxis. These are rare and probably result from hypersensitivity to a vaccine component, most likely residual egg protein. If influenza vaccines have any association with Guillain-Barré syndrome, it is on the order of one case per million vaccinees, well below the background rate in the population (see *Chapter 7: Addressing Concerns About Vaccines—Do Vaccines Cause Guillain-Barré Syndrome [GBS]?*).

In a retrospective study of 45,000 children 6 to 23 months of age, vaccination was not associated with any medically attended outcome, but several diagnoses, such as acute upper respiratory tract illness, otitis media, and asthma, were significantly *reduced*.[47] Some studies in adults show similar rates of systemic symptoms, such as fever, malaise, myalgia, and headache, between vaccinees and placebees. There is no evidence that IIV has any deleterious impact on HIV infection.

High-dose IIV-seasonal is somewhat more reactogenic than standard-dose.[39] Pain is reported by 36% of vaccinees and erythema by 15%; reactions are generally mild and resolve within 3 days. High fever is more common than standard-dose vaccine but experienced by only 1% of vaccinees.

In the Australian study of IIV-2009 H1N1,[40] 45% of subjects had local pain after the first dose, but this was characterized as severe in only 0.5%; 34% had redness and 17% swelling. Fever was seen in 24% but was ≤103.1°F (39.5°C) in 99.5%. In the adult study,[41] local discomfort was reported in 46% of subjects and systemic symptoms in 45%, but nearly all events were mild to moderate in intensity.

During the 2000 to 2001 season in Canada, a discrete oculo-respiratory syndrome was reported with IIV.[48] Symptoms were mild and self-limited, began within 24 hours of injection, and included hoarseness, sore throat, difficulty swallowing, cough, sore and/or itchy eyes, bilateral conjunctival erythema, facial edema, and nasal congestion. Microaggregates of unsplit virus were implicated as the cause.

■ LAIV

Children report rhinorrhea or congestion (20% to 75%), headache (2% to 46%), fever (up to 26%), vomiting (3% to 13%), abdominal pain (2%), and myalgias (up to 21%). Symptoms are more often associated with the first dose and are self-limited. In a randomized trial in 8352 children 6 to 59 months of age, rhinorrhea among first-time vaccinees was reported in 57% of LAIV recipients and in 46.3% of IIV recipients.[43] Temperature >100°F (37.8°C) was reported in 5.4% of LAIV and in 2% of IIV recipients. Among children <24 months of age, 3.2% of LAIV recipients and 2.0% of IIV recipients had medically significant wheezing after 1 dose.

Adult vaccinees report rhinorrhea (44%, vs 27% in placebees), headache (40% vs 38%), sore throat (28% vs 17%), tiredness (26% vs 22%), muscle aches (17% vs 15%), cough (14% vs 11%), and chills (9% vs 6%).

Serious adverse events are rare. Shedding of vaccine virus is common among children, with up to 80% shedding at least one strain from 1 to 21 days postvaccination. However, horizontal transmission appears to be rare—the estimated probability of a young child acquiring a vaccine virus from a vaccinated child in the day care setting is 0.6% to 2.4%. Up to 50% of adults may have viral antigen in nasal secretions for the first 7 days after vaccination. Person-to-person transmission among adults has not been assessed.

- *Contraindications for IIV*
  - Allergic reaction to previous dose of vaccine or any vaccine component, including eggs (risk of recurrent allergic reaction). Being able to eat eggs (even in baked goods) without adverse effects is a reasonable indication of a very low risk of anaphylaxis. Mild or local manifestations of allergy to eggs or feathers are not a contraindication. Skin testing can be done and desensitization may be possible.
- *Precautions for IIV*
  - Moderate or severe acute illness (difficulty distinguishing illness from vaccine reaction)
  - Personal history of Guillain-Barré syndrome within 6 weeks of a prior dose of influenza vaccine (risk of recurrent Guillain-Barré syndrome; family history not relevant)
- *Contraindications for LAIV*
  - Allergic reaction to previous dose of vaccine or any vaccine component, including eggs (risk of recurrent allergic reaction). Being able to eat eggs (even in baked goods) without adverse effects is a reasonable indication of a very low risk of anaphylaxis. Mild or local manifestations of allergy to eggs or feathers are not a contraindication.
  - Underlying medical conditions that place patients at high risk for complications and serve as an *indication* for influ-

enza vaccination, including asthma (or equivalent), chronic cardiopulmonary disease (except hypertension), diabetes, renal dysfunction, hemoglobinopathies, immunodeficiency, or immunosuppression (risk of exacerbating underlying condition or causing influenza-like disease)
- Children or adolescents receiving aspirin or other salicylates (risk of Reye syndrome)
- Pregnancy (theoretic risk to the fetus or attribution of birth defects to vaccination)
- Household or health care contacts of severely immunosuppressed individuals, eg, hematopoietic stem-cell transplant recipients who are confined to protective environments with regulated airflow, filtration, etc (risk of transmission of live virus to immunosuppressed person). Individuals who receive LAIV should avoid contact with severely immunosuppressed patients for 7 days; contact with patients who have lesser degrees of immunosuppression is acceptable. Health care personnel who work in the neonatal intensive care unit may receive LAIV.
- Individuals receiving influenza antivirals within 48 hours before or 2 weeks after vaccination (risk of decreased viral replication and poor immune response)
- *Precautions for LAIV*
  - Moderate or severe acute illness (difficulty distinguishing illness from vaccine reaction)
  - Personal history of Guillain-Barré syndrome within 6 weeks of a prior dose of influenza vaccine (risk of recurrent Guillain-Barré syndrome; family history not relevant)
  - Severe nasal congestion (interference with delivery of vaccine)
  - Use of nasal steroids is *not* a contraindication or precaution *per se*, but there are the theoretical risks of reduced immunogenicity and increased side effects. In addition, if the patient is being treated for nasal congestion, one should consider whether or not vaccine delivery to the nasal mucosa might be affected.

Recommendations

Influenza vaccine is given annually, usually beginning in October in the United States (in truth, vaccinations can begin as soon as vaccine is available). It is never too late in the season to vaccinate. In general, vaccination efforts should continue well into March. There is no preference for LAIV or IIV in otherwise healthy persons.

Every person ≥6 months of age should receive yearly influenza immunization. IIV may be used for anyone without a contraindication; LAIV should only be used for healthy persons 2 to 49 years of age. While asthma is a contraindication for LAIV, there are children in the 2- to 4-year age group who have had episodes of wheezing but who have not (yet) been diagnosed with asthma. The following screening question for parents has been suggested: "In the past 12 months, has a health care provider ever told you that your child had wheezing or asthma?" If the answer is yes, or if there is a wheezing episode documented in the medical record in the past 12 months, the child should receive IIV instead of LAIV.

Children <9 years of age who are receiving seasonal influenza vaccine for the first time, or who were vaccinated for the first time in the previous season and only received 1 dose, need 2 doses separated by 4 weeks; for the 2009 H1N1 vaccine, the age cut-off was <10 years. If the child reaches the age cut-off before the second dose is given, the second dose is not necessary. Recommendations for the 2010-2011 season should be available by the summer of 2010.

Within the context of a universal immunization program, there are some priority groups. For example, for some time it has been recommended that all persons ≥50 years of age, regardless of underlying conditions, receive IIV each year (there is no preference for high-dose versus standard dose preparations in persons ≥65 years of age). In addition, there is a particular focus on children 6 months to 4 years of age. The following high-risk groups should also be given priority (only IIV should be used):

- Women who will be pregnant during influenza season. There is no preference for products that are thimerosal free (see *Chapter 6: Vaccination in Special Circumstances— Pregnancy*)
- Patients with chronic conditions involving the following systems:
  - Pulmonary (eg, emphysema, chronic bronchitis, and asthma)
  - Cardiovascular, except for hypertension (eg, congestive heart failure)
  - Metabolic diseases (eg, diabetes mellitus)
  - Renal (eg, nephrotic syndrome, hemodialysis)
  - Hepatic (eg, cirrhosis)
  - Hematologic (eg, sickle cell disease, other hemaglobinopathies)
  - Immunologic (eg, immunosuppressive medications, congenital immunodeficiency, HIV infection)
  - Neurologic (eg, cognitive dysfunction, spinal cord injury, seizure disorder, neuromuscular disorder that compromises respiratory function or handling of secretions)
- Persons 6 months to 18 years of age on long-term aspirin therapy (to reduce the risk of Reye syndrome)

Persons in the following groups who are at increased risk for infection or who might spread influenza to high-risk persons should also be given priority (either IIV or LAIV may be used, depending on the age and presence or absence of contraindications):

- Household contacts of, and persons who provide care for, children <5 years of age (especially <6 months), adults ≥50 years of age, and persons with any of the high-risk conditions listed earlier. LAIV should not be used for those who have contact with severely immunosuppressed patients (eg, hematopoietic stem-cell transplant recipients who are confined to protective environments with regulated airflow, filtration, etc).
- Health care personnel (this includes physicians, nurses, residents, students, medical emergency response workers, and other workers in hospitals and clinics)
- Residents and employees of assisted-living residences, chronic or long-term care facilities, correctional facilities, nursing homes, and similar residential institutions
- Persons who provide essential community services
- Students living in dormitories
- Travelers (see *Chapter 6: Vaccination in Special Circumstances—Travel*)

REFERENCES

1. Morens DM, et al. *N Engl J Med*. 2009;361:225-229.
2. Taubenberger JK, et al. *Emerg Infect Dis*. 2006;12:15-22.
3. Johnson NPAS, et al. *Bull Hist Med*. 2002;76:105-115.
4. Kobasa D, et al. *Nature*. 2007;445:319-323.
5. Trifonov V, et al. *New Engl J Med*. 2009;361:115-119.
6. CDC. *MMWR*. 2009;58:521-524.
7. Cauchemez S, et al. *N Engl J Med*. 2009;361:2619-2627.
8. Writing Committee of the Second World Health Organization Consultation on Clinical Aspects of Human Infection with Avian Influenza A (H5N1) Virus, et al. *N Engl J Med*. 2008;358:261-273.
9. Louie JK, et al. *N Engl J Med*. 2010;362:27-35.
10. Libster R, et al. *N Engl J Med*. 2010;362:45-55.
11. CDC. *MMWR*. 2007;56(RR-6):1-54.
12. Glezen WP, et al. *N Engl J Med*. 1978;298:587-592.
13. Reichert TA, et al. *N Engl J Med*. 2001;344:889-896.
14. Poehling KA, et al. *N Engl J Med*. 2006;355:31-40.
15. Thompson WW, et al. *JAMA*. 2003;289:179-186.
16. Thompson WW, et al. *JAMA*. 2004;292:1333-1340.
17. CDC. *MMWR*. 2009;58:400-402.
18. Chan M. World now at the start of 2009 influenza pandemic. Available at: http://www.who.int/mediacentre/news/statements/2009/h1n1_pandemic_phase6_20090611/en/index.html. Accessed February 9, 2010.
19. CDC estimates of 2009 H1N1 influenza cases, hospitalizations and deaths in the United States, April-December 12, 2009. Centers

15

for Disease Control and Prevention Web site. http://www.cdc.gov /h1n1flu/estimates_2009_h1n1.htm. Accessed February 9, 2010.

20. CDC. *MMWR*. 2002;51(RR-3):1-32.

21. CDC. *MMWR*. 2004;53(RR-6):1-40.

22. CDC. *MMWR*. 2006;55(RR-10):1-42.

23. CDC. *MMWR*. 2008;57(RR-7):1-60.

24. CDC. *MMWR*. 2009;58(RR-8):1-52.

25. ACIP provisional recommendations for the use of influenza vaccines. Centers for Disease Control and Prevention Web site. http://www.cdc.gov/vaccines/recs/provisional/downloads/flu-vac -mar-2010-508.pdf. Accessed March 13, 2010.

26. CDC. *MMWR*. 2009;58(RR-10):1-8.

27. Nichol KL, et al. *N Engl J Med*. 1995;333:889-893.

28. Nichol KL. *Arch Intern Med*. 2001;161:749-759.

29. Maciosek MV, et al. *Am J Prev Med*. 2006;31:72-79.

30. Prosser LA, et al. *Emerg Infect Dis*. 2006;12:1548-1558.

31. Pearson ML, et al. *MMWR*. 2006;55(RR-2):1-16.

32. Treanor J. *N Engl J Med*. 2004;351:2037-2040.

33. Food and Drug Administration. Guidance for industry: clinical data needed to support the licensure of seasonal inactivated influenza vaccines. http://www.fda.gov/BiologicsBloodVaccines /GuidanceComplianceRegulatoryInformation/Guidances/Vaccines /ucm074794.htm. Accessed February 13, 2010.

34. CDC. *MMWR*. 2008;57:393-398.

35. Jefferson T, et al. *Lancet*. 2005;365:773-780.

36. Neuzil KM, et al. *Pediatr Infect Dis J*. 2001;20:733-740.

37. Clover RD, et al. *J Infect Dis*. 1991;163:300-304.

38. Ritzwoller DP, et al. *Pediatrics*. 2005;116:153-159.

39. Falsey AR, et al. *J Infect Dis*. 2009;200:172-180.

40. Nolan T, et al. *JAMA*. 2010;303:37-46.

41. Greenberg ME, et al. *N Engl J Med*. 2009;361:2405-2413.

42. Belshe RB, et al. *J Pediatr*. 2000;136:168-175.

43. Belshe RB, et al. *N Engl J Med*. 2007;356:685-696.

44. Rhorer J, et al. *Vaccine*. 2009;27:1101-1110.

45. Jefferson TO, et al. *Cochrane Database Syst Rev*. 2007;(2):CD001269.

46. Nichol KL, et al. *JAMA*. 1999;282:137-44.

47. Hambidge SJ, et al. *JAMA*. 2006;296:1990-1997.

48. Boulianne N, et al. *Can Commun Dis Rep*. 2001;27:85-90.

16
Japanese Encephalitis

The Pathogen

Japanese encephalitis (JE) virus (JEV) is a mosquito-borne flavivirus with a single-stranded RNA genome surrounded by a protein nucleocapsid and a lipid envelope. It is antigenically related to West Nile virus and St. Louis encephalitis virus.

Clinical Features

Only 1 in 250 to 1 in 1000 infections with JEV results in symptomatic illness.[1] The incubation period is 5 to 15 days. The most common clinical syndrome is acute encephalitis, followed by aseptic meningitis and undifferentiated febrile illness. Symptoms begin abruptly with fever, lethargy, headache, abdominal pain, nausea, and vomiting. Mental status changes, including disorientation, personality change, agitation, delirium, and abnormal movements are seen, classically resembling parkinsonism, with tremor, ataxia, choreoathetosis, cogwheel rigidity, mask-like facies, and extrapyramidal signs; progression to confusion, delirium, and coma are common.[2] Mutism is a presenting sign in some cases. Up to 75% of patients present with or develop seizures. One third of patients develop cranial nerve palsies and some develop generalized or asymmetric muscular weakness, flaccid or spastic paralysis, and clonus, and some cases resemble polio.

Analysis of the CSF shows moderate lymphocytic pleocytosis and moderately elevated protein. Imaging studies may show diffuse white matter edema, abnormal signal in the thalamus, and hemorrhage. Hyponatremia due to inappropriate secretion of antidiuretic hormone is a frequent complication. The case fatality rate is 20% to 30%; recovery may take months to years, and 30% to 50% of survivors have neurologic or psychiatric sequelae, including memory loss, motor and cranial nerve paresis, movement disorders, chronic seizures, cortical blindness, and behavioral disorders. JEV may cause intrauterine infection and miscarriage when it is acquired in the first or second trimester of pregnancy.

Epidemiology and Transmission

JEV is endemic throughout China, Southeast Asia, the Indian subcontinent, Indonesia, the Philippines, and Australia; approximately half of the world's population is potentially at risk.[3] In temperate areas, transmission generally occurs from May through September with periodic seasonal epidemics. In subtropical Asia, transmission is hyperendemic and the season is longer, from March through October. In tropical Asia, transmission occurs year-round without noticeable seasonable epidemics. In areas where the virus is endemic, almost all individuals will have been infected by early adulthood.

The virus is spread by *Culex* mosquitoes, which breed in ground pools (eg, rice paddies and ditches) in rural areas. These mosquitoes feed on aquatic birds and other animals that remain asymptomatic despite infection. Domestic pigs in particular have sustained viremia and serve as host to many feeding mosquitoes. Humans, horses, and domestic animals are incidental hosts. The risk of transmission is highest in rural areas, and the incidence of disease correlates with abundance of mosquitoes, proximity of pigs and birds, rainy season, and irrigation of agricultural fields. Most cases occur in children 2 to 10 years of age. Persons who travel extensively in or move to endemic areas acquire symptomatic infection at a rate of 1 per 50,000 persons per month.[4] The risk of disease in short-term travelers to developed or urban areas is <1 per million; the risk for travelers to rural areas during the season of risk is somewhere between 1 in 5000 to 1 in 20,000 travelers per week. The risk of infection increases with travel during the transmission season, exposure to rural areas, extended period of travel or residence, and outdoor activities, especially in the evenings when mosquitoes are active. Despite the known risks, only around 10% of at-risk travelers are vaccinated.[5]

Immunization Program

Residing in air-conditioned or screened-in areas, avoiding outdoor activities, and using permethrin-treated mosquito nets, insect repellents, and protective clothing can reduce the risk of infection. Societal changes, such as urbanization, less agriculture, use of pesticides, centralized pig rearing, and improved standards of living, may also contribute to lower disease rates. Since 1996, childhood immunization programs in China, Taiwan, Japan, and Korea have resulted in marked decreases in the number of reported cases. However, there are still 30,000 to 50,000 annual cases worldwide, mostly among children.

Until 2009, the only vaccine available in the United States was JE-MB, which was derived from mouse brain. The vaccine was highly immunogenic but was also reactogenic, and there were reports of a possible association with acute disseminated encephalomyelitis (ADEM), an autoimmune disease of the central nervous system. In 2009, JE-MB was replaced by JE-VC, which is derived from Vero cell culture, for use in adults. Enough doses of JE-MB for children 1 through 16 years of age are contained in the CDC stockpile to last until 2011.

Recommendations for use of JE vaccine were published in 1993[6] and were updated in 2010.[7]

Vaccines

Characteristics of the JE vaccines licensed in the United States are given in **Table 16.1**. These are inactivated, whole-virus vaccines made much the same way as the original Salk vaccine.[8]

Efficacy and/or Immunogenicity

Children 1 to 14 years of age were given JE-MB ($N = 21,628$), a bivalent vaccine that also contained the Beijing strain ($N = 22,080$), or tetanus toxoid as placebo ($N = 21,516$) in a clinical trial in Thailand. Subjects received 2 doses of vaccine 7 days apart. Efficacy of each vaccine was 91%. Based on this study, a 2-dose primary series is used in many parts of Asia. However, <80% of vaccinees in US trials developed protective antibody levels after 2 doses, and responses were short-lived. In contrast, >99% of subjects demonstrated adequate responses to regimens consisting of 3 doses over a 30-day period. The duration of protection after primary immunization is not well defined. In the Thai field trial, efficacy was maintained through 2 years of surveillance, but further follow-up data were not available. All 21 US Army personnel followed for 2 years after vaccination retained seroprotective antibody levels. In a Japanese study, individuals maintained seroprotective levels for 3 years after the primary series.

The immunogenicity of JE-VC was established in a blinded, randomized controlled trial involving 867 adults received either JE-VC at 0 and 28 days or JE-MB at 0, 7, and 28 days.[9] The proportion of subjects who achieved a plaque reduction neutralization titer of $\geq 1:10$, a recognized correlate of protection, was 96.4% in the JE-VC group and 93.8% in the JE-MB group, and the respective geometric mean titers were 243.6 and 102.0, meeting the study's predefined criteria for noninferiority (since the efficacy of JE-MB was already established, efficacy of JE-VC was inferred based on noninferior immunogenicity). In an intention-to-treat analysis of 181 JE-VC recipients, protective titers were maintained by 95% at 6 months and 83.4% at 12 months after vaccination. Booster doses were not evaluated.

TABLE 16.1 — Japanese Encephalitis Vaccines

Trade name	JE-Vax[a]	Ixiaro
Abbreviation	JE-MB (mouse brain-derived)	JE-VC (Vero cell-derived)
Manufacturer/distributor	Biken/Sanofi Pasteur	Intercell Biomedical/Novartis Vaccines and Diagnostics
Type of vaccine	Inactivated, whole agent	Inactivated, whole agent
Composition:		
Virus strain	Nakayama-NIH	SA^{14}-14-2
Propagation	Mouse brain	Vero cells
Inactivation	Formaldehyde	Formaldehyde
Adjuvant	None	Aluminum hydroxide (0.25 mg)
Preservative	Thimerosal (0.007%)	None
Excipients and contaminants	Gelatin (500 mcg) Formaldehyde (<100 mcg) Polysorbate 80 (<0.0007%) Mouse serum protein (<50 ng)	Formaldehyde ($\leq$200 ppm) Bovine serum albumin ($\leq$100 ng/mL) Host cell DNA ($\leq$200 pg/mL) Sodium metabisulphite ($\leq$200 ppm) Host cell proteins ($\leq$300 ng/mL) Protamine sulfate ($\leq$1 mcg/mL)
Latex	None	None
Labeled indications	Prevention of JE	Prevention of JE
Labeled ages	$\geq$1 years	$\geq$17 years

Dose	Age 1 to 2 years: 0.5 mL Age ≥3 years: 1 mL	0.5 mL
Route of administration	Subcutaneous	Intramuscular
Labeled schedule	Primary series: 0, 7, 30 days Abbreviated primary series: 0, 7, 14 days Booster dose in 2 years	0, 28 days[b]
Recommended schedule	Same	Same
How supplied (number in package)	1-dose vial (3), lyophilized, with diluent	Prefilled syringe (1)
Storage	Vaccine: refrigerate Diluent: Refrigerate Do not freeze Reconstituted vaccine: use within 8 hours	Refrigerate Do not freeze
Cost per dose ($US, 2009):		
Public	—	—
Private	260.00	167.00
Reference package insert	December 2005	January 2009

[a] No longer being manufactured as of 2006, but stockpiled vaccine should be available until 2011.
[b] Booster dose not evaluated

16

Injection site tenderness, redness, and swelling are reported in about 20% of JE-MB recipients. Systemic side effects, such as fever, headache, malaise, rash, chills, dizziness, myalgia, nausea, vomiting, and abdominal pain, are reported in 10%. Vaccinees may rarely experience generalized urticaria and angioedema, and the risk of severe hypersensitivity reactions is estimated at 10 to 260 cases per 100,000 vaccinees. Patients should be observed for 30 minutes after vaccination and warned about the possibility of delayed urticaria and angioedema of the extremities, face and oropharynx, airway, and especially the lips. Most such reactions occur within 10 days of vaccination, so travelers should remain in areas where they have access to medical care for that period of time. Persons with a history of idiopathic urticaria or urticaria after hymenoptera envenomation, drugs, or other provocations appear to be at increased risk. Moderate to severe neurologic symptoms have been reported at a rate of 0.1 to 2 cases per 100,000 vaccinees, but the WHO determined that there was no evidence of an increased risk of ADEM.

The total safety database for JE-VC includes over 3,500 adults who received at least 1 dose. About half of vaccinees experience injection site reactions, which is less than that seen after JE-MB. Pain and tenderness occur in about one-third, with erythema and induration in less than 10%. Headache occurs in about 30%, myalgia in about 15%, and fatigue or influenza-like illness in around 10%.

- *Contraindications*
  - Allergic reaction to previous dose of vaccine or any vaccine component (for JE-MB, this includes proteins of rodent or neural origin; for JE-VC, this includes protamine sulfate)
- *Precautions*
  - Moderate or severe acute illness
  - Pregnancy (theoretic risk to the fetus or attribution of birth defects to vaccination, although no deleterious effects from JE vaccine administered during pregnancy have been demonstrated and the risk of adverse fetal effects from an inactivated vaccine is extremely low; it is not clear why pregnancy is listed as a precaution for some inactivated vaccines but not others)
  - JE-MB: allergic reactions or urticaria attributed to any cause (eg, medications, other vaccines, insect bites)

Vaccination is not recommended for short-term travelers who will be restricted to urban areas or who are traveling outside of transmission season. Factors that should be considered in the decision to vaccinate include the incidence of JE in the location of intended stay, the conditions of housing, nature of activities, duration of stay, and the possibility of unexpected travel to high-risk areas. In general, vaccination *should be administered* to persons spending a month or longer in epidemic or endemic areas during the transmission season, especially if travel will include rural areas. Depending on the epidemic circumstances, vaccination *should be considered* for persons spending <30 days who are at particularly high risk, such as those engaging in extensive outdoor activities (eg, camping, hiking, fishing) in rural areas and those whose accommodations lack air conditioning, screens, or bed nets. Vaccination also should be considered for travel to areas with ongoing outbreaks and those who have uncertain or nonspecific itineraries.

No vaccine is available for use in infants <12 months of age. JE-MB is recommended for use in children 1 to 16 years of age and JE-VC for persons ≥17 years of age. Those who received 1 or 2 doses of JE-MB in the past should receive 2 doses of JE-VC if they remain at risk. The vaccine series should be completed at least one week before potential exposure, and travelers should take personal precautions to reduce exposure to mosquito bites. Current CDC advisories should be consulted with regard to disease activity in specific locales.

Laboratory workers with potential exposure to infectious JEV *should be vaccinated*. Periodic monitoring for neutralizing antibodies and/or administration of booster doses may be indicated.

16

REFERENCES

1. Thongcharoen P. *Southeast Asian J Trop Med Public Health.* 1989;20:559-573.

2. Ooi MH, et al. *Clin Infect Dis.* 2008;47:458-468.

3. Erlanger TE, et al. *Emerg Infect Dis.* 2009;15:1-7.

4. Shlim DR, et al. *Clin Infect Dis.* 2002;35:183-188.

5. Duffy M, Reed C, Edelson P, et al. Survey of US travelers to Asia to assess compliance with recommendations for Japanese encephalitis vaccine [presentation]. International Conference on Emerging Infectious Diseases; March 16-19, 2008, Atlanta, GA.

6. CDC. *MMWR.* 1993;42(RR-1):1-15.

7. Fischer M, et al. *MMWR.* 2010;59(RR-1):1-27.

8. Beasley DWC, et al. *Expert Opin Biol Ther.* 2008;8:95-106.

9. Tauber E, et al. *Lancet.* 2007;370:1847-1853.

Measles, Mumps, Rubella

The Pathogens

■ Measles

Measles (rubeola) virus is an enveloped, single-stranded RNA virus in the Paramyxoviridae family. There is only one antigenic type. Two proteins—the hemagglutinin, which mediates attachment, and the fusion protein, which facilitates cell-to-cell spread of the virus—are important in generating neutralizing antibodies. The virus infects the respiratory epithelium of the nasopharynx then spreads to regional lymph nodes, where replication leads to a primary viremia. Continued replication in the reticuloendothelial system leads to a secondary viremia about a week after infection; this leads to replication in the respiratory tract, skin, and viscera. Pathologic changes include lymphoid hyperplasia, mononuclear cell infiltration of the respiratory tract, and multinucleated giant cells.

■ Mumps

Mumps virus is an enveloped, single-stranded RNA virus in the Paramyxoviridae family. The virus contains a hemagglutinin and fusion protein, and there is only one antigenic type. Initial infection occurs in the respiratory epithelium of the nasopharynx, then spreads to regional lymph nodes, where replication leads to viremia and spread to glandular epithelia, including the salivary glands, testes, ovaries, and pancreas. Pathologic changes include interstitial edema and lymphocytic infiltration. Infarcts in the testes can lead to atrophy of the germinal epithelium. The virus also spreads to the CNS, where it infects the choroidal epithelium and ependymal lining of the ventricles, resulting in aseptic meningitis, and, in some cases, encephalitis.

■ Rubella

Rubella virus is an enveloped, single-stranded RNA virus in the Togavirus family. The virus has two major surface glycoproteins—E1 and E2. E1 is a hemagglutinin that engenders neutralizing antibodies. Infection occurs in the respiratory epithelium of the nasopharynx then spreads to regional lymph nodes, where replication leads to viremia. The virus then spreads throughout the body, including the respiratory tract, skin, lymph nodes, and body fluids. While postnatal infection is relatively benign, infection of the fetus, which occurs transplacentally, leads to a persistent infection and progressive generalized vasculitis, affecting organ development.

Clinical Features

■ Measles

Measles is characterized by a several-day prodrome of malaise, fever, anorexia, coryza, cough, and conjunctivitis. Temperature usually increases for 5 or 6 days and can be as high as 104°F (40°C). In uncomplicated cases, the temperature drops 2 to 3 days after the onset of exanthem. At some point between the second and fourth days after onset of symptoms, but before rash appears, characteristic Koplik's spots appear on the buccal mucosa. The rash generally appears around the ears and hairline 3 to 5 days into the illness and spreads downward and outward to cover the face, trunk, and extremities over the next 3 to 4 days. It is initially erythematous and maculopapular and tends to become confluent as it spreads, especially on the face and neck. The rash usually lasts about 5 days and resolves in the order of appearance.

Measles is most frequently complicated by diarrhea, middle ear infection, or bronchopneumonia. Encephalitis occurs in approximately one out of every 1000 cases, and survivors often have permanent brain damage. Death, usually from pneumonia or acute encephalitis, occurs in one to two out of every 1000 cases; the risk is greater for infants, young children, and adults than it is for older children and adolescents. Subacute sclerosing pan-encephalitis is a rare, fatal degenerative disease of the CNS that appears years after measles infection (5 to 10 per million cases) and is associated with persistent infection with a mutant form of the virus.

In developing countries, measles is often more severe, with case-fatality rates as high as 25%. Measles can be severe in persons with vitamin A deficiency, as well as in immunocompromised persons, particularly those who have leukemia, lymphoma, or HIV infection. In these patients, the typical rash may be absent and the patient may shed virus for several weeks.

■ Mumps

Mumps usually presents as bilateral, or less commonly unilateral, parotitis, which may be preceded by fever, headache, malaise, myalgia, and anorexia. Only 30% to 40% of mumps infections produce typical acute parotitis; 15% to 20% are asymptomatic and up to 50% are associated with respiratory or nonspecific symptoms. Parotitis occurs more commonly among children aged 2 to 9 years, and inapparent infection may be more common among adults. Serious complications can occur without evidence of parotitis.

Mumps is usually self-limited but complications do occur. Orchitis is the most common complication in postpubertal males, occurring in up to 50% of cases; half of patients are left with some degree of testicular atrophy, but sterility is rare. Aseptic meningitis is common, occurring asymptomatically in 50% to

60% of patients and associated with headache and stiff neck in up to 15%. Adults are at greater risk for this complication than children, and boys are more often affected than girls. Encephalitis is rare, occurring in <2 per 100,000 cases. Mumps was a leading cause of acquired sensorineural deafness in the prevaccine era, with an estimated incidence of one per 20,000 cases.

■ Rubella

Rubella is characterized by nonspecific signs and symptoms including transient, erythematous and sometimes pruritic rash, postauricular or suboccipital lymphadenopathy, arthralgia, and low-grade fever. Twenty-five percent to 50% of infections are subclinical. The disease is generally considered benign and self-limited.

The most severe effects of rubella occur in the fetuses of pregnant women who contract the infection during the first trimester of pregnancy. Infants born with congenital rubella syndrome may have deafness, cataracts, microophthalmia, cardiac defects, and CNS abnormalities.

Epidemiology and Transmission

■ Measles

Humans are the only natural hosts. In temperate climates, measles occurs primarily in late winter and spring. Transmission is primarily person-to-person via large respiratory droplets. Airborne transmission has been documented in closed areas (such as office examination rooms) for up to 2 hours after the presence of an infected person. Measles is highly contagious, with secondary household attack rates exceeding 90%. It is estimated that before the introduction of the first vaccine in 1963, there were 3 to 4 million cases of measles each year in the United States. That number had fallen to about 1500 by 1983.[1]

However, between 1989 and 1991, there were almost 56,000 reported cases and 123 deaths.[2] This resurgence was primarily due to pockets of low vaccine coverage in the population. Another contributing factor was the fact that infants <1 year of age were more susceptible than in previous eras—their mothers had vaccine-induced immunity rather than natural immunity, and their transplacental antibody inheritance was lower. Finally, primary vaccine failure may have contributed—2% to 5% of children fail to respond to a single dose of MMR.

Renewed efforts to vaccinate young children and the institution of a second vaccination at school entry effectively reversed the resurgence, such that by 2000, measles was considered to be no longer endemic in the United States.[3] This is not to say that importation-related outbreaks do not continue to occur. For example, from January through July of 2008, 131 measles cases were reported; 17 were directly imported from other countries and 99 were epidemiologically linked to imported cases. Most of the cases occurred during outbreaks in Illinois, New York, Washington, Arizona, and California, and 11% of the patients were hospitalized. Among the 123 US residents who got measles, 80% were under 20 years of age and 91% were either unvaccinated or had unknown vaccination status.[4] This experience underscores the importance of maintaining immunization rates despite the absence of endemic disease.

■ Mumps

Humans are the only natural hosts. Mumps incidence peaks in winter and spring, but disease has been reported throughout the year. Transmission occurs through airborne droplet nuclei or direct contact with saliva. Contagiousness is similar to that of influenza and rubella but less than that for measles and chickenpox. The infectious period is considered to be from 3 days before to 4 days after the onset of active disease.

In 1964 there were 212,000 cases in the United States; by 1983, after the vaccine had been licensed for 16 years, the number had fallen to 3000. There was a resurgence of disease among teenagers in the late 1980s that peaked a few years before the measles resurgence. A major contributing factor was the fact that this cohort of teenagers had missed the universal infant vaccination recommendation. The resurgence was reversed by institution of the second MMR vaccine at school entry, and the number of cases reached a low of 258 in 2004. However, 2006 saw a multistate outbreak of 6584 cases, mostly in college students and other young adults, many of whom had 2 doses of the vaccine. Contributing factors may have been failure of 2 doses to produce immunity in some persons and waning immunity from childhood vaccination.[5] Another large outbreak in New York and New Jersey began in June 2009.[6] The index case was an 11-year-old boy who had acquired mumps in the United Kingdom and attended a tradition-observant Jewish summer camp after returning to the United States. By January 2010, 1521 cases had been reported, most of which had occurred in the same Jewish community; 75% of cases had received 2 doses of vaccine.

■ Rubella

Humans are the only natural hosts. In temperate climates, rubella occurs in late winter and early spring. There is no carrier state per se, but infants with congenital rubella syndrome may shed large quantities of virus for up to a year. Rubella is only moderately contagious and spreads from person to person via airborne droplet nuclei shed from the respiratory tract. Transmission by subclinical cases, which constitute 20% to 50% of all infections, can occur. The disease is most contagious when the rash is erupting, but virus may be shed from 7 days before to

7 days after rash onset. Between 1964 and 1965, there were >12 million cases of rubella in the United States and 20,000 babies were born with congenital rubella syndrome.[7] After vaccination was initiated in 1969, the number of cases declined dramatically, such that by 2004, rubella was considered to be no longer endemic in the United States.[8] Disease, however, is still seen, especially in immigrants from Latin America.

Immunization Program

The rationale for measles and mumps immunization is to prevent complications and death due to those diseases in children and adults. The rationale for rubella immunization is to prevent infection in pregnant women, thereby preventing congenital rubella syndrome. The first live-attenuated measles vaccine was licensed in 1963; mumps vaccine was licensed in 1967, and rubella vaccine in 1969. The first MMR vaccine was licensed in 1971; in 1979, a rubella vaccine grown in human diploid fibroblasts (RA 27/3) was licensed and replaced the duck embryo-passaged strain that was in MMR. Since 1980, MMR has been the preferred vaccine against these three diseases. A single dose was recommended for all children at 15 months of age until 1989, when the measles resurgence discussed above prompted recommendations for a routine second dose at 4 to 6 years of age.[9] In 1998, the age for the first dose was changed to 12 to 15 months, and the preference for MMR (as opposed to the corresponding component vaccines) was reiterated.[1] In 2005, MMRV was licensed, and, in the context of a general preference for combination vaccines, preferred over separate MMR plus VAR.[10] In 2006, in response to the mumps resurgence discussed above, the 2-dose requirement was extended to mumps immunization (practically speaking, this had already occurred because of the 2-dose measles recommendation and the use of MMR).[11] In 2008, because of concerns over febrile seizures, the general preference for MMRV was retracted[12]; in 2009, clarifications regarding the use of MMRV were posted, confirming no preference for MMRV versus MMR plus VAR for the first dose but generally preferring MMRV for the second dose.[13] Updated evidence of immunity requirements for health care personnel were released in 2009.[14]

Use of MMR in the United States has been remarkably successful, leading to the elimination of endemic transmission of measles and rubella and drastically reducing the annual number of reported cases of mumps. However, since 1998 these successes have been threatened by the false belief that MMR vaccine causes autism (see *Chapter 7: Addressing Concerns About Vaccines— Does MMR Cause Autism?*).

Vaccines

Characteristics of the MMR vaccine licensed in the United States are given in **Table 17.1**. This vaccine is a mixture of live-attenuated strains of measles, mumps, and rubella viruses. Each was attenuated by serial passage in tissue culture, much the same way as was the Sabin polio vaccine.

Efficacy and/or Immunogenicity

■ Measles

Antibodies develop in approximately 95% of children vaccinated at 12 months of age and 98% of children vaccinated at 15 months of age. Studies show that >99% of persons who receive 2 doses of vaccine (separated by at least 1 month) at ≥1 year of age develop serologic evidence of measles immunity. Although vaccine-induced antibody titers are lower than those following natural disease, immunity is probably lifelong in most people. Individuals who lose antibody over time have demonstrable anamnestic responses to revaccination, indicating that they are most likely still protected. A small percentage of vaccinated individuals may lose protection after several years.

■ Mumps

More than 97% of vaccinees develop protective antibody titers, albeit lower than those following natural infection. In postlicensure studies conducted between 1973 and 1989, efficacy of a single dose was 75% to 91%, and efficacy of 2 doses during the 2006 outbreak in the United States was estimated at 76% to 88%.[15] A study published in 2008 showed that 94% of university students and staff had antibody to mumps virus after having received 2 doses of vaccine.[16] The level of antibody was lower among those vaccinated ≥15 years earlier as compared with those vaccinated in the preceding 5 years, but seronegative subjects mounted anamnestic responses after repeat vaccination. Whereas antibody titers have been shown to wane with time,[17] cellular responses have been shown to persist beyond 15 years.[18]

■ Rubella

At least 95% of vaccinees ≥12 months of age develop protective antibody titers. Vaccine-induced rubella antibodies have persisted in >90% of vaccinees at least 15 years after receipt of the RA 27/3 vaccine. Lifelong protection against clinical reinfection, asymptomatic viremia, or both usually results from a single dose of vaccine early in childhood. In some cases, vaccinees exposed to natural rubella develop an asymptomatic increase in antibody titer (reinfection with wild-type rubella virus has been observed in persons with previous natural rubella). Infection of vaccinees is rarely associated with viremia or pharyngeal shedding, and person-to-person transmission has not been reported. Among vaccinated women, the risk of congenital rubella syndrome from rubella infection during pregnancy is extremely low.

Safety

Five to 15% of vaccinees develop fever $\geq 103°F$ (39.4°C) and about 5% develop a mild morbilliform rash, usually within 7 to 10 days. Transient lymphadenopathy sometimes occurs following MMR, and parotitis has been reported rarely. Arthralgia, which is reported in up to 25% of susceptible adult women given MMR, is attributed to the rubella component; persistent or recurrent joint symptoms have been reported but are rare. It should be mentioned that the incidence of joint problems after immunization is lower than that after natural infection at the same age.

One case of immune thrombocytopenic purpura, defined as a platelet count $\leq 50,000$ per microliter with clinical bleeding, occurs for every 40,000 doses; this is much less than the incidence after natural measles or rubella. [19] The risk of febrile seizures is increased 2- to 3-fold in the second week after vaccination, but there is no association with subsequent seizures or neurodevelopmental disabilities.[20] Most allergic reactions are minor and consist of a wheal and flare or urticaria at the injection site, and anaphylactic reactions are extremely rare. The vaccine does not contain significant amounts of egg protein and can safely be given to patients with allergies to eggs, chickens, and feathers without prior skin testing and without incremental dosing.

The viruses in MMR are not transmitted from person-to-person after vaccination and therefore the vaccine can be given to contacts of immunosuppressed and pregnant individuals.

- *Contraindications*
    - Allergic reaction to previous dose of vaccine or any vaccine component (risk of recurrent allergic reaction; this includes reactions to gelatin and neomycin)
    - Severe immunodeficiency or immunosuppression (risk of disease caused by live virus)
    - Pregnancy (theoretic risk of live virus vaccine to the fetus or attribution of birth defects to vaccination). ACIP recommends that vaccinated women avoid pregnancy for one month; the package insert says 3 months (ACIP recommendations are usually followed in practice).
- *Precautions*
    - Moderate or severe acute illness (difficulty distinguishing illness from vaccine reaction)
    - History of thrombocytopenia or thrombocytopenic purpura (risk of recurrent thrombocytopenia)
    - Recent receipt of antibody-containing blood product (risk of impaired response to vaccine)

371

TABLE 17.1 — Measles, Mumps, and Rubella Vaccine[a]

Trade name	M-M-R$_{II}$
Abbreviation	MMR
Manufacturer/distributor	Merck
Type of vaccine	Live-attenuated, classical
Composition	Measles virus, Moraten strain (derived from the Edmonston B strain), propagated in chick embryo cells, at least 1000 TCID$_{50}$
	Mumps virus, Jeryl Lynn strain (actually consists of two distinct strains), propagated in chick embryo cells, at least 12,500 TCID$_{50}$
	Rubella virus, RA 27/3 strain, propagated in human diploid lung fibroblast (WI-38) cells, at least 1000 TCID$_{50}$
Adjuvant	None
Preservative	None
Excipients and contaminants	Sorbitol (14.5 mg)
	Sodium phosphate
	Sucrose (1.9 mg)
	Sodium chloride
	Hydrolyzed gelatin (14.5 mg)
	Recombinant human albumin (≤0.3 mg)
	Fetal bovine serum (<1 ppm)
	Neomycin (25 mcg)
	Buffer and media ingredients
Latex	None
Labeled indications	Prevention of measles, mumps, and rubella
Labeled ages	≥12 months
Dose	0.5 mL
Route of administration	Subcutaneous
Labeled schedule	12 to 15 months of age
	Revaccination before school entry
Recommended schedule	12 to 15 months of age
	Revaccination at 4 to 6 years of age
How supplied (number in package)	1-dose vial (10), lyophilized, with diluent

Continued

TABLE 17.1 — *Continued*

Trade name	M-M-R$_{II}$
Abbreviation	MMR
Storage:	
Vaccine	Refrigerate
	Protect from light
Diluent	Refrigerate or room temperature,
	Do not freeze
Reconstituted vaccine	Refrigerate for up to 8 hours
	Protect from light
Cost per dose ($US, 2009):	
Public	18.30
Private	48.31
Reference package insert	September 2009

^a The components of MMR (Attenuvax [measles], Mumpsvax [mumps], Meruvax II [rubella], and M-M-Vax [measles and mumps]) are licensed by Merck as separate vaccines. However, as of 2008 they are no longer available in the United States. MMR is also available in combination with VAR (ProQuad; Merck).

   – Active, untreated tuberculosis (risk of exacerbation of tuberculosis). Measles vaccine virus replication can suppress the response to a tuberculin skin test. If not given before or on the same day as a tuberculin skin test, MMR should be delayed 4 weeks after the tuberculin skin test is done. Note that the package insert states that persons with active, untreated tuberculosis should not be vaccinated.

   – MMRV: personal, sibling or parent history of seizures (risk of febrile seizure)

Recommendations

All persons who do not have evidence of immunity to measles, mumps, and rubella should be vaccinated with MMR. The criteria for immunity to these diseases are given in **Table 17.2**. For children, the first dose is usually given at 12 to 15 months of age and the second dose at 4 to 6 years of age. The second dose may be given any time ≥28 days following the first dose. High-risk adults who lack evidence of immunity should receive 2 doses of MMR separated by ≥28 days (those who have a history of 1 dose in the past should have a second dose); low-risk adults who lack evidence of immunity should receive at least 1 dose. Women who might become pregnant and who lack evidence of immunity should receive 1 dose of MMR (pregnancy should be deferred at least one month after vaccination). Rubella vaccine may be given

TABLE 17.2 — Immunity to Measles, Mumps, and Rubella

Criteria[a]	Persons to Whom the Criteria Apply		
	Measles	Mumps	Rubella
Birth before 1957	Everyone except health care personnel[b]	Everyone except health care personnel[b]	Everyone except health care personnel[b] and women who might become pregnant
Personal history of clinical disease	Persons with a history of *physician-diagnosed* disease except health care personnel[b]	Persons with a history of *physician-diagnosed* disease except health care personnel[b]	Not considered reliable evidence of immunity in anyone
Personal history of laboratory-confirmed disease	Everyone	Everyone	Everyone
Written history of at least 1 dose of vaccine	Children 1 year of age to school-aged Low-risk adults	Children 1 year of age to school-aged Low-risk adults	Anyone ≥1 year of age
Written history of 2 doses of vaccine	School-aged children (grades K-12) High-risk adults (health care personnel[b], international travelers, students at postsecondary educational institutions)	School-aged children (grades K-12) High-risk adults (health care personnel[b], international travelers, students at postsecondary educational institutions)	Not required

| Positive virus-specific IgG antibody test | Everyone | Everyone | Everyone |

[a] Any one criterion is considered sufficient.

[b] Unvaccinated health care personnel born before 1957 who lack laboratory evidence of immunity should be vaccinated. Technically speaking, two doses of measles and mumps vaccine, but only one dose of rubella vaccine, are required. Practically speaking, this means two doses of MMR separated by $\geq$28 days. A personal history of physician-diagnosed measles or mumps is not sufficient proof of immunity for health care personnel.

Adapted from Watson JC, et al. *MMWR.* 1998;47(RR-8):1-57, CDC. *MMWR.* 2006;55:629-630, and Centers for Disease Control and Prevention Web site. http://www.cdc.gov/vaccines/recs/provisional/downloads/mmr-evidence-immunity-Aug2009-508.pdf. Accessed February 5, 2010.

17

after anti-Rho(D) immune globulin administration, but testing for seroconversion should be performed 6 to 8 weeks later.

During measles outbreaks, when the likelihood of exposure is high, measles vaccine can be given to infants as young as 6 months of age. Doses given before the first birthday, however, *do not count* in the series, and these children should receive 2 subsequent doses according to the usual schedule. Although measles vaccination is not a requirement for entry into any country, measles and mumps are still endemic in many parts of the world. Persons who lack evidence of immunity and are planning travel to these areas should receive 2 doses of MMR (separated by $\geq$28 days) before leaving. Infants 6 to 12 months of age who will be traveling anywhere outside the United States should receive 1 dose, but should be revaccinated according to the routine schedule when they reach 12 months of age (vaccination of infants <6 months of age is not necessary because most will be protected by maternal antibodies).

Measles vaccine given within 72 hours of exposure to measles may prevent infection, but this is not true for mumps and rubella vaccines. Immunocompromised individuals who are exposed to measles should receive intramuscular immune globulin, 0.5 mL/kg (maximum 15 mL), within 6 days of exposure. The AAP recommends immune globulin prophylaxis for *all* HIV-infected children and adolescents exposed to measles, regardless of vaccination status, degree of symptoms, and level of immune suppression (the dose for asymptomatic HIV-infected persons is 0.25 mL/kg, maximum 15 mL); the ACIP specifies prophylaxis only for *symptomatic* HIV infection. Susceptible household contacts of measles cases, especially those <1 year of age, should receive immune globulin as well (0.25 mL/kg, maximum 15 mL). Immune globulin is not recommended for postexposure prophylaxis against rubella or mumps.

REFERENCES

1. Watson JC, et al. *MMWR*. 1998;47(RR-8):1-57.
2. The National Vaccine Advisory Committee. *JAMA*. 1991;266:1547-1552.
3. CDC. *MMWR*. 2004;53:713-716.
4. CDC. *MMWR*. 2008;57:893-896.
5. Dayan GH, et al. *N Engl J Med*. 2008;358:1580-1589.
6. High P, et al. *MMWR*. 2010;59 125-129.
7. CDC. *MMWR*. 2005;54:279-282.
8. Reef SE, et al. *Clin Infect Dis*. 2006;43(suppl 3):S126-S132.
9. CDC. *MMWR*. 1989;38(S-9):1-18.
10. CDC. *MMWR*. 2005;54:1212-1214.
11. CDC. *MMWR*. 2006;55:629-630.
12. CDC. *MMWR*. 2008;57:258-260.
13. Centers for Disease Control and Prevention Web site. ACIP provisional recommendations for use of measles, mumps, rubella and varicella (MMRV) vaccine. http.//www.cdc.gov/vaccines/recs/provisional/default.htm#acip. Accessed February 5, 2010.
14. Centers for Disease Control and Prevention Web site. ACIP provisional recommendations for measles-mumps-rubella (MMR) 'evidence of immunity' requirements for healthcare personnel. http://www.cdc.gov/vaccines/recs/provisional/downloads/mmr-evidence-immunity-Aug2009-508.pdf. Accessed February 5, 2010.
15. Marin M, et al. *Vaccine*. 2008;26:3601-3607.
16. Date AA, et al. *J Infect Dis*. 2008;197:1662-1668.
17. LeBaron CW, et al. *J Infect Dis*. 2009;199:552-560.
18. Vandermeulen C, et al. *J Infect Dis*. 2009;199:1457-1460.
19. France EK, et al. *Pediatrics*. 2008;121:e687-e692.
20. Vestergaard M, et al. *JAMA*. 2004;292:351-357.

17

18   *Neisseria meningitidis*

The Pathogen

N meningitidis is a gram-negative bacterium that typically takes the appearance of intracellular diplococci on Gram's stain. The organism produces a polysaccharide capsule that is the basis for classification into serogroups, the most important of which in causing disease are A, B, C, W-135, and Y. The capsule contributes to virulence by inhibiting complement-mediated lysis, phagocytosis by neutrophils, and the action of antimicrobial peptides.[1] Pathogenicity is enhanced by the production of endotoxin. *N meningitidis* often colonizes the nasopharynx, and disease results from bacteremia and spread to distant sites such as the meninges. Colonization occurs through the interaction between host cell receptors and bacterial adhesions, which undergo antigenic and phase variation that facilitate evasion of host immunity.[2] Certain genetic polymorphisms, particularly those involving the complement and coagulation systems, contribute to disease outcome.[3]

Clinical Features

Meningococcemia (bloodstream infection with *N meningitidis*) is characterized by the sudden onset of fever, lethargy, myalgia, rash, and vomiting, followed by altered mental status, high fever or hypothermia, tachypnea, and hypotension.[4] Initially, the rash may be macular or maculopapular, but there is rapid transition to petechiae and/or purpura. *Purpura fulminans* is characterized by rapid progression to disseminated intravascular coagulation, hypotension, shock, and possibly death within hours despite antimicrobial therapy and supportive measures. Death is common, and survivors may lose extensive areas of skin or extremities due to ischemia. Some individuals experience transient meningococcal bacteremia that resolves spontaneously without treatment.

Meningitis presents with fever, vomiting, headache and photophobia. It is distinguished from other forms of pyogenic meningitis by the association with petechial or purpuric rash in two thirds of patients. Neurologic sequelae include deafness, cranial nerve palsies, hydrocephalus, and developmental delay. Meningococcus also causes pneumonia, myocarditis, pericarditis, arthritis, conjunctivitis, endophthalmitis, urethritis, and pharyngitis. Immune mediated arthritis, cutaneous vasculitis, and pericarditis can occur late in the course of infection, after antibiotic therapy is instituted. *Chronic meningococcemia* occurs rarely and is characterized by recurrent episodes of fever, chills, rash, arthralgias, and headache over a 6- to 8-week period.

Epidemiology and Transmission

Humans are the only natural hosts and transmission occurs by direct person-to-person contact or via respiratory droplets. Whereas asymptomatic carriage of *N meningitidis* in the general population is common, <5% of individuals carry pathogenic strains. In contrast, nasopharyngeal colonization with invasive strains approaches 50% in closed settings where a case has occurred. The secondary attack rate in households is 3% to 4%, and the risk to household members is 500 to 800 times the risk in the general population (this is why chemoprophylaxis is used for close contacts).

Data from 1998 to 2007 indicate that the highest incidence of invasive meningococcal disease, 5.4 per 100,000, occurs in infants <1 year of age.[5] A second peak, 0.78 per 100,000, occurs in adolescence and young adulthood, when intimate contact with other people increases. The overall incidence of disease decreased 64% from 1998 to 2007; this was likely the result of natural epidemiological cycles as well as environmental factors such as less smoking and crowding and possibly increased antibiotic use. Disease occurs predominantly in late winter and early spring, and outbreaks may parallel increases in influenza activity. Risk factors include active and passive smoking, respiratory illness, steroid use, new residence, new school, lower socioeconomic status, and household crowding. Individuals with congenital or acquired immunodeficiency, especially complement deficiency (classically terminal component deficiency), asplenia, antibody deficiency, and HIV infection are also at increased risk. During outbreaks, alcohol use and patronizing bars and nightclubs are implicated as risk factors.

Epidemics caused by serogroup A most commonly occur in the meningitis belt of sub-Saharan Africa, central Asia, the Indian subcontinent, and Saudi Arabia. Such epidemics are rare in developed countries. In the United States, the vast majority of cases are sporadic, but localized outbreaks have increased. In the 1980s, most US cases were due to serogroups B and C, and only 2% were due to serogroup Y. By the 1990s, serogroups B, C, and Y each accounted for about one third of cases.[6] Between 1998 and 2007, serogroup B accounted for 31% of invasive disease overall but 57% of cases <1 year of age; overall, serogroup C accounted for 28% and serogroup Y 34% of cases.[5]

Prior to the initiation of a universal adolescent immunization program in the United States, up to 2800 cases of invasive disease occurred each year. The overall case-fatality rate was close to 10% and was higher (around 20%) in adolescents than in young children (around 5%).[7] Up to 20% of survivors had some form of permanent disability; that proportion approaches 60% in teenage survivors.[8] Half of patients had meningitis, making meningococcus the most common cause of bacterial meningitis in persons 2 to 18 years of age.

Since licensure in 1981, MPSV4 was used in persons with medical conditions that placed them at high risk for meningococcal disease, as well as in persons traveling to endemic areas and laboratory workers and for outbreak control. The vaccine was never recommended for universal use for a number of reasons, including the limited duration of protection, absence of herd-immunity effects, and the low incidence of disease in the general population. In the late 1990s, studies showed that college freshmen living in dormitories were at increased risk for meningococcal disease, of the order of 2- to 5-fold higher than the general population.[9] Upward of 80% of these cases were caused by serotypes A, C, W-135, or Y. In 2000, it was recommended that all college students be informed about the risk of meningococcal disease, and that MPSV4 be made available to those who requested it.[10] It was estimated that vaccination of all college freshmen living in dormitories would prevent 16 to 30 cases and one to three deaths, at a cost of $617,000 to $1.85 million per case prevented and $6.8 to $20.4 million per death prevented.

The licensure of MCV4-D in 2005 prompted reassessment of the meningococcal prevention strategy in the United States. Meningogoccal conjugate vaccines were expected to result in more effective and longer-lived antibody responses, as well as the potential to reduce nasopharyngeal colonization and result in herd immunity. Moreover, the reality of herd effects was borne out in the experience with serogroup C conjugate vaccines in the United Kingdom, where a universal immunization program for children 12 months to 17 years of age initiated in 1999 resulted in dramatic declines in disease among both vaccinated and unvaccinated persons, as well as decreases in nasopharyngeal carriage.[11,12] It was estimated that a universal MCV4 program in the United States for children 11 years of age plus a catch-up campaign for adolescents would (assuming herd effects) prevent >5000 cases over a 10-year period, at a cost of $532,000 per case prevented and $5.9 million per death prevented.[13]

These estimates make routine MCV4 vaccination more costly per health outcome than the programs for prevention of disease due to *H influenzae* type b and *S pneumoniae*. Nevertheless, rec-

381

ommendations for universal immunization of adolescents at 11 to 12 years of age, with limited catch-up of adolescents at 15 years of age, were released in 2005[13]; the idea was to provide protection against the exposures that would occur in high school (more aggressive catch-up was not recommended because of anticipated supply issues). It was felt that immunization at 11 to 12 years of age would anchor the recommended routine preadolescent health care visit and would lay a foundation for the adolescent vaccination platform, which has since been rounded out with Tdap and the HPV vaccine. MCV4-D also was recommended as a replacement for MPSV4 in high-risk persons within the labeled age group, from 11 to 55 years of age, and the recommendation for college freshmen living in dormitories was strengthened from "educate" to "vaccinate."

In June 2007, when supply was sufficient, catch-up of all adolescents 11 to 18 years of age with MCV4-D was recommended.[14] In October 2007, with the extension of the label down to 2 years of age, the recommendation was made to substitute MCV4-D for MPSV4 in high-risk children.[15] In February 2008, the decision was made *not* to recommend universal immunization of children 2 to 10 years of age, for the following reasons: 1) it was not clear that immunization at younger ages would provide protection when it would be needed most, ie, at high school entry; 2) the burden of disease in that age group was lower than in infants and adolescents, and a smaller proportion of cases were due to vaccine serogroups; and 3) vaccinating children at 2 years of age would be much less cost-effective than vaccinating children at 11 years of age.[16]

In June 2009, the ACIP recommended routine revaccination of persons who remain at high risk.[17] MCV4-CRM was licensed in February 2010 for use in persons 11 to 55 years of age, and updated recommendations were issued.[18]

Vaccines

Characteristics of meningococcal vaccines licensed in the United States are given in **Table 18.1**. One consists of pure polysaccharide and the other two are protein-polysaccharide conjugates.[19] Biologic differences between conjugate and polysaccharide vaccines are discussed in *Chapter 1: Introduction to Vaccinology—The Germinal Center Reaction.*

Efficacy and/or Immunogenicity

Serogroup A polysaccharide vaccines induce an antibody response in infants as young as 3 months of age, but responses are not comparable to those in adults and efficacy declines within 3 years. Serogroup C polysaccharide is poorly immunogenic in children <18 months of age. In children <5 years of age, antibodies to serogroups A and C wane by 3 years after receipt of a single dose. In healthy adults, antibody concentrations after polysaccharide vaccine decrease with time but may be detectable for as long as 10 years after vaccination.

Serogroup C polysaccharide vaccine demonstrated 90% efficacy a study among US Army troops between 1969 and 1970. During an epidemic of serogroup C disease in Sao Paulo, Brazil, in 1974, efficacy was 67% among children 24 to 36 months of age. During an epidemic of serogroup A disease in Finland in 1975 and 1976, efficacy of serogroup A vaccine in a controlled trial was 100%, as it was in a New Zealand study in 1985 and 1986. Administration of serogroup C vaccine to all US troops since 1972 as resulted in the elimination of serogroup C disease in this population. During a mass immunization campaign among persons 6 months to 20 years of age in Quebec in 1992 and 1993, 1.6 million doses of vaccine were distributed; 24% of these contained serogroups A, C, W-135, and Y and 76% contained serogroups A and C only. Protection against serogroup C was 65% in the first 2 years but 0% in the next 3 years. Efficacy was strongly related to age, ranging from 83¾% for ages 15 to 20 years to 41% for ages 2 to 9 years.

Some studies suggest that multiple doses of serogroup A and C polysaccharides (but not conjugated polysaccharides) can cause immunologic hyporesponsiveness, which means that the response to subsequent doses is reduced.[20,21] The clinical significance of this phenomenon has not been addressed.

Licensure of MCV4-D was based on immunologic non-inferiority to MPSV4 rather than demonstrated efficacy. In a randomized trial of adolescents who received either MCV4-D ($N=423$) or MPSV4 ($N=423$), the percentage of subjects in each group achieving a ≥4-fold rise in bactericidal antibody titer was approximately ≥90% for serogroups A, C, and W-135; responses to serogroup Y were lower but similar for both vaccines (81.8% and 80.1%, respectively). The percentage of subjects achieving a *rabbit complement assay* serum bactericidal titer of ≥1:128—the presumed protective level with this assay—was >98% for all serogroups for each vaccine. In a similar study of adults, those who received MCV4-D ($N=1280$) less often had ≥4-fold rises in antibody as compared with those who received MPSV4 ($N=1098$); however, the percentage achieving titers ≥1:128 were similar and the criteria for noninferiority were met. Again, 4-fold responses for serogroup Y were lower than for other serogroups (73.5% and 79.4%, respectively).

In a study involving children 2 to 3 years of age, antibody responses to each serogroup were higher among MCV4-D recipients ($N=48$ to 52) than MPSV4 recipients ($N=50$ to 53). The percentage of MCV4-D subjects achieving a *human complement*

TABLE 18.1 — *N meningitidis* Vaccines

Trade name	Menactra	Menveo	Menomune—A/C/Y/W-135
Abbreviation	MCV4-D	MCV4-CRM	MPSV4
Manufacturer/distributor	Sanofi Pasteur	Novartis	Sanofi Pasteur
Type of vaccine	Inactivated, engineered subunits	Inactivated, engineered subunits	Inactivated, purified subunits
Composition	Group-specific polysaccharides (4 mcg each) from *N meningitidis* serogroups A, C, Y, and W-135, conjugated to diphtheria toxoid (48 mcg)	Group-specific polysaccharides (serogroup A, 10 mcg; serogroups C, Y, W-135, 5 mcg each) from *N meningitidis*, conjugated to CRM$_{197}$, a nontoxic mutant diphtheria toxin (32.7 to 64.1 mcg)	Group-specific polysaccharides (50 mcg each) from *N meningitidis* serogroups A, C, Y, and W-135
Adjuvant	None	None	None
Preservative	None	None	Thimerosal (25 mcg mercury) or none
Excipients and contaminants	Formaldehyde (<2.66 mcg)	Formaldehyde (<0.3 mcg)	Lactose (2.5 to 5 mg)
Latex	Vial stopper contains dry natural rubber	None	Vial stopper contains dry natural rubber

Labeled indications	Prevention of invasive meningococcal disease due to serogroups A, C, Y, and W-135	Prevention of invasive meningococcal disease due to serogroups A, C, Y, and W-135	Prevention of invasive meningococcal disease due to serogroups A, C, Y, and W-135
Labeled ages	2 to 55 years	11 to 55 years	≥2 years
Dose	0.5 mL	0.5 mL	0.5 mL
Route of administration	Intramuscular	Intramuscular	Subcutaneous
Labeled schedule	1 dose	1 dose	1 dose
Recommended schedule	1 dose Consider revaccination (see text)	1 dose Consider revaccination (see text)	1 dose Consider revaccination (see text)
How supplied (number in package)	1-dose vial (5) Prefilled syringe (1, 5)[a]	1-dose vial (5), lyophilized serogroup A, with diluent containing serogroups C, Y and W-135	Preservative-free formulation: 1-dose vial (1), lyophilized, with diluent Thimerosal-containing formulation: 10-dose vial (1), lyophilized, with diluent

Continued

TABLE 18.1 — *Continued*

Trade name	Menactra	Menveo	Menomune—A/C/Y/W-135
Abbreviation	MCV4-D	MCV4-CRM	MPSV4
Storage	Refrigerate Do not freeze	Vaccine and diluent: Refrigerate Do not freeze Protect from light Reconstituted vaccine: Use immediately Room temperature for up to 8 hours	Vaccine: Refrigerate Do not freeze Diluent: Refrigerate Do not freeze Reconstituted vaccine: Use immediately 10-dose vial, refrigerate for up to 35 days
Cost per dose ($US, 2009):			
Public	79.75	—	—
Private	98.52	—	252.00
Reference package insert	May 2009	February 2010	January 2009

a This presentation is not available in the United States as of March 2010.

assay serum bactericidal titer of ≥1:8—the presumed protective level for this assay—was 73% for serogroup A, 63% for C, 63% for W-135, and 88% for Y. Similarly, responses were higher among children 4 to 10 years of age who received MCV4-D (*N* = 84) as compared with those who received MPSV4 (*N* = 84). The percentage of MCV4-D subjects achieving a serum bactericidal titer (human complement assay) of ≥1:8 was 81% for serogroup A, 79% for C, 85% for W-135, and 99% for Y.

Prelicensure trials showed that 75% and 86% of teenagers vaccinated with MCV4-D retained protective levels of antibody against meningococcus serogroups C and Y, respectively, 3 years later. Among children vaccinated between 2 and 10 years of age, 55% and 94% retained protective levels of antibody against serogroups C and Y, respectively, 5 years out. All individuals in these studies revaccinated with MCV4-D achieved protective antibody titers.[17]

Licensure of MCV4-CRM was based on immunologic noninferiority to MCV4-D rather than demonstrated efficacy. In a randomized, controlled Phase 3 trial, 2663 subjects received MCV4-CRM and 876 received MCV4-D; the primary endpoint was seroresponse rates, defined as a postvaccination titer of ≥1:8 (human complement assay) in those with no prevaccination antibody, or a ≥4-fold increase in titer. The seroresponse rate for each serogroup among adolescents who received MCV4-CRM (*N* = 1075) was noninferior to that of MCV4-D recipients (*N* = 359). For serogroups A, W-135, and Y, the seroresponse rates were statistically superior (75% vs 66%, 75% vs 63%, and 68% vs 41%, respectively), and the geometric mean titers for all serogroups were statistically superior.[22] The seroresponse rate for each serogroup among adults who received MCV4-CRM (*N* = 963) also was noninferior to that of MCV4-D recipients (*N* = 321), and in fact the responses were statistically superior for serogroups C, W-135, and Y.

Safety

Among teenagers receiving MPSV4, solicited adverse events include localized pain (29%), redness (6%), and induration (5%), none of which are severe. Systemic symptoms include fatigue (25%), headache (29%), and malaise (17%), and <1% of reactions are severe. Moderate to severe fever is seen in <1% of vaccinees. Solicited adverse events are more common among adults.

Pain is reported in about half of adolescent and adult MCV4-D recipients and is of moderate severity in <15%. Induration or erythema occur in 10% to 20% but is moderate or severe in <5%. Headache occurs in 36% to 41%, fatigue 30% to 35%, malaise 22% to 24%, and fever 2% to 5%. One percent or less of these reactions is considered severe. The reactogenicity of MCV4-CRM is comparable.

See *Chapter 7: Addressing Concerns About Vaccines—Do Vaccines Cause Guillain-Barré Syndrome [GBS]?* for a discussion of Guillain-Barré syndrome following receipt of MCV4-D.

- *Contraindications*
  - Allergic reaction to previous dose of vaccine or any vaccine component (risk of recurrent allergic reaction; for MCV, this includes reactions to any diphtheria toxoid-containing vaccine, since these vaccines contain either diphtheria toxoid or CRM_{197}, a mutant diphtheria toxin)
- *Precautions*
  - Moderate or severe acute illness (difficulty distinguishing illness from vaccine reaction)
  - MCV: personal history of Guillain-Barré syndrome (GBS; risk of recurrent GBS; family history not relevant). The MCV4-D package insert lists GBS as a contraindication, but ACIP considers this to be a precaution. The MCV4-CRM package insert states that data are not available to assess the risk.

Recommendations

All adolescents should be vaccinated against *N meningitidis*. The usual schedule is 1 dose of MCV4 at 11 to 12 years of age, but adolescents ≤18 years of age who have not been vaccinated should receive a dose at the earliest opportunity. There is no preference for MCV4-D or MCV4-CRM.

In all situations where vaccination against *N meningitidis* is called for, MCV4 is preferred over MPSV4 if the individual is 2 to 55 years of age (only MCV4-D is licensed in children 2 to 10 years of age). At ≥56 years of age, MPSV4 is used. In addition to age-based routine use, MCV4 *is recommended* for the following persons or situations.

- College freshmen living in dormitories
- Microbiologists routinely exposed to *N meningitidis*
- Military recruits
- Travelers to or residents of countries in which *N meningitidis* is hyperendemic or epidemic
- Persons with persistent complement (especially late component) deficiencies, properdin deficiency, or Factor D deficiency
- Persons with anatomic or functional asplenia (in elective situations, such as planned splenectomy, vaccination should occur at least 2 weeks earlier, if possible)

Immunization also is used for outbreak control. In general, outbreaks are defined as ≥3 cases in 3 months, resulting in a primary attack rate of ≥10 cases per 100,000 population. For short-term protection of infants 3 to 23 months of age during outbreaks of serogroup A, 2 doses of MPSV4 may be given 3 months apart.

Immunization *should be considered* for persons with HIV infection, although the risk of meningococcal disease is not as great as the risk for invasive pneumococcal disease. In addition, anyone who wants to reduce his or her risk of meningococcal disease should be offered vaccination.

Individuals who were previously vaccinated (with either MPSV4 or MCV4) because they were at increased risk for meningococcal disease should be revaccinated with an age-appropriate meningococcal vaccine if they remain at increased risk. The preferred product for revaccination of persons 2 to 55 years of age is MCV4 (as of February 2010, only MCV4-D was licensed for use in children 2 to 10 years of age); for those ≥56 years of age, it is MPSV4. For children who were first vaccinated at 2 through 6 years of age, the first revaccination should be given 3 years later. For example, a sickle cell patient who received MPSV4 at 2 years of age should receive a dose of MCV4-D at 5 years of age. For persons ≥7 years of age, a minimum of 5 years should elapse. For example, a 41-year-old who received MPSV4 at 36 years of age before relocating to sub-Saharan Africa should receive MCV4 (either MCV4-D or MCV4-CRM) if he intends to remain there. Revaccination with MCV4 would be indicated every 5 years until 56 years of age, at which point the preferred product would switch to MPSV4. College freshmen who were previously vaccinated with MCV4 *do not* routinely need revaccination; those who were previously vaccinated with MPSV4 ≥5 years previously *should be* revaccinated with MCV4.

18

REFERENCES

1. Lo H, et al. *Lancet Infect Dis*. 2009;9:418-427.
2. Carbonnelle E, et al. *Vaccine*. 2009;27S:B78-B89.
3. Wright V, et al. *Vaccine*. 2009;27S:B90-B102.
4. Rosenstein NE, et al. *N Engl J Med*. 2001;344:1378-1388.
5. Cohn AC, et al. *Clin Infect Dis*. 2010;50:184-191.
6. Rosenstein NE, et al. *J Infect Dis*. 1999;180:1894-1901.
7. Kaplan SL, et al. *Pediatrics*. 2006;118:e979-e984.
8. Borg J, et al. *Pediatrics*. 2009;123:e502-e509.
9. Bruce MG, et al. *JAMA*. 2001;286:688-693.
10. CDC. *MMWR*. 2000;49(RR-10):13-20.
11. Balmer P, et al. *J Med Microbiol*. 2002;51:717-722.
12. Maiden MCJ, et al. *Lancet*. 2002;359:1829-1830.
13. Bilukha OO, et al. *MMWR*. 2005;54(RR-7):1-21.
14. CDC. *MMWR*. 2007;56:794-795.
15. CDC. *MMWR*. 2007;56:1265-1266.
16. CDC. *MMWR*. 2008;57:462-465.
17. CDC. *MMWR*. 2009;58:1042-1043.
18. CDC. *MMWR*. 2010;59:273.
19. Snape MD, et al. *Lancet Infect Dis*. 2005;5:21-30.
20. MacDonald NE, et al. *JAMA*. 1998;280:1685-1689.
21. Borrow R, et al. *Vaccine*. 2000;19:1129-1132.
22. Jackson LA, et al. *Clin Infect Dis*. 2009;49:e1-e10.

19 Polio

The Pathogen

Poliovirus is small, nonenveloped, single-stranded RNA virus in the Picornaviridae family. Initial replication occurs in the pharynx, lower gastrointestinal tract, and associated lymph nodes. This leads to primary viremia that seeds peripheral sites, including the viscera and skeletal muscle. Most infections are contained at this point and are therefore subclinical. In a minority of individuals, replication at peripheral sites leads to secondary viremia and nonspecific symptoms such as fever and malaise; in about one in 100 infections, the CNS is involved, either through hematogenous spread or axonal transport from muscle. Once in the CNS, poliovirus can cause self-limited aseptic meningitis, but more importantly can replicate in and destroy anterior horn cells of the spinal cord, leading to lower motor-neuron paralysis.

Clinical Features

Approximately 95% of poliovirus infections are asymptomatic. Minor, nonspecific illness with low-grade fever and sore throat occurs in 4% to 8% of infected people; aseptic meningitis, sometimes with paresthesias, occurs in 1% to 2% of patients a few days after these symptoms resolve. The CSF may show mild pleocytosis with lymphocytic predominance. Less than 1% of patients experience rapid onset of asymmetric flaccid paralysis and areflexia; the proximal lower extremity muscles are most often involved, and some patients have cranial nerve involvement. Prior to the availability of modern assisted ventilation, most deaths occurred from respiratory failure. In the past, patients who survived the acute illness but failed to recover respiratory muscle function lived out the remainder of their lives in iron lungs; today, tracheostomy and positive-pressure ventilation are used. Somewhat more than half of patients who develop limb paralysis have permanent functional deficits. Adults who contracted paralytic polio during childhood may develop postpolio syndrome, characterized by muscle pain and exacerbation of weakness 30 to 40 years later.

Epidemiology and Transmission

Humans are the only natural hosts and transmission occurs by the fecal-oral route, although pharyngeal secretions may be involved. Communicability is greatest shortly before and after onset of clinical illness, but patients may be contagious in the absence of symptoms and fecal excretion may persist for weeks. Immunodeficient patients can excrete the virus for >6 months.

Infection is more common in infants and young children and occurs at an earlier age among children living in poor hygienic conditions. The risk of paralytic disease increases with age. In temperate climates, poliovirus infections are most common during the summer and autumn. In the tropics, the seasonal pattern is variable with a less-pronounced peak of activity.

The last reported indigenous case of polio in the United States occurred in 1979, and the only identified imported case of paralytic polio since 1986 occurred in a child transported here for medical care in 1993. Since 1979, all other cases of polio, an average of eight per year between 1980 and 1996, were caused by OPV-derived strains. While OPV has not been used in the United States since 2000, infections with OPV-derived strains still occur. In 2005, four unimmunized children in an Amish community in Minnesota were found to be infected with an OPV-derived strain of poliovirus.[1] The index case was an infant with severe combined immunodeficiency disease, and the other three children were otherwise healthy siblings in a separate household. Genetic analysis suggested that the strain had been imported by someone vaccinated with OPV in another country. Vaccine-derived poliovirus that has reverted to virulence can emerge because of continuous replication in immunodeficient individuals or continuous circulation in unimmunized populations. The latter phenomenon was highlighted during an outbreak of paralytic polio in the Caribbean in 2000 to 2001, which was caused by a strain of OPV that had reverted to virulence in areas of very low vaccine coverage.[2]

Immunization Program

Because of widespread vaccination, worldwide eradication of polio is now on the horizon. In the United States, the annual number of wild-type cases fell from >18,000 to zero in about 2 decades. In 1988, the World Health Assembly resolved to eradicate polio through the Global Polio Eradication Initiative. As a result, the number of cases worldwide has been reduced from 350,000 in 1988 to 1597 in 2009.[3] The number of countries that have never succeeded in interrupting wild poliovirus transmission has been reduced from 125 to just 4: Afghanistan, India, Nigeria, and Pakistan.

In 2006 alone, Global Polio Eradication Initiative partners immunized 375 million children in 36 countries with 2.1 billion doses of vaccine, and the technical feasibility of polio eradication was affirmed.[4] We may soon be living in a world free of circulating wild-type polioviruses.[5] After global eradication, however, it will be difficult to decide when or if polio immunization should be discontinued. Live-attenuated vaccine strains could still be circulating. In addition, reservoirs of wild-type virus could still exist (eg, in laboratories that have frozen stool specimens from the polio era), and infectious virus that can be used for bioterrorism can be reconstructed from the genetic material of the virus.

OPV was the vaccine of choice for children in the United States since the early 1960s because it induced optimal intestinal immunity, was relatively inexpensive, was painless, required little training to administer, and contributed to immunity at the population level through fecal-oral spread. For these same reasons, OPV continues to be used in the worldwide eradication effort. However, the continued use of OPV, with the attendant five to ten cases of vaccine-associated polio per year, was felt to be unjustified in the United States in the absence of wild-type disease. IPV was known to be highly effective, incapable of causing polio, and was used routinely in several countries that controlled or eliminated polio. Accordingly, expanded use of IPV was recommended beginning in 1997,[6] and as of January 2000, the recommendation was made to substitute IPV for OPV in the United States.[7]

In 2009, the ACIP updated the polio recommendations, emphasizing the importance of a dose at ≥ 4 years of age (regardless of the number of previous doses), extending the minimum interval from Dose 3 to Dose 4 to 6 months, and clarifying the schedule when combination vaccines containing IPV are used.[8]

Vaccines

Characteristics of the polio vaccines licensed in the United States are given in **Table 19.1**. These are inactivated, whole-virus vaccines made much the same way as the original Salk vaccine.

Efficacy and/or Immunogenicity

Ninety-percent or more of vaccinees develop protective antibody to all three serotypes after 2 doses, and $\geq 99\%$ are immune after 3 doses. Protection against paralytic disease correlates with the presence of serum antibody. IPV appears to induce less mucosal immunity than does OPV, so persons who receive IPV are more readily infected in the gastrointestinal tract with wild poliovirus. Thus a person immunized with IPV could become infected in an endemic area and shed virus upon return to the United States. The infected person would be protected from paralytic polio, but the wild virus shed in the stool could be transmitted to a contact. The duration of immunity from IPV is not known with certainty but is probably many years after a complete series.

TABLE 19.1 — Polio Vaccine[a]

Trade name	IPOL[b]
Abbreviation	IPV
Manufacturer/distributor	Sanofi Pasteur
Type of vaccine	Inactivated, whole agent
Composition:	
Virus strain and amount	Type 1 (Mahoney), 40 D antigen units
	Type 2 (MEF-1), 8 D antigen units
	Type 3 (Saukett), 32 D antigen units
Propagation	Vero (African Green Monkey kidney) cells
Inactivation	Formalin
Adjuvant	None
Preservative	2-phenoxyethanol (0.5%) and formaldehyde ($\leq$0.02%)
Excipients and contaminants	Neomycin (<5 ng)
	Streptomycin (<200 ng)
	Polymyxin B (<25 ng)
	Calf serum protein (<1 ppm)
Latex	None
Labeled indications	Prevention of poliomyelitis
Labeled ages	$\geq$6 weeks
Dose	0.5 mL
Route of administration	Intramuscular or subcutaneous
Labeled schedule	2, 4, 6 to 18 months, 4 to 6 years of age
Recommended schedule	Same
How supplied (number in package)	10-dose vial (1)
	Prefilled syringe (10)
Storage	Refrigerate
	Do not freeze
Cost per dose ($US, 2009):	
Public	11.51
Private	23.90
Reference package insert	December 2005

[a] An IPV that is very similar to IPOL is available in combination with DTaP and HepB (Pediarix; GlaxoSmithKline). This IPV is not licensed or distributed separately in the United States. Pediarix is usually given at 2, 4, and 6 months of age. The same IPV is available in combination with DTaP (Kinrix; GlaxoSmithKline). Kinrix is indicated for the booster doses of DTaP and IPV at 4 to 6 years of age. The IPV in Pediarix and Kinrix is considered interchangeable with IPOL.

[b] An IPV that is very similar to IPOL (Poliovax; Sanofi Pasteur) is also available in combination with DTaP and Hib (Pentacel; Sanofi Pasteur). Pentacel is usually given at 2, 4, 6, and 15 to 18 months of age.

Safety

Minor local reactions, such as pain and redness, may occur following IPV. No serious adverse events have been associated with use of the currently available vaccine.

- *Contraindications*
  - Allergic reaction to previous dose of vaccine or any vaccine component (risk of recurrent allergic reaction)
- *Precautions*
  - Moderate or severe acute illness (difficulty distinguishing illness from vaccine reaction)
  - Pregnancy (theoretic risk to the fetus or attribution of birth defects to vaccination, although no deleterious effects from IPV vaccine administered during pregnancy have been demonstrated and the risk of adverse fetal effects from an inactivated vaccine is extremely low; it is not clear why pregnancy is listed as a precaution for some inactivated vaccines but not others)

Recommendations

All children should be vaccinated against polio. The primary series of IPV consists of 3 doses, usually given at 2, 4, and 6 to 18 months of age. Dose 4 is given around the time of school entry, at 4 to 6 years of age. The final dose should be given at ≥4 years of age; therefore, if Dose 4 is given at <4 years of age, another dose should be given at 4 to 6 years of age. Routine immunization of US adults ≥18 years of age is not recommended. However, a 3-dose series of IPV (0, 1 to 2, and 6 to 12 months) *is* recommended for *previously unvaccinated adults* in the following circumstances (an accelerated schedule consisting of doses at 0, 1, and 2 months can be used if necessary):

- Travel to countries where polio is epidemic or endemic
- Members of a community experiencing wild-type poliovirus disease
- Health care workers who will come into close contact with patients potentially excreting wild-type poliovirus
- Laboratory workers who will come in contact with specimens that may contain poliovirus

Adults who have received a primary series of at least 3 doses who are at increased risk of exposure to polio should receive a single supplemental dose of IPV (this does not need to be repeated). Those who have had <3 doses (of either OPV or IPV) should complete the primary series of 3 doses using IPV, regardless of the interval since the last dose and the type of vaccine that was previously given.

19

REFERENCES

1. CDC. *MMWR*. 2005;54:1053-1055.
2. CDC. *MMWR*. 2001;50:855-856.
3. Wild poliovirus weekly update. Global Polio Eradication Initiative Web site. http://www.polioeradication.org/casecount.asp. Accessed February 5, 2010.
4. Global Polio Eradication Initiative. Annual Report 2006. http://www.polioeradication.org/content/publications/AnnualReport2006_ENG.pdf. Accessed February 5, 2010.
5. Hull HF. *Lancet Infect Dis*. 2001;1:299-303.
6. CDC. *MMWR*. 1997;46(RR-3):1-25.
7. Prevots DR, et al. *MMWR*. 2000;49(RR-5):1-22.
8. CDC. *MMWR*. 2009;58:829-830.

20   Rabies

The Pathogen

Rabies virus is an enveloped, bullet-shaped, single-stranded RNA virus in the Rhabdoviridae family, genus *Lyssavirus*. The virion surface is covered with glycoprotein (G-protein) spikes, which mediate attachment to the heavily sialated gangliosides on neuronal cells. Attachment also may occur at nicotinic acetylcholine receptors in muscle, facilitating entry into peripheral nerves. The virus moves by retrograde axoplasmic flow from the site of inoculation to neuronal cell bodies, where it replicates and spreads to the brain; from there it may spread further to other organs, such as salivary and lacrimal glands. Gross pathologic changes in the brain include vascular congestion and edema, and the characteristic cellular abnormality is eosinophilic cytoplasmic neuronal inclusions called *Negri bodies*. The clinical severity of the disease is disproportionate to the degree of histopathologic derangement.

Clinical Features

Rabies presents in four sequential stages: the incubation period, prodrome, acute neurologic phase, and coma/death.[1] Two thirds of patients present with a *furious form*, characterized by fluctuating consciousness, phobic spasms, dilated pupils, and hypersalivation. The other one third present with a *paralytic form*, which is differentiated from Guillain-Barré syndrome by the presence of fever, intact sensation, and urinary incontinence. The incubation period is typically a few weeks to 2 months but may be many years. Animal bites to the head usually result in shorter incubation periods than bites to the extremities.

There are no symptoms during the *incubation phase*, but the *prodrome*, which lasts 2 to 10 days, is characterized by fever, headache, malaise, fatigue, anorexia, anxiety, agitation, irritability, insomnia, or depression, and pain, pruritus, or paresthesia at the site of the bite. The *acute neurologic phase*, which lasts 2 to 12 days, is characterized by hyperactivity, disorientation, hallucinations, bizarre behavior, aggressiveness, seizures, paralysis, aerophobia, hyperventilation, and cholinergic manifestations, including hypersalivation, lacrimation, mydriasis, and hyperpyrexia. Agitation may be precipitated by tactile, auditory, visual, or other stimuli, and hydrophobia, characterized by painful spasms of the pharynx and larynx, may be precipitated by eating or drinking or even the sight of liquids. Paralysis occurs in 20% of cases. At the end of the neurologic phase, the patient may become comatose. Death from respiratory or cardiac arrest usually occurs within 7 days, although with supportive care, coma may last for months. There are only a handful of reported survivors, most of whom have neurologic sequelae. Successful treatment of a 15-year-old girl from Wisconsin was reported in 2005; the strategy included therapeutic coma, using gamma-aminobutyric acid receptor agonists along with N-methyl-D-aspartate receptor antagonists.[2]

Epidemiology and Transmission

All mammals can be infected with rabies, but only carnivorous mammals and bats are considered true reservoirs. Transmission from animals to humans occurs by exposure to saliva, usually through an animal bite, scratch, or contact with mucous membranes. Infection by aerosol has been reported in laboratories that handle the virus and in caves inhabited by bats (here, direct infection of the olfactory apparatus is implicated). Rabies can also be transmitted by allografts. In nature, dogs, wolves, foxes, coyotes, jackals, raccoons, skunks, weasels, bats, and mongooses are most commonly infected. However, in some areas of the world, dogs and cats account for the majority of animal rabies and the greatest number of exposures to humans. In the United States, where domestic animal rabies is well controlled through animal vaccination, most human exposures come from contact with wild animals, such as skunks, raccoons, and bats. Silver-haired bats have become a particular problem because the strains they carry may infect human skin more easily and their bites may be too small to see. Small rodents (eg, squirrels, rats, and mice) and lagomorphs (eg, rabbits and hares) rarely carry rabies.

Most animal exposures in the United States involve dogs, cats, and rodents; the vast majority of these exposures carry a very low risk for rabies transmission, even though postexposure prophylaxis is commonly given.[3] Insectivorous bats are now the most common source of human infection in the United States.[4,5] In at least half of cases, there is no known bite—in some cases, the bite may simply have been imperceptible or might have occurred during sleep; in others, transmission could have occurred through a scratch or bat saliva coming into contact with a mucous membrane or break in the skin.

Oral vaccination of wildlife has proven effective in preventing spread of enzootic disease. Traditional approaches have utilized bait seeded with live-attenuated rabies strains. A recent approach uses a vaccinia recombinant expressing the G protein of rabies virus.

There are an estimated 50,000 human rabies cases each year worldwide; only one or two of these occur in the United States. The long incubation period makes rabies uniquely suited to postexposure prophylaxis through both vaccination and passive immunization with human rabies immune globulin (HRIG); in this respect, rabies is similar to hepatitis B.[6] The common occurrence of animal contacts combined with the near certainty of death if rabies occurs leads to frequent consideration of postexposure prophylaxis. However, postexposure prophylaxis is considered *urgent*, not *emergent*—in other words, the time frame in which to administer prophylaxis is hours, not minutes, and in some cases may be days (eg, if signs of rabies develop in an animal during quarantine).

Postexposure prophylaxis is cost saving (from the societal perspective) when given to persons bitten by test-positive rabid animals or untested reservoir or vector animals. For other risk situations, the cost-effectiveness of postexposure prophylaxis varies widely. For example, it costs $2.9 million per life saved to administer prophylaxis after a bite from an untested cat, $403 million per life saved after a bite from an untested dog, and $4 billion per life saved after a lick from an untested dog (2004 dollars).[7] Although it still stands, the recommendation to administer postexposure prophylaxis after bedroom exposure to a bat while sleeping (without direct evidence of physical contact) has been called into question—approximately 2.7 million persons would need to be treated in this context to prevent a single case of rabies.[8] About 23,000 courses of postexposure prophylaxis are given each year in the United States, most of which are given without guidance from public health authorities.[9]

Pre-exposure vaccination of persons likely to encounter the virus can simplify postexposure treatment by eliminating the need for HRIG and reducing the number of vaccine doses needed. It also protects people who may have unapparent exposures or whose postexposure therapy might be delayed. Pre-exposure vaccination is particularly important for persons who are at high risk of exposure, but who may be in situations where modern prophylaxis is not available.

Recommendations for prevention of human rabies were published in 1999[10] and updated in 2008.[7] In 2010, based on new data from pathogenesis studies, animal models, clinical observations, and epidemiologic surveillance, the recommended vaccine series was reduced from 5 to 4 doses for otherwise healthy persons.[11]

20

Characteristics of the rabies vaccines licensed in the United States are given in **Table 20.1**. These are inactivated, whole-virus vaccines made much the same way as the original Salk vaccine.

HRIG is used in conjunction with vaccination for postexposure prophylaxis. Two preparations are available in the United States. They consist of IgG derived from pooled plasma of human donors who have been hyperimmunized with RAB; they are therefore polyclonal (contain a variety of antibodies, including antibodies to other organisms). Both products are initially purified by cold ethanol fractionation and then formulated for IM administration.

- *HyperRAB S/D* (Talecris Biotherapeutics) is treated with a solvent (tri-n-butyl phosphate), a detergent (sodium cholate), and heat in order to inactivate potential blood borne viruses. The immune globulin is then purified by precipitation, filtration, ultrafiltration, and diafiltration. The final product is 15% to 18% protein at a pH of 6.4-7.2 with 0.21-0.32 M glycine and no preservative; the average potency is 150 IU/mL. It is supplied in 2 mL- (300 IU) and 10 mL- (1,500 IU) vials that should be stored in the refrigerator (do not freeze).
- *Imogam Rabies—HT* (Sanofi Pasteur) is stabilized with 0.3 M glycine then heat-treated in order to inactivate potential bloodborne viruses. The final product is 10% to 18% protein at a pH of 6.8 and has no preservative; the minimum potency is 150 IU/mL. It is supplied in 2 mL- (300 IU) and 10-mL (1,500 IU) vials that should be stored in the refrigerator (do not freeze).

Efficacy and/or Immunogenicity

Essentially all persons given pre- or postexposure prophylaxis achieve seroprotective concentrations of antibody.[12] Multiple studies have demonstrated that postexposure prophylaxis with cell culture-derived vaccine and HRIG provide absolute protection against rabies—in fact, there has never been a failure of properly administered postexposure prophylaxis in the United States.

Safety

Local reactions to RAB-HDC occur in 60% to 90% of vaccinees, with local pain occurring in 21% to 77%. Mild systemic symptoms, such as fever, headache, dizziness, and gastrointestinal complaints, occur in 7% to 56%. Systemic hypersensitivity, including urticaria, pruritic rash, and angioedema, may be seen in up to 6% of persons receiving booster doses. This is thought to be mediated by IgE antibodies to human albumin that is chemically altered by betapropiolactone.

Local reactions to RAB-PCEC occur in 11% to 57% of vaccinees, with local pain occurring in 2% to 23%. Mild systemic symptoms are seen in 0% to 31%. From 1997 to 2005, the reporting rate to VAERS for adverse events was 30 per 100,000 doses distributed, and for serious adverse events it was 3 per 100,000 doses distributed.[13]

Local reactions to HRIG include pain, tenderness, erythema, and induration. Systemic reactions are reported in 75% to 81% of recipients.

- *Contraindications*
  - In the event of exposure to rabies, there are no contraindications to vaccination or use of HRIG.
- *Precautions*
  - Allergic reaction to previous dose of vaccine or any vaccine component (risk of recurrent allergic reaction)
  - *Immunosuppression*: Immunosuppressive agents should not be administered during postexposure prophylaxis unless absolutely essential. If possible, pre-exposure prophylaxis should be postponed until immunocompromising conditions are resolved. When an immunosuppressed person is given pre- or postexposure prophylaxis, antibody titers should be checked (a rapid fluorescent focus inhibition test that demonstrates complete virus neutralization at a serum dilution of 1:5 is considered to be indicative of protection).
  - Patients with selective IgA deficiency may be at increased risk for anaphylactic reactions to HRIG because it may contain minute amounts of IgA.

Recommendations

Table 20.2 gives recommendations for pre-exposure prophylaxis. Table 20.3 lists the situations where postexposure prophylaxis should be considered, and Table 20.4 gives the postexposure regimens. Cell culture-derived rabies vaccines are considered interchangeable, although situations where one would need to complete a series with one vaccine that was initiated with a different vaccine should be very rare.

TABLE 20.1 — Rabies Vaccines[a]

Trade name	Imovax Rabies	RabAvert	
Abbreviation	RAB-HDC	RAB-PCEC	
Manufacturer/distributor	Sanofi Pasteur	Novartis	
Type of vaccine	Inactivated, whole agent	Inactivated, whole agent	
Composition:			
Virus strain	PM-1503-3M	Flury LEP	
Propagation	Human diploid (MRC-5) cells	Purified chick embryo cells (fibroblasts)	
Inactivation	Beta-propiolactone	Beta-propiolactone	
Antigen content	$\geq$2.5 IU	$\geq$2.5 IU	
Adjuvant	None	None	
Preservative	None	None	
Excipients and contaminants	Albumin (<100 mg)	Polygeline (processed bovine gelatin) (<12 mg)	
	Neomycin sulfate (<150 mcg)	Human serum albumin (<0.3 mg)	
	Phenol red (20 mcg)	Potassium glutamate (1 mg)	
		Sodium EDTA (0.3 mg)	
		Ovalbumin (<3 ng)	
		Neomycin (<1 mcg)	
		Chlorotetracycline (<20 ng)	
		Amphotericin B (<2 ng)	
Latex	None	None	

Labeled indications	Pre-exposure (primary series and booster dose) and postexposure prophylaxis	Pre-exposure (primary series and booster dose) and postexposure prophylaxis
Labeled ages	All ages	All ages
Dose	1 mL	1 mL
Route of administration	Intramuscular	Intramuscular
Labeled schedule:		
Pre-exposure	0, 7, and 21 or 28 days	0, 7, and 21 or 28 days
	Periodic booster doses	Periodic booster doses
Postexposure (unvaccinated)[b]	0, 3, 7, 14, 28 days	0, 3, 7, 14, 28 days
Postexposure (previously vaccinated)	0, 3 days	0, 3 days
Recommended schedule:		
Pre-exposure	See **Table 20.2**	See **Table 20.2**
Postexposure	See **Table 20.4**	See **Table 20.4**
How supplied (number in package)	1-dose vial (1), lyophilized, with diluent	1-dose vial (1), lyophilized, with diluent
Storage:		
Vaccine	Refrigerate	Refrigerate
	Do not freeze	Protect from light
Diluent	Refrigerate	Refrigerate
	Do not freeze	Protect from light
Reconstituted vaccine	Use immediately	Use immediately

Continued

20

403

TABLE 20.1 — *Continued*

Trade name	Imovax Rabies	RabAvert
Abbreviation	RAB-HDC	RAB-PCEC
Cost per dose ($US, 2009):		
Public	—	—
Private	283.00	479.00
Reference package insert	December 2005	October 2006

[a] Two vaccines are no longer available in the United States: Rabies Vaccine Adsorbed (BioPort) and Imovax Rabies I.D. (Sanofi Pasteur).
[b] HRIG should also be given to exposed, previously unvaccinated persons (see **Table 20.4**).

REFERENCES

1. Plotkin SA. *Clin Infect Dis*. 2000;30:4-12.

2. Willoughby RE Jr, et al. *N Engl J Med*. 2005;352:2508-2514.

3. Moran GJ, et al. *JAMA*. 2000;284:1001-1007.

4. Messenger SL, et al. *Clin Infect Dis*. 2002;35:738-747.

5. De Serres G, et al. *Clin Infect Dis*. 2008;46:1329-1337.

6. Rupprecht CE, et al. *N Engl J Med*. 2004;351:2626-2635.

7. Manning SE, et al. *MMWR*. 2008;57(RR-3):1-28.

8. De Serres G, et al. *Clin Infect Dis*. 2009;48:1493-1499.

9. Christian KA, et al. *Vaccine*. 2009;27:7156-7161.

10. Arguin PM, et al. *MMWR*. 1999;48(RR-1):1-23.

11. Rupprecht CE, et al. *MMWR*. 2010;59(RR-2):1-9.

12. Rupprecht CE, et al. *Vaccine*. 2009;27:7141-7148.

13. Dobardzic A, et al. *Vaccine*. 2007;25:4244-4251.

20

TABLE 20.2 — Indications for Pre-exposure Rabies Prophylaxis

Intensity of Exposure	Nature of Exposure[a]	Examples	Vaccination
Continuous	Continuous Possible high concentration of virus May go unrecognized Bite, nonbite, aerosol	Rabies research laboratory workers[b] Rabies biologics production workers	3-dose primary series[c] Serology every 6 months Booster dose if titer[d] <1:5
Frequent	Episodic with recognized source May go unrecognized Bite, nonbite, aerosol	Rabies diagnostic laboratory workers[b] Spelunkers Veterinarians and staff Animal-control and wildlife workers in enzootic areas All persons who frequently handle bats	3-dose primary series[c] Serology every 2 years Booster dose if titer[d] <1:5
Infrequent	Episodic with recognized source Bite or nonbite	Veterinarians, animal-control, and wildlife workers in nonenzootic areas Veterinary students Travelers to enzootic areas where immediate access to medical care is limited	3-dose vaccine series[c]
Rare	Episodic with recognized source Bite or nonbite	General US population (including epizootic areas)	Not necessary

[a] See **Table 20.3** for explanation of types of exposure.
[b] Judgment of relative risk and monitoring of immunization status is the responsibility of the laboratory supervisor.
[c] 1 mL intramuscularly on days 0, 7, and 21 or 28.
[d] Rapid fluorescent focus inhibition test.

Adapted from Manning SE, et al; Advisory Committee on Immunization Practices Centers for Disease Control and Prevention. *MMWR*. 2008;57(RR-3):1-28.

TABLE 20.3 — Indications for Postexposure Rabies Prophylaxis

Animal[a]	Animal Evaluation and Disposition	Recommendations
Dog, cat, ferret	Healthy and quarantined for 10-day observation period[b]	Do not begin prophylaxis routinely Institute prophylaxis at first sign of rabies in the animal[c]
	Rabid or suspected rabid	Institute prophylaxis immediately[c]
	Unknown or not available for observation	Consult public health officials[d]
Skunk, raccoon, fox, other carnivore (eg, coyote, bobcat, wild-animal hybrid), bat	Regard as rabid[e]	Consider immediate prophylaxis[c]
Livestock, horse, small rodent (eg, squirrel, chipmunk, rat, mouse, hamster, guinea pig, gerbil), large rodent (eg, woodchuck or groundhog, beaver), lagomorph (eg, rabbit, hare), other mammal[f]	Consider individually	Consult public health officials[d]

[a] *Bite* exposures occur when there has been any penetration of the skin by teeth. *Nonbite* exposures include scratches, abrasions, open wounds, or mucous membranes contaminated with saliva or other potentially infectious material (eg, brain or neural tissue). Contact between intact skin and saliva does not constitute an exposure; neither does casual petting or handling or contact with blood, urine, or feces. However, any potential contact with a bat deserves evaluation because bat bites are small and can go unrecognized. Exposure is assumed to have occurred if a person in the same room as a bat might have been unaware that a bite or direct contact had occurred. Examples include a sleeping person who awakens to find a bat in the room or finding a bat in the room with an unattended child, mentally disabled person, or intoxicated person (awake or asleep). *Aerosol* exposure is rare but has been reported in laboratories that handle the virus and in caves infested with millions of bats. *Human-to-human* transmission occurs almost exclusively through tissue or organ transplantation.

[b] The animal should be quarantined and observed for 10 days. This usually takes place under the supervision of the local health department, which specifies approved facilities (private or government) and monitors the animal's behavior. If signs of rabies develop (eg, aggressive or combative behavior, irritability, hyperreaction to stimuli, or paralysis), the animal should be euthanized and the brain sent for detection of rabies virus antigens by direct fluorescent antibody test (this is usually done at the state lab).

[c] **Table 20.4** gives the recommended prophylaxis regimens. If prophylaxis is initiated but the animal is found not to have rabies by direct fluorescent antibody testing of the brain, prophylaxis may be discontinued.

[d] The epidemiology of rabies is complex and varies from region to region. Local and state public health officials should be consulted to determine the likelihood of exposure in specific situations.

[e] These animals should be regarded as rabid unless proved negative by immunofluorescence testing of the brain (this is usually done at the state lab). Prophylaxis should be initiated unless the brain is known to be negative or expeditious testing is under way. Prophylaxis should be considered more urgent if the exposure was from an animal species in the area known to carry rabies; if the animal exhibited abnormal behavior or signs of illness, had an unexplained wound, attacked *without provocation* (bites that result from attempts to feed or handle an apparently healthy animal should generally be regarded as *provoked*); or if the person's wounds were severe or involved the head and neck. Every effort should be made by properly trained officials to obtain the animal for euthanization and testing; quarantine for observation is *not* recommended because signs of rabies in wild animals cannot be interpreted reliably.

[f] Bites of small rodents and lagomorphs almost never require prophylaxis. Large rodents, such as woodchucks, could survive an attack by a rabid animal and go on to develop rabies. This should be considered in areas where raccoon rabies is prevalent.

Adapted from Manning SE, et al; Advisory Committee on Immunization Practices Centers for Disease Control and Prevention. *MMWR.* 2008;57(RR-3):1-28, and Rabies exposure: When should I seek medical attention? Centers for Disease Control and Prevention Web site. http://www.cdc.gov/rabies/exposure/index.html. Accessed March 24, 2010.

20

TABLE 20.4 — Postexposure Rabies Prophylaxis Regimens

Vaccination Status	Treatment[a]	Regimen
Not previously vaccinated	Wound cleansing	Immediately cleanse all wounds thoroughly with soap and water
		Use a virucidal agent like povidone-iodine solution if available
	HRIG	Administer 20 IU/kg (0.133 mL/kg)[b]
		Infiltrate the full dose around the wound and give any remaining volume intramuscularly at another site[c]
		Do not exceed the recommended dose[d]
		Use separate syringes for HRIG and vaccine
	Rabies vaccine	*Healthy individual*: administer 1 mL intramuscularly on days 0, 3, 7, and 14[e]
		Immunosuppressed individual: administer 1 mL intramuscularly on days 0, 3, 7, 14, and 28[e]
Previously vaccinated[f]	Wound cleansing	Immediately cleanse all wounds thoroughly with soap and water
		Use a virucidal agent like povidone-iodine solution if available
	HRIG	Not recommended
	Rabies vaccine	Administer 1 mL intramuscularly on days 0 and 3[e]

[a] Postexposure prophylaxis should be initiated regardless of the time that has elapsed since the exposure. State or local health departments should be contacted for patients whose postexposure prophylaxis was initiated outside of the United States, because the regimens and products used may be suboptimal. For bites, the need for tetanus immunization and prophylactic antibiotics should be assessed. Wound closure should be avoided if possible.

[b] HRIG should be given at the same time the vaccine series is initiated. If not given on the day of the first dose of vaccine (day 0), it may be given up to and including day 7. Beyond this it is not indicated because the vaccine is presumed to have induced antibodies at that point.

c The intramuscular site, if used, should be different from the site where the first dose of vaccine is given. Subsequent doses of the vaccine may be given in the same muscle where the HRIG was given, if that is a preferred site for vaccination.

d Exceeding the dose of HRIG may suppress the antibody response to vaccination.

e In 2010, the recommended number of doses was reduced from 5 to 4 for otherwise healthy persons (the package inserts still say 5 doses; in this situation, ACIP recommendations are usually followed). The deltoid area is the only acceptable site for adults and older children. The anterolateral thigh can be used for young children (see **Table 4.3**), and the dose is the same as for adults. The gluteal area should never be used. The series does not need to be reinitiated because of minor interruptions of the vaccine schedule—just pick up where you left off, maintaining the intervals between doses specified in the schedule. If major deviations occur, and for all immunosuppressed individuals, test for antibody after completing the series (a rapid fluorescent focus inhibition test that demonstrates complete virus neutralization at a serum dilution of 1:5 is considered to be indicative of protection).

f This includes: 1) persons who received a full pre- or postexposure series of one of the currently licensed cell culture-derived vaccines or of Rabies Vaccine Adsorbed (which is no longer available in the United States); and 2) persons who received another type of rabies vaccine and had a documented antibody response. Serologic testing at the time of exposure is not recommended.

Adapted from Rupprecht CE, et al; Advisory Committee on Immunization Practices Centers for Disease Control and Prevention. *MMWR.* 2010;59(RR-2):1-9.

20

21   Rotavirus

The Pathogen

Rotavirus is a nonenveloped virus with a wheel-like appearance in the Reoviridae family. The genome is divided into 11 double-stranded RNA segments, most of which encode only one viral protein. Infection of the gastrointestinal tract causes diarrhea by several mechanisms: increased fluid secretion due to the effects of a virus-encoded enterotoxin (NSP4) and stimulation of the enteric nervous system, and increased osmotic load caused by destruction of villus epithelial cells, decreased absorption of salt and water, and decreased disaccharidase activity. Protection against disease is mediated by immune responses to the G, or coat, protein (also known as VP7) and the P, or spike, protein (also known as VP4). Any given rotavirus strain has a specific G type, designated by a serotype number (as in "G1") and a P type, designated by a serotype number (as in "P1a") and/or a genotype number in brackets (as in "P[8]"). Certain combinations of G and P types are found more commonly than others, eg, G1P[8] and G2P[4].

Clinical Features

The incubation period is 1 to 4 days. Illness begins abruptly with fever and vomiting, and diarrhea ensues shortly thereafter. There may be >20 daily episodes of vomiting and/or diarrhea during the peak of the illness. Severe vomiting may lead to dehydration even before the diarrhea begins, and associated symptoms include irritability and lethargy. The illness lasts for about a week and appears to be more severe than other forms of gastroenteritis in infants. For example, in one study of outpatients with acute gastroenteritis, children with rotavirus more often had fever (60% vs 43%) as well as both vomiting *and* diarrhea (75% vs 50%) when compared with those with other etiologies; more days of work were lost by the parents (median of 2 vs 0) and more days of day care were lost by the children (median of 3 vs 1).[1]

Risk factors for hospitalization include low birth weight, child-care attendance, and absence of breast-feeding.[2] Common complications of severe rotavirus infection include isotonic dehydration, electrolyte disturbances, metabolic acidosis, and temporary milk intolerance. Rare complications include necrotizing enterocolitis and hemorrhagic gastroenteritis. Immunocompromised patients may develop particularly severe or fatal illness and may shed virus in the stool for months.[3] When infected, adults are usually asymptomatic, but outbreaks in nursing homes have led to symptomatic disease and fatalities in the elderly.

Epidemiology and Transmission

Transmission occurs from person to person through the fecal-oral route, airborne droplets, and contaminated fomites. Infected children shed as many as 100 billion viral particles per milliliter of stool. Since the infectious dose is around 10,000 particles, it only takes one ten-millionth of a milliliter of stool to transmit the infection. This makes rotavirus one of the more contagious forms of gastroenteritis. Because rotavirus is not spread through contaminated food or water, improvements in sanitation and public hygiene do not affect the incidence of disease; this explains why the proportion of severe gastroenteritis caused by rotavirus is the same in developed countries as it is in developing countries.

Virtually all children experience at least one rotavirus infection by 5 years of age. Before institution of a universal immunization program, rotavirus caused up to 410,000 office visits, 272,000 emergency department visits, 70,000 hospitalizations, and 60 deaths each year in the United States.[4] Rotavirus hospitalizations occurred at a frequency of 22.5 per 10,000 children <3 years of age, emergency department visits at 301 per 10,000, and outpatient visits at 312 per 10,000.[5] The numbers worldwide are staggering—2 million hospitalizations and approximately 25 million outpatient visits. First infections and those occurring in infants are the most severe, and it is worth noting that rotavirus causes about 10% of all first-time pediatric hospital admissions in the United States. Deaths, while unusual in the United States and other developed countries, are common in developing countries, with annual worldwide mortality estimated at 527,000 (29% of all diarrheal deaths among children <5 years of age).[6] Reinfection is common but results in mild or no disease, and repeated reinfections reduce the likelihood of subsequent infections. Outbreaks and nosocomial spread occur frequently in day care centers, pediatric hospital wards, and nurseries.

In the tropics, rotavirus may occur at any time of the year. In the United States, annual epidemics begin in the late fall in the Southwest and spread to the North and East by the end of winter or early spring. From 1996 to 2005, G1P[8] strains accounted for 78.5% of infections, G2P[4] for 9.2%, G9P[8] 3.6%, G3P[8] 1.7%, and G4P[8] 0.8%.[7] This is similar to the distribution of serotypes globally, although G9P[8] is more common in some regions outside the United States and other strains are seen in the Eastern Mediterranean and Africa.[8] The predominant types vary from year to year and within geographic regions.

The first vaccine against rotavirus, rhesus rotavirus vaccine, tetravalent (RRV-TV), was licensed in 1998 under the trade name RotaShield (Wyeth, acquired by Pfizer in 2009). The vaccine included a G3-like rhesus rotavirus strain that was naturally attenuated for humans, as well as three rhesus-human reassortants representing serotypes G1, G2, and G4 (each strain also expressed the rhesus P[3]). The vaccine was administered PO at 2, 4, and 6 months of age, was 70% to 95% effective at preventing severe rotavirus gastroenteritis, and was recommended for all infants in the United States.[9]

Within a year of licensure, RRV-TV was found to be associated with intussusception (see *Chapter 2: Vaccine Infrastructure in the United States—The Safety Net in Action*). The attributable risk was estimated at about one in 10,000 vaccinees, with most cases occurring in the first 2 weeks after Dose 1, the time when viral replication peaks.[10] RRV-TV was withdrawn in 1999; the mechanism whereby it caused intussusception is still not clear, but may have been related to certain biologic characteristics of the native rhesus rotavirus strain.

The disease burden continued to justify a vaccination program, as did the cost of rotavirus disease—>$1 billion each year in the United States alone in direct medical and societal costs. It was estimated that a universal vaccination program instituted in a single US birth cohort—assuming only 70% coverage and looking at outcomes over 5 years—would reduce the number of domiciliary episodes of rotavirus gastroenteritis by 48%, office visits by 60%, emergency department visits by 64%, hospitalizations by 66%, and deaths by 44%. The cost per case averted would be $138, cost per serious case averted would be $3024, and cost per year of life saved would be $197,190 (2004 dollars).[11]

RV5 was licensed in February 2006. Prelicensure clinical trials demonstrated safety, efficacy, and importantly, no association with intussusception, and the vaccine was recommended for all infants in the United States.[4] By May 2008, coverage for 1 dose in infants 3 months of age was estimated to be 56% and coverage for 3 doses in children 13 months of age was estimated to be 34%.[12] In the prevaccine era, the average rotavirus season started in December and lasted 26 weeks. The 2007-2008 season started in early March and lasted 14 weeks; the 2008-2009 season started in late January and lasted 17 weeks.[13] The median percentage of tests that was positive for rotavirus at sentinel laboratories dropped from 25% to around 10%. In addition, many centers reported dramatic reductions in hospitalizations due to rotavirus disease. These data indicate substantial impact of the vaccination program, and, given the fact that vaccine uptake was incomplete, suggest that herd immunity is operative.

415

RV1 was licensed in April 2008, and updated recommendations for prevention of rotavirus disease were published in 2009.[14] No preference for RV1 or RV5 was expressed, and a harmonized dosing schedule was recommended, despite differences in the labeled dosing schedules.

Vaccines

Characteristics of the rotavirus vaccines licensed in the United States are given in **Table 21.1**. Both are live-attenuated vaccines that are given PO. RV5 is a mixture of five different reassortant viruses, each of which is a (naturally attenuated) bovine rotavirus strain that has been engineered to express a different immunogenic protein (G1, G2, G3, G4, or P[8]) from human rotavirus. RV1 is a single human rotavirus strain (G1P[8]) that was attenuated by serial passage in tissue culture, much the same way as was the Sabin polio vaccine.

Efficacy and/or Immunogenicity

Prelicensure studies of RV5 involved >70,000 infants in many countries throughout the world; half of the subjects were enrolled in the United States, a third in Finland, and the rest in Latin America, Europe, and Taiwan. Detailed information about efficacy came from about 7000 of these infants. The pivotal trial, a placebo-controlled study called the **R**otavirus **E**fficacy and **S**afety **T**rial (REST), consisted of a large-scale safety study ($N = 69,625$), a detailed safety substudy ($N = 9605$), and an efficacy substudy ($N = 5673$); efficacy against rotavirus-related hospitalizations and emergency department visits was determined in the entire cohort.[15] Efficacy against rotavirus gastroenteritis of any severity due to serotypes G1 through G4 during the first season after vaccination was 74%, and against severe disease was 98% (efficacy was still 98% against severe disease when the data were looked at without regard to serotype). Efficacy against disease of any severity was 71% through two seasons; in the second season alone, efficacy was 63% against disease of any severity and 88% against severe disease. Emergency department visits due to rotavirus serotypes G1 through G4 were reduced by 94% during the 2 years following Dose 3, and hospitalizations were reduced by 96%; in a separate post hoc analysis, efficacy against hospitalizations and emergency department visits due to G9P[8] strains was 100%.

A postlicensure study utilizing a national health insurance claims database compared 33,140 infants who received 3 doses of RV5 to 26,167 unimmunized controls. Effectiveness was estimated at 100% against rotavirus hospitalizations and emergency department visits and 96% against outpatient visits.[16]

Prelicensure studies of RV1 also involved >70,000 infants (efficacy was evaluated in about 24,000). Two pivotal trials were done—3994 infants were enrolled in a European trial[17] and 63,225 in a trial in Latin America and Finland.[18,19] Efficacy in the European study against rotavirus gastroenteritis of any severity through one season was 87% and through two seasons was 79%; the respective efficacies against severe disease were 96% and 90%. Hospitalizations were reduced by 100% through one season and 96% through two seasons. In the Latin America/Finland study, efficacy against severe rotavirus gastroenteritis through one season was 85% and through two seasons was 81%; hospitalizations were reduced by 85% and 83%, respectively. Type-specific efficacy was evaluated in about 4000 infants. The vaccine was highly effective against G1P[8] strains. For non-G1 strains, efficacy through one season against any severity of disease ranged from 76% for G9P[8] to 90% for G3P[8] but was not significant for G2P[4] (very few cases occurred). Efficacy through two seasons against any severity of disease ranged from 58% for G2P[4] to 85% for G3P[8]. Efficacy through one season against severe disease ranged from 95% for G9P[8] to 100% for G3P[8] and G4P[8] but was not significant for G2P[4] (again, very few cases occurred). Efficacy through two seasons against severe disease ranged from 85% for G9P[8] to 95% for G4P[8].

In an integrated analysis of all randomized, double-blind, placebo-controlled, Phase 2 and 3 studies of RV1, efficacy against severe disease caused by G1P[8] strains (which share both G and P types with the vaccine) was estimated at 87.4%.[20] Efficacy against severe disease caused by G2P[4] strains was estimated at 71.4%; since these strains share neither G nor P types with the vaccine, these data indicate significant cross-protection.

Safety

In REST, 11 cases of intussusception occurred within 42 days of any dose of RV5—six among vaccinees and five among placebees, a difference that was not statistically significant.[15] No clustering of cases was seen after any dose. By August 2007, over 9 million doses of RV5 had been distributed in the United States and there were 160 reports of intussusception in VAERS.[21] Assuming 75% reporting and 75% administration of distributed vaccine, the number of VAERS reports was about half that expected in the first 21 days after vaccination, providing further reassurance that RV5 does not cause intussusception. Prelicensure trials showed a slight excess of vomiting (6.7% vs 5.4%) and diarrhea (10.4% vs 9.1%) after Dose 1 and a slight excess of diarrhea (8.6% vs 6.4%) after Dose 2.

In the Latin America/Finland study of RV1, 13 cases of intussusception occurred within 31 days of any dose of RV1—six

TABLE 21.1 — Rotavirus Vaccines

	Rotarix	RotaTeq
Trade name	Rotarix	RotaTeq
Abbreviation	RV1 (rotavirus vaccine, monovalent)	RV5 (rotavirus vaccine, 5-valent)
Manufacturer/distributor	GlaxoSmithKline	Merck
Type of vaccine	Live-attenuated, classical	Live-attenuated, engineered
Composition:		
Virus strain	Human rotavirus strain 89-12, serotype G1P1[8]	5 naturally attenuated bovine rotavirus reassort-ants expressing the following serotypes: Human G1, bovine P7[5] Human G2, bovine P7[5] Human G3, bovine P7[5] Human G4, bovine P7[5] Bovine G6, human P1[8]
Propagation	Vero (African Green Monkey kidney) cells	Vero (African Green Monkey kidney) cells
Amount	10⁶ median cell culture infective dose	2.0 to 2.8 × 10⁶ infectious units of each virus
Adjuvant	None	None
Preservative	None	None
Excipients and contaminants	Lyophilized vaccine: Amino acids Dextran Dulbecco's Modified Eagle Medium Sorbitol Sucrose	Sucrose Sodium citrate Sodium phosphate monobasic monohydrate Sodium hydroxide Polysorbate 80 Cell culture media

	Diluent: Calcium carbonate Xanthan	Fetal bovine serum (trace)
Latex	Tip cap and plunger of oral applicator contain dry natural latex rubber	None
Labeled indications	Prevention of rotavirus gastroenteritis caused by serotype G1 and non-G1 serotypes G3, G4, and G9	Prevention of rotavirus gastroenteritis caused by serotypes G1, G2, G3, and G4
Labeled ages	6 to 24 weeks	6 to 32 weeks
Dose	1 mL	2 mL
Route of administration	PO[a]	PO[a]
Labeled schedule:		
Dose 1	6 to 20 weeks of age	6 to 12 weeks of age
Dose 2	≥4 weeks after Dose 1 but <24 weeks of age	≥4 weeks after Dose 1 but not >32 weeks of age
Dose 3	—	≥4 weeks after Dose 2 but not >32 weeks of age
Recommended schedule[b]:		
Dose 1	2, 4 months of age	2, 4, 6 months of age
Dose 2	6 weeks to 14 weeks 6 days of age	6 weeks to 14 weeks 6 days of age
Dose 3	≥4 weeks after Dose 1 but <8 months 0 days of age	≥4 weeks after Dose 1 but <8 months 0 days of age
	—	>4 weeks after Dose 2 but <8 months 0 days of age
How supplied (number in package)	1-dose vial (10), lyophilized, with diluent in prefilled oral applicator	1-dose squeezable, plastic tube (10)

Continued

21

419

TABLE 21.1 — *Continued*

Trade name	Rotarix	RotaTeq
Abbreviation	RV1 (rotavirus vaccine, monovalent)	RV5 (rotavirus vaccine, 5-valent)

Storage	Vaccine:
	  Refrigerate
	  Do not freeze
	  Protect from light
	Diluent:
	  Room temperature
	  Do not freeze
	Reconstituted vaccine:
	  Refrigerate or room temperature for up to 24 hr
	  Do not freeze
		Refrigerate
		Do not freeze
		Protect from light
		Administer as soon as possible after removing from refrigerator

Cost per dose ($US, 2009):		
Public	83.25	57.20
Private	102.50	69.59
Reference package insert	May 2009	December 2009

a The dose should not be repeated if it is spit out or regurgitated.
b The series should be completed with the same product, but vaccination should not be deferred if the same product is unknown or not available. If any dose in the series is RV5 or unknown, a total of 3 doses should be given.

among vaccinees and seven among placebees, a difference that was not statistically significant.[18] There were no confirmed cases within the 14-day period following Dose 1, which was the highest risk period for RRV-TV. Solicited adverse events occurred at similar rates among RV1 recipients and placebo recipients. RV1 was, however, associated with slightly increased unsolicited reports of irritability (11.4% vs 8.7%) and flatulence (2.2% vs 1.3%) when compared with placebo. An integrated safety summary of 8 randomized, double-blind trials involving a total of 71,209 infants demonstrated no differences in solicited adverse events or serious adverse events, including intussusception and death, between vaccinees and placebees.[22]

RV1 is shed in about 50% of vaccinees, more commonly after Dose 1; horizontal transmission has been documented.[23] RV5 is shed in about 10% of vaccinees after Dose 1 but very rarely after subsequent doses; horizontal transmission has not been documented.

- *Contraindications*
  - Allergic reaction to previous dose of vaccine or any vaccine component (risk of recurrent allergic reaction). The oral applicator for RV1 contains latex, so infants with severe latex allergy should receive RV5. Some experts recommend RV5 for infants with spina bifida or bladder extrophy in order to minimize the risk of sensitization; however, if only RV1 is available, it should be given.
  - Severe combined immunodeficiency disease (risk of disease caused by live virus[24])
- *Precautions*
  - Moderate or severe acute illness (difficulty distinguishing illness from vaccine reaction)
  - Moderate or severe acute gastroenteritis (risk of impaired immune response)
  - Immunodeficiency or immunosuppression (risk of disease caused by live virus). Adverse events are unlikely in HIV-infected infants because the vaccine strains are considerably attenuated, and the vast majority of HIV-exposed infants in the United States will not have HIV infection.
  - Previous intussusception (risk of recurrent intussusception).

Recommendations

All infants should be vaccinated against rotavirus. There is no preference for one vaccine over the other. Vaccination *is recommended* in the following circumstances:

- Infants who have already had an episode of rotavirus gastroenteritis
- Breast-feeding

- Premature infants who are clinically stable and are being or have been discharged from the nursery (those who are remaining in the nursery or neonatal intensive care unit *should not* be vaccinated)
- Infants living in the home of immunocompromised or pregnant individuals (standard precautions should be followed to minimize the potential for transmission)
- Infants who have received antibody-containing blood products (there is the theoretical risk that passively acquired antibodies could inactivate a dose of the vaccine, but this should not be an issue since it is a multiple-dose series)
- Infants with pre-existing gastrointestinal conditions such as malabsorption syndromes, Hirschsprung's disease, short-gut syndrome (for these conditions, ACIP considers the benefits to outweigh the theoretic risks). The RV1 package insert lists as a contraindication uncorrected congenital malformation of the gastrointestinal tract that would predispose to intussusception.

The series should be completed with the same product, but vaccination should not be deferred if the same product is not available (if a mixed schedule is used, or if a previous product is unknown, a total of 3 doses should be given). It is not necessary to repeat a dose if the infant spits up. Standard precautions should be used for infants who are hospitalized after vaccination.

REFERENCES

1. Coffin SE, et al. *Pediatr Infect Dis J*. 2006;25:584-589.
2. Dennehy PH, et al. *Pediatr Infect Dis J*. 2006;25:1123-1131.
3. Saulsbury FT, et al. *J Pediatr*. 1980;97:61-65.
4. Parashar UD, et al. *MMWR*. 2006;55(RR-12):1-13.
5. Payne DC, et al. *Pediatrics*. 2008;122:1235-1243.
6. Parashar UD, et al. *J Infect Dis*. 2009;200(suppl 1):S9-S15.
7. Gentsch JR, et al. *Clin Infect Dis*. 2009;200:S99-S105.
8. CDC. *MMWR*. 2008;57:1255-1257.
9. CDC. *MMWR*. 1999;48(RR-2):1-23.
10. Peter G, et al. *Pediatrics*. 2002;110:e67.
11. Widdowson MA, et al. *Pediatrics*. 2007;119:684-697.
12. CDC. *MMWR*. 2008;57:697-700.
13. Panozzo CA, et al. *MMWR*. 2009;58:1146-1149.
14. Cortese MM, et al. *MMWR*. 2009;58(RR-2):1-25.
15. Vesikari T, et al. *N Engl J Med*. 2006;354:23-33.
16. Wang FT, et al. *Pediatrics*. 2010;125:e208-e213.
17. Vesikari T, et al. *Lancet*. 2007;370:1757-1763.
18. Ruiz-Palacios GM, et al. *N Engl J Med*. 2006;354:11-22.
19. Linhares AC, et al. *Lancet*. 2008;371:1181-1189.
20. De Vos B, et al. *Pediatr Infect Dis J*. 2009;28:261-266.
21. Haber P, et al. *Pediatrics*. 2008;121:1206-1212.
22. Cheuvart B, et al. *Pediatr Infect Dis J*. 2009;28:225-232.
23. Anderson EJ. *Lancet Infect Dis*. 2008;8:642-649.
24. Patel NC, et al. *N Engl J Med*. 2010;362:314-319.

21

22   Smallpox

The Pathogen

Variola virus is a very large, brick-shaped, enveloped DNA virus in the genus *Orthopoxvirus* that replicates in the cytoplasm and is closely related to vaccinia, cowpox, and monkeypox. Direct organ damage by viral infection is unusual, as is secondary bacterial infection. Instead, death results from toxemia associated with circulating immune complexes and viral antigens. Encephalitis can occur and is similar to the acute perivascular demyelination syndromes that may complicate measles and varicella infection, or smallpox vaccination.

Clinical Features

Initial infection takes place at mucosal surfaces of the oropharynx or respiratory tract. Three to 4 days later, viremia leads to visceral dissemination, but the patient remains asymptomatic. Secondary viremia leads to a marked prodromal illness, which begins 12 to 14 days after infection and is characterized by high fever, malaise, headache, backache, prostration, chills, vomiting, delirium, and/or abdominal pain. Rash begins 1 to 4 days into the prodrome and is coincident with a decrease in fever; maculopapular lesions initially appear in the mouth and on the face and forearms, spreading to the trunk and legs. The lesions evolve slowly into vesicles and pustules, which are characteristically deep-seated, round, firm, and discrete, although some may coalesce. Eventually, the lesions develop an umbilicated appearance with a central dimple. Fever usually continues until scabs form, about 2 weeks into the illness. Scars are evident after the scabs separate.

Variola major refers to the typical smallpox syndrome, which is easily recognized and accounts for the vast majority of cases; mortality rates approximate 30%. *Hemorrhagic smallpox* follows a shorter incubation period and is characterized by an extreme prodrome, the development of dusky erythema, and the eruption of petechiae and hemorrhage into skin and mucous membranes. Pregnant women are disproportionately affected and the syndrome is uniformly fatal. In *malignant (flat) smallpox*, the onset is equally abrupt, but the initial confluent lesions never evolve into pustules, instead remaining flat, soft, and velvety. Mortality approaches 100% as well. *Modified smallpox* occurs in previously vaccinated persons, and although the prodrome may be severe, the lesions are fewer in number, more superficial, and evolve more rapidly; death is rare. *Variola minor (alastrim)*, caused by a less-pathogenic strain of the virus, is differentiated by fewer constitutional symptoms, sparse rash, and excellent prognosis. *Variola sine eruptione* is asymptomatic or self-limited with fever and flu-like symptoms; it occurs in previously vaccinated persons or infants with maternal antibodies.

Failure to diagnose the first wave of cases during a smallpox attack would have grave consequences. For this reason, and given the fact that most practicing physicians today have never seen a case, attention has focused on recognizing the clinical signs and symptoms and differentiating smallpox from other conditions that bear similarities, most notably chickenpox. **Table 22.1** provides clues to accurate and timely diagnosis. Suspected cases should immediately be reported to state or local health departments. The CDC also maintains a 24/7 Emergency Operations Center that is available to health care providers at 770-488-7100.

Epidemiology and Transmission

Natural smallpox has been *eradicated* from the face of the earth, but the variola virus itself is not extinct, existing as it is in US and Russian government laboratory freezers (see *Chapter 1: Introduction to Vaccinology—Goals of Immunization Programs*). The possibility exists that the virus could get into the wrong hands and be used as a weapon of bioterrorism.[1]

Certain features of smallpox make it attractive as a weapon, including the small infectious dose, high mortality rate, absence of natural and vaccine-induced immunity at the population level, lack of established therapy, historical fear and panic related to the disease, and person-to-person spread, which would amplify the effect of a primary release by generating secondary and tertiary cases. Epidemic disease in developed countries today would have the potential for great devastation because of the high point prevalence of atopic skin disease and relative immunoincompetency resulting from immunosuppressive therapy, chronic conditions, HIV infection, and aging.

Fortunately, variola virus is labile, and <90% remains viable for 24 hours after aerosol release in the presence of ultraviolet light. Transmission occurs through direct contact with body fluids and inhalation of aerosols and droplet nuclei expelled from the oropharynx of infected persons. Close contact is usually required, and secondary attack rates vary from about 40% to 90% under these circumstances. Distant airborne transmission is rare, but fomites such as bedding or clothing can transmit the virus. Transmission does not occur through insects or animals. Patients are most infectious 7 to 10 days after the rash develops; since this occurs after a debilitating prodromal illness, patients are likely to be easily recognized and bedridden at the time they are most contagious. Transmission from subclinical cases is of little epidemiologic importance.

Immunization Program

Until 1972, smallpox vaccine was given in the United States at 1 year of age. This program was abandoned because of global eradication. The remaining interest in smallpox vaccination resides in protecting laboratory workers and preparing for the possibility of bioterrorism.

Universal pre-event vaccination would constitute an absolute deterrent to a smallpox attack and could be conducted under controlled conditions.[2,3] However, this approach is not favored by scientists because the overall risk of an attack is considered to be low, the population at risk cannot be determined, and the risks of vaccination are substantial. The strategy of *surveillance and containment*, or *ring vaccination*, involves the isolation of suspected and confirmed cases and the identification, vaccination, and monitoring of their contacts. Vaccination can be extended to household contacts of contacts as well, or other people with indirect exposure, and the strategy can be supplemented by local quarantine and travel restrictions. This strategy, which was highly successful during the global eradication campaign, is workable because vaccination is effective if given soon after exposure. Ring vaccination, however, might not work as well in a largely nonimmune, highly mobile population experiencing a multisite intentional aerosol release of virus. In addition, the logistical complexity of this approach is daunting, especially in the face of the potential for public panic. *Universal postevent vaccination* would be logistically difficult and would provide little additional benefit to ring vaccination, although the CDC National Pharmaceutical Stockpile has protocols for simultaneous delivery of vaccine to every state and territory within 24 hours of an event. The current US vaccination plan combines limited pre-event vaccination with ring vaccination.[4]

As of June 2001, pre-event vaccination was recommended only for laboratory and health care personnel involved in orthopox research.[5] Certain groups were targeted for postevent vaccination, including people with primary exposure, close contacts of cases (face-to-face, household, or <2 meters distance), medical personnel with potential patient contact, clinical laboratory personnel, and ancillary personnel with potential exposure to infectious waste. The earliest vaccinations were to be targeted to persons who had been vaccinated in the past. In the wake of the anthrax attacks of October 2001, supplemental recommendations were

TABLE 22.1 — Diagnosis of Smallpox

Clinical Finding	Smallpox[a]	Chickenpox[b]
Major Criteria		
Prodrome	Fever ≥101°F (38.3°C) beginning 1 to 4 days before rash and at least one of the following: prostration, headache, backache, chills, vomiting, severe abdominal pain	None or mild
Lesion morphology	Deep-seated, firm, round, well-circumscribed vesicles or pustules, may be umbilicated or confluent	Superficial vesicles (resembling dewdrops on a rose petal)
Lesion development	Same stage of development on any one part of the body	Crops at different stages of development on any one part of the body
Minor Criteria		
Distribution	Centrifugal (concentrated on face and distal extremities)	Centripetal (concentrated on trunk)
Initial lesions	Oral mucosa, palate, face, forearms	Face or trunk
General appearance	Toxic or moribund	Well
Evolution	Slow (from macules to papules to pustules over days)	Rapid (from macules to papules to vesicles to pustules to crusts in <24 hours)
Palms and soles	Involved	Spared

a If the patient has all three major criteria, the risk of smallpox is high and authorities should be notified immediately. If the patient has a febrile prodrome and one other major criterion or ≥4 minor criteria, the risk is moderate and urgent evaluation is indicated. Other conditions to be considered in the differential diagnosis include disseminated herpes zoster or herpes simplex, impetigo, drug eruptions, erythema multiforme, Stevens-Johnson syndrome, enterovirus infection, scabies, secondary syphilis, bullous pemphigoid, and molluscum contagiosum. Cowpox and monkeypox resemble smallpox but can only be acquired directly from the respective animals. The differential diagnosis of hemorrhagic smallpox includes meningococcemia, hemorrhagic varicella, Rocky Mountain spotted fever, ehrlichiosis, and gram-negative sepsis.

b Other clues to the diagnosis of chickenpox include absence of a personal history of varicella or varicella vaccination and exposure to chickenpox or shingles. Most cases will occur in children because most adults are immune. The lesions are usually intensely pruritic and scarring is unusual.

Adapted from Centers for Disease Control and Prevention Web site. Evaluating patients for smallpox. http://www.bt.cdc.gov/agent/smallpox/diagnosis/pdf/spox-poster-full.pdf. Accessed February 6, 2010.

made to vaccinate smallpox response teams in each state and smallpox health care teams at predesignated isolation and care facilities, and, eventually, at each acute care hospital.[6]

The federal plan announced in December 2002 called for voluntary vaccination of up to 500,000 health and safety workers constituting local Smallpox Response Teams.[7] By mid-2003 it was clear that the federal plan to vaccinate civilians was proceeding much slower than anticipated; in all, only 40,000 civilians had been vaccinated, and the CDC had effectively ceased efforts to vaccinate additional people. The concomitant DOD plan called for stepwise, compulsory vaccination, first involving up to 5000 members of smallpox epidemic response teams, then 10,000 to 25,000 medical team members, then up to 500,000 mission-critical forces. As of January 2005, >700,000 service members had been vaccinated.

Vaccines

The origin of vaccinia virus is not clear, but it appears to be a hybrid between cowpox and smallpox that is not found in nature. In October 2002, the FDA relicensed Dryvax (Smallpox Vaccine, Dried, Calf Lymph Type), a product manufactured by Wyeth (acquired by Pfizer in 2009) until 1982, but held in storage at the CDC since then. Relicensure was intended to facilitate administration of the vaccine outside of investigational protocols. Dryvax was a lyophilized preparation of the New York City Board of Health strain of vaccinia harvested from lymph contained in skin lesions that develop after scarification of calves. As of December 2002, two lots of Dryvax with a total of 2.7 million doses were approved for release. In 2002, approximately 85 million doses of a similar vaccine (in liquid formulation) that had been in cold storage since the 1950s were discovered by Sanofi Pasteur and donated to the CDC for further study. Since studies indicated that Dryvax could be diluted up to 1:5 without diminution in the response rate in naïve subjects, it was estimated that sufficient doses were on hand in the event of an emergency.

A new, second-generation, cell culture derived smallpox vaccine called ACAM2000 was licensed in August 2007 and will replace Dryvax in the Strategic National Stockpile.[8] Characteristics of this vaccine are given in **Table 22.2**. ACAM2000 consists of live vaccinia virus that was plaque purified from Dryvax.

Handling and administration of smallpox vaccine is different from all other vaccines, as summarized below.
- *Reconstitution*
  - Wear gloves, use aseptic technique, and avoid contact of the vaccine with skin, eyes, and mucous membranes.
  - Bring the vaccine up to room temperature.

TABLE 22.2 — Smallpox Vaccine

Trade name	ACAM2000[a]
Abbreviation	—
Manufacturer/distributor	Sanofi Pasteur (formerly Acambis)
Type of vaccine	Live-attenuated, classical
Composition	Vaccinia, New York Board of Health strain
	Propagated in African green monkey kidney cells
	2.5 to 12.5×10^5 PFU/dose
Adjuvant	None
Preservative	None
Excipients and contaminants	HEPES (pH 6.5 to 7.5) (6 to 8 mM)
	Human serum albumin (2%)
	Sodium chloride (0.5% to 0.7%)
	Mannitol USP (5%)
	Neomycin (trace)
	Polymyxin B (trace)
	Glycerin USP (50% v/v)
	Phenol USP (0.25% v/v)
Latex	None
Labeled indications	Prevention of smallpox
Labeled ages	All ages
Dose	15 punctures *(see text)*
Route of administration	Percutaneous (scarification)
Labeled schedule	1 dose
	Booster doses every 3 years (for persons at continued high risk of exposure)
Recommended schedule	See text
How supplied (number in package)	100-dose vial, lyophilized, with diluent, bifurcated needles, and tuberculin syringe for reconstitution
Storage:	Vaccine: freeze
	Diluent: room temperature
	Reconstituted vaccine: may be used at room temperature for 6 to 8 hours and may be refrigerated for up to 30 days
Reference package insert	August 2007

[a] ACAM2000 is not commercially available but rather will be purchased by the federal government for inclusion in the Strategic National Stockpile. Dryvax (Smallpox Vaccine, Dried, Calf Lymph Type; Pfizer [formerly Wyeth]) is no longer available in the United States. Any remaining lots of Dryvax should have been destroyed by March 31, 2008.

22

- Lift up the cap seals on the vaccine and diluent vials.
- Wipe off the rubber stopper with alcohol and allow it to dry.
- Draw up 0.3 mL of diluent in the 1-mL tuberculin syringe fitted with a 25-gauge 5/8-inch needle that is provided with the vaccine.
- Transfer the contents of the syringe to the vaccine vial.
- Gently swirl without letting the liquid get on the rubber stopper. The reconstituted vaccine is clear to slightly hazy, colorless to straw-colored, and free from particulates.

• *Administration*
- Providers must be properly educated on administration technique and must provide vaccinees with an FDA-approved Medication Guide.
- Wear gloves, use aseptic technique, and avoid contact of the vaccine with skin, eyes, and mucous membranes.
- Preparation of the skin with alcohol is not required (this may inactivate the virus). Use soap and water if the site is grossly contaminated. If alcohol is used, the skin must be allowed to dry thoroughly before inoculation.
- Remove the vaccine vial cap (maintain sterile conditions for later recapping).
- Remove the bifurcated needle from its individual wrapping. Dip the bifurcated needle into the reconstituted vaccine and withdraw. A sufficient amount of liquid (approximately 0.0025 mL) is retained between the prongs by capillary action.
- Hold the needle between the thumb and first finger, perpendicular to the vaccinee's skin. Lay your wrist on the vaccinee's arm below the deltoid region. Use your other hand to pull the skin taught from underneath.
- Deposit the drop of vaccine on the skin. Using firm strokes from the wrist, make 15 rhythmic perpendicular insertions through the drop into the skin within a 5-mm area. A trace of blood should be visible after each puncture. *Do not* reinsert the needle into the vial between punctures or after the whole procedure.
- Discard the bifurcated needle immediately in a leak-proof, puncture-proof biohazard waste container. When ready for disposal, the vaccine vial, stopper, diluent syringe, and vented needle should be placed in a similar container. The container can be disposed of in the usual way.
- Absorb excess vaccine and blood with sterile gauze and discard in a biohazard container.
- Close the vaccine vial by reinserting the cap and return it to the refrigerator.
- Cover the site with gauze and adhesive tape. If the vaccinee will have direct patient contact, cover the gauze with a semipermeable dressing such as OpSite (Smith & Nephew)

or Tegaderm (3M) (some of these products are supplied with attached gauze pads). Semipermeable dressings should not be used alone because they macerate the skin.

- **Postvaccination Care**
  - Vaccinees should make sure a layer of clothing covers the dressing and should exercise meticulous hand hygiene after touching the site or dressings.
  - Change the dressing every 3 to 5 days or more often if exudates accumulate (dressings can be discarded in the household trash if sealed in a plastic bag).
  - Avoid rubbing and scratching.
  - Do not put salves or ointments on the site.
  - Keep the site dry. Showering or bathing can continue. If the site is uncovered it should not be touched. The site should be blotted dry with gauze, which should then be discarded in a sealed plastic bag in the household trash. If a towel is used for drying the site, it should not be used on the rest of the body.
  - Separately wash clothing or other material that comes into contact with the site, using hot water with detergent and/or bleach.

- **Assessing Response**
  - The subject should return for examination in 7 days.
  - A red, pruritic papule should form 2 to 5 days after vaccination. This becomes vesicular then pustular and reaches a maximum size by 8 to 10 days. The pustule dries and forms a scab, which separates by 14 to 21 days, leaving a pitted scar.
  - Failure to develop a skin lesion as described indicates failure of vaccination, and revaccination should be considered, unless the vaccinee had been previously vaccinated (pre-existing immunity can modify the cutaneous reaction). Images of appropriate primary and revaccination responses are shown in the package insert, and images of normal and adverse reactions can be viewed on the CDC Web site.[9]

22

Efficacy and/or Immunogenicity

Studies with Dryvax suggest that protection persists for at least 5 years after primary vaccination. Antibody levels steadily decline 5 to 10 years following vaccination, and although detectable cellular responses may persist, it must be assumed that immunity to smallpox wanes. Revaccination even one time results in boosted antibody levels that may persist for 30 years.

Two randomized, multicenter studies were conducted comparing ACAM2000 to Dryvax. One study looked at 1647 persons who had been vaccinated over 10 years earlier; 1242 received ACAM2000 and 405 received Dryvax. Successful revaccination was slightly less common in the ACAM2000 group, but antibody titers were not inferior. The second study looked at 1037 vaccinia-naïve subjects; 780 received ACAM2000 and 257 received Dryvax. In this case, vaccination success rates were not inferior, although antibody titers were lower. Overall, ACAM2000 was noninferior to Dryvax where it counts most—major cutaneous reaction in vaccinia-naïve subjects and strength of antibody response in vaccinia-experienced subjects (whose pre-existing immunity might have modified the cutaneous reaction).

Safety

Smallpox vaccine is the most reactogenic and dangerous of all licensed vaccines. By definition, successfully vaccinated persons develop a pustule at the inoculation site that lasts several weeks. Many experience additional local reactions and associated systemic complaints. In about one third of patients, these symptoms may lead to missed work, school, or recreational activities, or to trouble sleeping. Common side effects for ACAM2000 include itching, soreness, fever, headache, rash, and fatigue. As with Dryvax, transmission to individuals who are pregnant, immunocompromised, or have chronic skin problems can lead to serious complications. In order to prevent serious adverse events, a Risk Minimization Action Plan has been implemented for ACAM2000. This includes provision of an FDA-approved Medication Guide to recipients, education of health care providers, expedited adverse event reporting, and a strategy for risk management evaluation.

Potential complications of vaccination include inadvertent inoculation, generalized vaccinia, erythema multiforme, eczema vaccinatum, post-vaccinal encephalitis or encephalomyelitis, progressive vaccinia, contact vaccinia, and fetal infection. In 2005, the safety of the post-9/11 civilian and military smallpox vaccination program (in which Dryvax was used) was reviewed.[7] Nearly 800,000 vaccinees were included. No cases of eczema vaccinatum, progressive vaccinia, fetal vaccinia, or workplace contact transmission were reported, suggesting that education and screening procedures were successsful. Anticipated reactions included 43 cases of generalized vaccinia, later determined to be hypersensitivity reactions, and 2 cases of encephalitis. Inadvertent infection of the skin occurred in 62 vaccinees and 50 contacts of vaccinees. Cardiac ischemic events (including 3 fatal myocardial infarctions) occurred in 33 persons, which was below the expected background rate. A total of 107 cases of myopericarditis were reported. Among military personnel alone, the observed incidence within 30 days of vaccination (16.11 per 100,000) was 7.5-fold higher than the background rate (for unknown reasons, the increased risk was seen among primary vaccinees in the military program but among revaccinees in the civilian program). A causal relationship was further suggested by temporal clustering as well as wide geographic and cross-seasonal distribution. The risk of myocarditis and/or pericarditis after vaccination with ACAM2000 is estimated to be 1 in 175 previously unvaccinated adults.

- *Contraindications (postexposure)*
  - In the event of exposure to smallpox, there are no contraindications to vaccination.
- *Contraindications (pre-event, applies to potential vaccinees and their household or sexual contacts)*—most of these involve risk of disease caused by live virus
  - *Eczema, atopic dermatitis, other acute, chronic, or exfoliative skin conditions*: burns, impetigo, chickenpox, contact dermatitis, shingles, herpes, severe acne, psoriasis, Darier's disease (keratosis follicularis), even if currently inactive. Two screening questions have been suggested (a *yes* to either question means *no* vaccine): Have you or a member of your household ever been diagnosed with eczema or atopic dermatitis? Have you or a family member ever had an itchy, red, scaly rash that lasts for >2 weeks and often comes and goes?
  - *Immunodeficiency or immunosuppression*: solid organ or bone marrow transplantation, generalized malignancy, leukemia, lymphoma, agammaglobulinemia, autoimmune disease, treatment with radiation, antimetabolites, alkylating agents, corticosteroids (in similar doses to those outlined in *Chapter 6: Vaccination in Special Circumstances—Medication–Induced Immunosuppression*), chemotherapy agents or organ transplant medications, and HIV infection (routine testing is not recommended, but should be done in persons with risk factors, those who are unsure of their status and those who are concerned that they could have HIV infection)
  - *Pregnancy*: currently pregnant or planning to become pregnant in the next 4 weeks (vaccinated women should be counseled not to become pregnant for 4 weeks). For reassurance, women can perform a urine pregnancy test on the first morning void on the day of vaccination. Routine pregnancy testing is not recommended. Inadvertent vaccination during pregnancy is not ordinarily a reason to terminate the pregnancy, although the mother should be aware of the extremely rare occurrence of fetal vaccinia.
- *Contraindications (pre-event, applies to potential vaccinees only)*
  - Allergic reaction to previous dose of vaccine or any vaccine component (risk of recurrent allergic reaction)

22

435

- Infants <12 months of age (risk of disease caused by live virus; ACIP advises against pre-event vaccination of persons <18 years of age)
- Breast-feeding (risk of disease caused by live virus)
- Cardiac risk, including underlying heart disease with or without symptoms, persons with three or more risk factors such as hypertension, diabetes, hypercholesterolemia, first-degree relative under age 50 years with heart disease, and smoking (risk of myocarditis). Verbal screening for risk factors is recommended. Special follow-up for persons with risk factors who have already been vaccinated is not recommended.
- *Precautions (postexposure)*
  - In the event of exposure to smallpox, there are no precautions to vaccination.
- *Precautions (pre-event)*
  - Moderate or severe acute illness (difficulty distinguishing illness from vaccine reaction)
  - Inflammatory eye disease requiring steroid therapy (risk of disease from live virus)

Vaccinia immune globulin (VIG), a polyclonal immune globulin product made from blood of recently vaccinated blood donors, can be used to treat complications of vaccination. As of 2008, there are 2700 treatment doses of VIG available at the CDC, enough to treat expected complications from >27 million vaccinations. The usual dose is 0.6 mL/kg intramuscularly, and indications include progressive vaccinia, eczema vaccinatum, severe generalized vaccinia, and inadvertent inoculation resulting in a large number of lesions, toxicity, or significant pain. Cidofovir may help limit viral replication. Both VIG and cidofovir are available through CDC under an investigational new-drug protocol. Civilian providers seeking access should first contact their state health department.

The Public Readiness and Emergency Preparedness Act, enacted in December 2005, provides compensation to persons for serious physical injuries or deaths resulting from pandemic, epidemic, or security countermeasures in the event of designated public health emergencies. Smallpox vaccine injuries are covered under this program.[10]

Recommendations

For those who receive pre-event vaccination today, a single dose is recommended, with booster doses every 10 years. Revaccination every 3 years should be considered for workers with occupational exposure to orthopox viruses. The vaccine will completely prevent or significantly modify smallpox if given 3 to 4 days postexposure; vaccination 4 to 7 days postexposure probably modifies the severity of the disease.

As of 2003, the US Civilian Smallpox Preparedness and Response Program called for all acute care hospitals to establish Smallpox Health Care Teams. These teams should provide hospital-based in-room evaluation and management for the first 7 to 10 days, using 8- to 12-hour shifts. Team members should include the following:

- Emergency department and intensive care unit staff, including physicians and nurses
- General medical and primary care staff
- House staff
- Medical subspecialists, including infectious disease specialists, experienced physicians, dermatologists, ophthalmologists, pathologists, surgeons, and anesthesiologists
- Infection control professionals
- Respiratory therapists
- Radiology technicians
- Security personnel
- Housekeeping staff

Clinical laboratory workers are not included because clinical specimens are expected to contain low levels of virus and standard precautions are considered to be protective. Although emergency medical technicians (EMTs) should not routinely be vaccinated, hospital-based EMTs could be vaccinated if included on the response teams. Designated vaccinated staff should examine all vaccinated health care personnel each day after vaccination, assess vaccine take, and change the dressings if indicated. Persons handling the vaccine should also be vaccinated.

Routine leave for vaccinated health care personnel is not recommended. However, leave is indicated for systemic illness, extensive lesions that cannot be covered, or inability to adhere to infection control precautions. Institutions should take a phased in, staggered approach to vaccination, beginning with groups of previously vaccinated persons. Rigorous screening for contraindications is recommended, but routine pregnancy and HIV testing is not.

Revaccination of persons who were initially vaccinated under the civilian program is recommended only on an "out-the-door" basis, ie only after there is determination of a credible threat to public health and prior to engaging in activities involving a risk for exposure to smallpox.[11] Revaccination is recommended every 10 years, however, for persons who routinely administer vaccine to others.

Smallpox vaccination is recommended for laboratory workers who directly handle cultures or animals infected with non-highly attenuated vaccinia viruses or vaccinia recombinants, as well as

437

other orthopoxviruses that infect humans (eg, monkeypox and cowpox). Vaccination should also be considered for health care personnel who may contact materials contaminated with such viruses.

Smallpox vaccine may be administered simultaneously with all inactivated vaccines and live vaccines except for VAR, in which case ≥4 weeks should separate the 2 inoculations. Tuberculin skin tests should be deferred at least 1 month following smallpox vaccination to minimize the risk of false-negatives. Blood donation by vaccinees (as well as persons with contact vaccinia) should be deferred until the scab spontaneously separates or 21 days postvaccination, whichever is later.

Under all circumstances, *pre-event* vaccination of civilians is voluntary. A complete information packet for potential vaccinees is available at the CDC Web site.[4]

REFERENCES

1. Henderson DA, et al. *JAMA*. 1999;281:2127-2137.
2. Halloran ME, et al. *Science*. 2002;298:1428-1432.
3. Bozzette SA, et al. *N Engl J Med*. 2003;348:416-425.
4. Emergency preparedness and response: smallpox. Centers for Disease Control and Prevention Web site. http://www.bt.cdc.gov /agent/smallpox. Accessed February 6, 2010.
5. Rotz LD, et al. *MMWR*. 2001;50(RR-10):1-25.
6. Wharton M, et al. *MMWR*. 2003;52(RR-7):1-16.
7. Poland GA, et al. *Vaccine*. 2005;23:2078-2081.
8. CDC. *MMWR*. 2008;57:207-208.
9. Smallpox vaccination and adverse events training module. Centers for Disease Control and Prevention Web site. http://www.bt.cdc.gov /training/smallpoxvaccine/reactions. Accessed February 6, 2010.
10. Countermeasures Injury Compensation Program. Health Resources and Services Administration Web site. http://www.hrsa.gov/coun termeasurescomp. Accessed February 6, 2010.
11. CDC interim guidance for revaccination of eligible persons who participated in the US Civilian Smallpox Preparedness and Response Program. Centers for Disease Control and Prevention Web site. http://www.bt.cdc.gov/agent/smallpox/revaxmemo.asp. Accessed February 6, 2010.

23

Streptococcus pneumoniae

The Pathogen

S pneumoniae is a facultatively anaerobic, catalase-negative gram-positive bacterium that looks like lancet-shaped diplococci on Gram's stain. The organism produces a polysaccharide capsule that is the basis for serotyping (there are >90 known serotypes, although most invasive disease is caused by <20 of these). The capsule contributes to virulence by inhibiting complement-mediated lysis and phagocytosis by neutrophils. Other virulence factors include pneumolysin and pneumococcal surface protein A. *S pneumoniae* often colonizes the nasopharynx—disease results from contiguous spread to respiratory tract structures such as the middle ear space, hematogenous seeding of distant sites such as the meninges, or from bacteremia without focal infection. Resistance to penicillin and other antibiotics has increased dramatically since the early 1990s.

Clinical Features

Prior to the conjugate-vaccine era, bacteremia without focal infection accounted for 70% of invasive disease in those <2 years of age; bacteremic pneumonia accounted for another 12% to 16%.[1] With the disappearance of invasive *H influenzae* type b disease from the United States in the 1990s, *S pneumoniae* became the leading cause of bacterial meningitis among children <5 years of age (collectively, bacteremia, meningitis, and infection of other normally sterile body sites is referred to as *invasive pneumococcal disease* or IPD). *S pneumoniae* was also a common cause of noninvasive respiratory syndromes including acute otitis media (AOM), where it accounted for 28% to 55% of cases. By age 12 months, 62% of children had at least one episode of AOM, making this one of the more common reasons for sick visits to pediatric offices. Complications of otitis media include mastoiditis and suppurative intracranial infection.

Pneumonia is the most common presentation of pneumococcal disease in adults. Classically, there is abrupt onset of fever and a single episode of rigor. Other symptoms include pleuritic chest pain, productive cough yielding mucopurulent, rusty sputum, dyspnea, tachypnea, hypoxia, tachycardia, malaise, and weakness. Nausea, vomiting, and headaches occur less frequently. Complications include empyema, pericarditis, and abscess. Pneumococcal meningitis also occurs in adults. Symptoms include headache, lethargy, vomiting, irritability, fever, nuchal rigidity, cranial nerve signs, seizures, and coma. The spinal fluid profile and neurologic complications are similar to those seen in other forms of bacterial meningitis. One quarter of patients with pneumococcal meningitis also have pneumonia.

Mortality is highest in patients with bacteremia or meningitis, in patients with underlying medical conditions, and in the very young and the very old. In some high-risk groups, mortality from bacteremia is as high as 40% despite antibiotic therapy.

Epidemiology and Transmission

Humans are the only natural hosts and transmission occurs by direct person-to-person contact or via respiratory droplets. Spread within the household is facilitated by crowding and occurs more often in the late winter and early spring, when respiratory viral disease is more prevalent. In general, higher rates of nasopharyngeal carriage lead to higher rates of disease.

It is estimated that 1 million children worldwide die from IPD each year. In 1999, the year before the introduction of PCV7 in the United States, the overall incidence of IPD was 24 per 100,000 population.[2] The rate was as high as 205 per 100,000 in children 1 year of age and as low as 4 per 100,000 in children between 5 and 17; adults ≥65 years of age had a rate of 62 per 100,000. It was estimated that there were a total of 64,400 cases of IPD and 7300 deaths. The most common serious clinical syndrome was bacteremic pneumonia (54%), followed by bacteremia without a focus (38%) and meningitis (5%), and pneumococcus was estimated to cause over one third of community-acquired and one half of hospital-acquired pneumonia cases in adults. In addition, an estimated 5 million cases of AOM due to pneumococcus occurred each year in children <5 years of age. Children with functional or anatomic asplenia, particularly those with sickle cell disease, and children with HIV infection were at particularly high risk for IPD, with rates in some studies >50 times those in age-equivalent children without these conditions. Alaska Native, American Indian, and African American children were also at increased risk. The reason for this is not known, but the same racial and ethnic predilection was seen for invasive *H influenzae* type b disease. Day care attendance was associated with a 2- to 3-fold increase in the risk of IPD and AOM among children <5 years of age.

Immunization Program

A 14-valent pneumococcal polysaccharide vaccine was licensed in the United States in 1977. In 1983, this was replaced by PPSV23 (Pneumovax 23 [Merck] and Pnu-Immune 23 [Lederle]; only the former is still available), which was recommended for all persons ≥65 years of age as well as high-risk persons from 2 to 64 years of age.[3] PCV7 was introduced in 2000 and was recommended for all infants, with a booster dose in the second year of life.[1] At that time, PCV7 covered 80% of the serotypes causing IPD in young children in the United States. By 2005, universal infant immunization had resulted in a 77% reduction in IPD among children <5 years of age.[4] The largest percentage decline was among children 1 year of age. During 2001-2005, 62,000 children <5 years of age were spared IPD—59% through direct effects of the vaccine and the remainder through indirect effects (herd immunity as the result of decreased nasopharyngeal carriage rates). Rates of pneumococcal meningitis hospitalization in children <2 years of age declined from 7.7 per 100,000 in the prevaccine era to 2.6 per 100,000 in 2001-2004 (there was also a 33% decrease among adults ≥65 years of age).[5]

By 2004, all-cause pneumonia admission rates had declined by 39% in children <2 years of age; admissions for pneumococcal pneumonia declined 65%[6] and outpatient visits for otitis media declined by 20%.[7] Rates of infection due to drug-resistant strains also declined[8]; possible mechanisms for this include direct effects on vaccine serotypes, which are disproportionately resistant, as well as global decreases in antibiotic use.[9] Considering only direct effects of PCV7 on IPD, pneumonia, and otitis media in children <5 years of age, PCV7 is estimated to have cost $201,000 per life-year saved, with a net cost of $145 per child vaccinated (2006 dollars).[10] However, with the inclusion of indirect effects in all age groups, PCV7 was estimated to be cost saving, to the tune of $503 per child vaccinated. Studies demonstrated significant decreases in nasopharyngeal carriage of vaccine serotypes among vaccinated children and their adult contacts, but there was an increase in colonization with nonvaccine serotypes.[11,12] This was accompanied by relative increases in IPD due to those serotypes (so called *replacement disease*), particularly serotype 19A.[13]

Declines in IPD due to vaccine serotypes also were seen among older persons as a result of herd immunity (**Figure 1.7**). In fact, by 2003 the incidence of IPD caused by PCV7 serotypes declined 50% among persons ≥50 years of age, with no change in disease caused by the 14 serotypes contained in PPSV23 that are not in PCV7.[14] In 2008, ACIP extended the recommendations for PPSV23 to include adults 19 to 64 years of age who smoke or have asthma.[15] Most studies show that routine vaccination of adults ≥65 years of age is cost-effective, at <$50,000 per life-year or QALY gained.[16]

PCV7 was routinely used from 2000 through 2009. In 2008, ACIP recommended including a dose of PCV7 for all incompletely immunized children 24 to 59 months of age.[17] PCV13, which covers 6 additional pneumococcal serotypes, was licensed in February 2010. Shortly thereafter, ACIP recommended replacing PCV7 with PCV13 in the routine schedule.[18] In addition, recommendations were made for supplemental dosing in children who had already completed the PCV7 series, as well as for dosing of high-risk children. As of 2007, 64% of IPD occurring in children <5 years of age was caused by serotypes contained in PCV13 but not in PCV7 (mostly, serotypes 3, 7F, and 19A); of the estimated 4600 cases that occurred that year, 2900 were potentially preventable by PCV13.[19]

Vaccines

Characteristics of pneumococcal vaccines licensed in the United States are given in **Table 23.1**. PPSV23 is a 23-valent pure polysaccharide vaccine. PCV7 and PCV13 are protein-polysaccharide conjugate vaccines. Biologic differences between conjugate and polysaccharide vaccines are discussed in *Chapter 1: Introduction to Vaccinology—The Germinal Center Reaction* and are summarized in **Table 1.3**.

Efficacy and/or Immunogenicity

After 4 doses of PCV7, virtually all healthy infants develop antibody to all seven serotypes. PCV7 also is immunogenic in infants and children with sickle cell disease and HIV infection. In a controlled clinical trial involving nearly 40,000 children, the vaccine reduced IPD caused by vaccine serotypes by 97%; there was also an 89% reduction in IPD caused by all serotypes, including those not in the vaccine.[20] The vaccine also reduced X-ray-confirmed pneumonia by 73%. Children who received PCV7 had 7% fewer episodes of AOM and underwent 20% fewer tympanostomy tube placements than unvaccinated children. In a Finnish study, efficacy against AOM caused by vaccine-related serotypes was 57%, but there was an increase of 33% in otitis episodes caused by nonvaccine serotypes.[21] Despite this, there was a net reduction of 34% in AOM caused by *S pneumoniae*. In a 2009 meta-analysis of clinical trials in children <24 months of age, efficacy against IPD due to vaccine serotypes was approximately 90% and efficacy against otitis media due to vaccine serotypes was just over 50%.[22] Efficacy against radiographically confirmed pneumonia (serotypes largely unknown) was about 30%. A case-control study done after licensure demonstrated that ≥1 dose of PCV7 was 96% effective in preventing IPD in healthy children 3 to 59 months of age and 81% effective in those with coexisting disorders.[23] Effectiveness also was demonstrated against serotype 6A, which is not in the vaccine but is closely related to 6B, which is in the vaccine.

PCV13 was compared with PCV7 in a noninferiority trial involving over 600 infants.[18] The proportion of subjects achieving

≥0.35 mcg/mL of anticapsular antibody to the 7 shared serotypes after 3 doses was similar (generally above 90%) in PCV13 recipients as compared to PCV7 recipients. While the prespecified noninferiority criteria were not met for 6B and 9V, the differences were marginal and the functional (opsonophagocytic) antibody levels elicited were similar. For the 6 nonshared serotypes, responses to PCV13 were noninferior to the least immunogenic PCV7 serotype (6B), except serotype 3, for which, however, opsonophagocytic antibodies were detected. After 4 doses, the geometric mean concentration of antibody was higher than after 3 doses for all 13 serotypes. Noninferiority criteria were met for all serotypes except 3, but opsonophagocytic antibody titers ≥1:8 to all 13 serotypes were seen in >90% of vaccinees. On the basis of these data, PCV13 was given indications for the prevention of IPD and otitis media caused by the 7 serotypes shared with PCV7, as well as an indication for prevention of IPD caused by the additional 6 serotypes.

Protective efficacy of pneumococcal polysaccharide vaccines was initially demonstrated in healthy gold miners in South Africa. Postlicensure case-control studies estimate the efficacy of PPSV23 in preventing serious pneumococcal disease in immunocompetent persons to be 56% to 81%, and a meta-analysis suggested efficacy against bacteremic pneumococcal pneumonia in low-risk, but not high-risk, adults.[24] A surveillance study demonstrated 57% overall effectiveness against IPD caused by vaccine serotypes; effectiveness was 65% to 84% in persons with underlying high-risk conditions and 75% in immunocompetent adults ≥65 years of age.[25] A recent Cochrane Review placed the efficacy of PPSV23 at 80% based on randomized controlled trials and 52% based on observational studies.[26] Antibody levels decline 5 to 10 years after vaccination, and may decline faster in the elderly. At least one study suggested that protection can last as long as 9 years. PPSV23 does not reduce nasopharyngeal carriage and does not protect children from otitis media.

Safety

Local reactions to PCV7, which are more common after Dose 4, occur in 10% to 20% of recipients. Fewer than 3% of local reactions are considered to be severe (eg, tenderness that interferes with limb movement). In clinical trials, fever >100.4°F (38°C) within 48 hours of any dose of the primary series was reported in 15% to 24% of children. However, in these studies, DTwP was administered simultaneously with each dose and may have been responsible for the fever. In a study in which DTaP was given at the same visit as the booster dose of PCV7, 11% of recipients developed a temperature >102.2°F (39°C). During the first 2 years after licensure, adverse events were reported to

TABLE 23.1 — *S pneumoniae* Vaccines

Trade name	Pneumovax 23	Prevnar	Prevnar 13
Abbreviation	PPSV23	PCV7 (PCV7-CRM)	PCV13 (PCV13-CRM)
Manufacturer/distributor	Merck	Pfizer (formerly Wyeth)	Pfizer (formerly Wyeth)
Type of vaccine	Inactivated, purified subunits	Inactivated, engineered subunits	Inactivated, engineered subunits
Composition	Capsular polysaccharides (25 mcg each) from *S pneumoniae* serotypes 1, 2, 3, 4, 5, 6B, 7F, 8, 9N, 9V, 10A, 11A, 12F, 14, 15B, 17F, 18C, 19A, 19F, 20, 22F, 23F, 33F	Capsular polysaccharides from *S pneumoniae* serotypes 4, 9V, 14, 18C, 19F, and 23F (2 mcg each), and serotype 6B (4 mcg), conjugated to CRM_{197}, a nontoxic mutant diphtheria toxin (20 mcg)	Capsular polysaccharides from *S pneumoniae* serotypes 1, 3, 4, 5, 6A, 7F, 9V, 14, 18C, 19A, 19F, 23F (2.2 mcg each) and 6B (4.4 mcg each), conjugated to CRM_{197}, a nontoxic mutant diphtheria toxin (34 mcg)
Adjuvant	None	Aluminum phosphate (0.125 mg aluminum)	Aluminum phosphate (0.125 mg aluminum)
Preservative	Phenol (0.25%)	None	None
Excipients and contaminants	None reported	None reported	Polysorbate 80 (100 mcg) Succinate buffer (295 mcg)
Latex	None	None	None

Labeled indications	Prevention of pneumococcal disease caused by vaccine serotypes	Prevention of IPD and otitis media caused by vaccine serotypes	Prevention of IPD caused by all 13 vaccine serotypes; Prevention of otitis media caused by the PCV7 serotypes
Labeled ages	≥2 years	Infants and toddlers	6 weeks to 71 months
Dose	0.5 mL	0.5 mL	0.5 mL
Route of administration	Intramuscular or subcutaneous	Intramuscular	Intramuscular
Labeled schedule	1 dose	2, 4, 6, 12 to 15 months of age	2, 4, 6, 12 to 15 months of age; Substitute for PCV7 in routine schedule; 1 dose for children 15 to 71 months of age who have received 4 doses of PCV7
Recommended schedule	1 dose; Revaccination in 5 years	2, 4, 6, 12 to 15 months of age; 1 dose for children 24 to 59 months of age with incomplete schedules	2, 4, 6, 12 to 15 months of age; Substitute for PCV7 in routine schedule; See text for supplemental dosing in healthy children with or without complete PCV7 schedules and in high-risk children

Continued

23

445

TABLE 23.1 — *Continued*

	Pneumovax 23	Prevnar	Prevnar 13
Trade name			
Abbreviation	PPSV23	PCV7 (PCV7-CRM)	PCV13 (PCV13-CRM)
How supplied (number in package)	1-dose vial (10) 5-dose vial (1, 10)	Prefilled syringe (10)	Prefilled syringe (10)
Storage	Refrigerate Do not freeze	Refrigerate Do not freeze	Refrigerate Do not freeze
Cost per dose ($US, 2009):			
Public	18.34	71.04	91.75
Private	32.99	83.88	108.75
Reference package insert	June 2009	July 2009	February 2010

VAERS at a rate of 13.2 per 100,000 doses distributed; most of these were fever, injection site reactions, fussiness, rashes, and urticaria.[27] The proportion of reports that were serious was similar to other vaccines. Importantly, the number of passively reported adverse events declined dramatically in later years despite increased vaccine uptake (this pattern is seen with many other vaccines and pharmaceuticals).[28]

The safety of PCV13 was evaluated in over 4700 vaccinees across 13 clinical trials. Injection site reactions, fever, decreased appetite, irritability, and sleep disturbance were seen in over 20% of subjects. The incidence and severity of these reactions was similar to those in PCV7 recipients.

For persons ≥65 years of age receiving PPSV23, overall injection-site adverse experiences occur in about 50% after primary vaccination and in 80% after revaccination; moderate-severe pain and/or significant induration occur in about 10% of primary vaccinees and in 30% of revaccinees. Systemic adverse experiences such as fatigue, myalgia, and headache, are reported after primary vaccination in approximately 22% and after revaccination in 33%.

- *Contraindications*
    - Allergic reaction to previous dose of vaccine or any vaccine component (risk of recurrent allergic reaction; for PCV7 and PCV13, this includes reactions to any diphtheria toxoid-containing vaccine, since these vaccines contain CRM_{197}, a mutant diphtheria toxin)
- *Precautions*
    - Moderate or severe acute illness (difficulty distinguishing illness from vaccine reaction)

Recommendations

All children should be vaccinated against *S pneumoniae*. The primary series of PCV consists of doses at 2, 4, and 6 months of age, with a booster dose given at 12 to 15 months of age. For previously unimmunized infants, all 4 doses should be PCV13; unvaccinated older children should also be immunized, but the number of doses depends on the age at which the series is initiated (**Table 23.2**). Those who have already started the series with PCV7 should transition to PCV13 (**Table 23.3**). A single (supplemental) dose of PCV13 is recommended for the following: children 14 to 59 months of age (14 to 71 months of age if high-risk) who have completed a PCV7 schedule, and healthy children 24 to 59 months of age with any incomplete PCV7 or PCV13 schedule, including those who have never been immunized. High-risk children 24 to 71 months of age who are either previously unimmunized or have received <3 doses of PCV7 or PCV13 before 24 months of age should receive 2 doses of PCV13 separated by 8 weeks. High-risk children 6 to 18 years of age

447

TABLE 23.2 — PCV13 Schedule for Infants and Children With No Previous PCV Vaccination

Age at First Dose (Months)	Primary Series[a]	Booster Dose[b]
2 to 6	3 doses	12 to 15 months
7 to 11	2 doses	12 to 15 months
12 to 23	2 doses	—
24 to 59 (healthy)	1 dose	—
24 to 71 (high-risk[c])	2 doses	—
≥5 years (healthy)	—	—
6 to 18 years (high-risk[c])	1 dose	—

[a] The minimum interval between doses for infants <12 months of age is 4 weeks. The minimum interval between doses for children ≥12 months of age is 8 weeks.

[b] The minimum interval between the last dose and the booster dose is 8 weeks.

[c] PCV13 should be given even if the patient has previously received PPSV23 (the minimum interval between a previous dose of PPSV23 and PCV13, and between doses of PCV13 at this age, is 8 weeks). High-risk conditions are summarized in the text.

Adapted from CDC. *MMWR*. 2010;59:258-261.

should receive a single dose of PCV13, regardless of previous pneumococcal vaccine history.

PPSV23 may be used to boost immunity in high-risk children ≥2 years of age who are already caught up on PCV. One dose is given ≥8 weeks after the last dose of PCV, and one-time revaccination in 5 years is recommended for the highest-risk patients.

All adults ≥65 years of age should be vaccinated against *S pneumoniae*. One dose of PPSV23 is usually given at 65 years of age, and routine revaccination is not recommended (those who received a dose before 65 years of age should receive a second dose if ≥5 years have elapsed since the first dose). Adults at high risk for IPD should receive PPSV23, with one-time revaccination in 5 years for those at highest risk.

Risk categories for IPD in children and adults are summarized below:

• *Increased risk*
  – Chronic heart disease, including cyanotic congenital heart disease, congestive heart failure, and cardiomyopathy
  – Chronic lung disease, including cystic fibrosis
  – Diabetes
  – Alcoholism
  – Cirrhosis
  – CSF leak
  – Cochlear implant

TABLE 23.3 — Transition Schedule From PCV7 to PCV13 by Vaccination History

Infant Series			Booster	Supplemental Dose
2 Months	4 Months	6 Months	≥12 Months[a]	14 to 59 Months[b]
PCV7	PCV13	PCV13	PCV13	—
PCV7	PCV7	PCV13	PCV13	—
PCV7	PCV7	PCV7	PCV13	—
PCV7	PCV7	PCV7	PCV7	PCV13

[a] Children 12 to 23 months of age who have received 2 or 3 doses of PCV before 12 months of age and at least 1 dose of PCV13 at ≥12 months of age do not need further doses.

[b] The age range for a supplemental dose is 14 to 71 months of age for children with high-risk conditions. This dose is given even if the patient has previously received PPSV23 (the minimum interval between a previous dose of PPSV23 and PCV13 is 8 weeks). High-risk conditions are summarized in the text.

Adapted from CDC. *MMWR*. 2010;59:258-261.

23

- Asymptomatic HIV infection
  - Asthma (adults; children only if treated with prolonged high-dose oral steroids)
  - Cigarette smoking (adults only)
- *Highest risk*
  - Chronic renal failure
  - Nephrotic syndrome
  - Functional, congenital, or surgical asplenia, including sickle cell disease and other hemoglobinopathies
  - Symptomatic HIV infection
  - Immunosuppressive conditions, including Hodgkin disease, leukemia, lymphoma, multiple myeloma, generalized malignancy, solid organ or bone marrow transplantation, long-term high-dose corticosteroid therapy, chemotherapy, and radiation therapy
  - Congenital immunodeficiency, including humoral or cellular deficiency, complement deficiency (particularly C1, C2, C3, and C4), and phagocyte disorders excluding chronic granulomatous disease

In elective situations such as planned splenectomy, placement of a cochlear implant, or initiation of chemotherapy or immunosuppressive medication, vaccination should occur at least 2 weeks before the procedure, if possible. Routine use of PPSV23 is not indicated for otherwise healthy Alaska Native or American Indian persons, although public health authorities may recommend vaccination in special situations. Women who are at high risk for pneumococcal disease should be vaccinated before pregnancy, but may be vaccinated during pregnancy if necessary.

PPSV23 is often used to assess the adequacy of polysaccharide antibody responses in persons ≥2 years of age who are suspected of having immune deficiency. A serum specimen is drawn, the vaccine is administered, and a second serum specimen is obtained 3 to 4 weeks later. The specimens are then tested in parallel for serotype-specific antibodies. Increases in antibody to PCV serotypes represent anamnestic responses if the patient was previously immunized; antibodies to the other serotypes represent de novo responses to polysaccharide antigen.

Optimizing pneumococcal immunization can be tricky given the switch from PCV7 to PCV13 and use of PPSV23 in some patients. **Table 23**.4 gives some likely scenarios and recommended actions.

TABLE 23.4 — Pneumococcal Vaccination Scenarios

Condition	Current Age	Vaccination History	Action
Healthy	6 months	PCV7 at 2 and 4 months of age	PCV13 now PCV13 at 12 months of age
Healthy	24 months	PCV7 at 2, 4, 6, and 12 months of age	PCV13 now
Sickle cell disease	24 months	PCV7 at 2, 4, 6, and 12 months of age	PCV13 now PPSV23 in 8 weeks Repeat PPSV23 at 7 years of age
Sickle cell disease	24 months	PCV7 at 2 months and 12 months of age	PCV13 now PCV 13 at 26 months of age PPSV23 at 28 months of age Repeat PPSV23 at 7 years of age
Congenital asplenia	36 months	PCV7 at 2, 4, 6, and 12 months of age PPSV23 at 24 months of age	PCV13 now Repeat PPSV23 at 8 years of age
Nephrotic syndrome	12 years	None	PCV13 now PPSV23 8 weeks later Repeat PPSV23 at 17 years of age
Symptomatic HIV infection	35 years	None	PPSV23 now Repeat PPSV23 at 40 years of age

23

451

REFERENCES

1. CDC. *MMWR*. 2000;49(RR-9):1-35.
2. ABCs report: *Streptococcus pneumoniae*, 1999. Centers for Disease Control and Prevention Web site. http://www.cdc.gov/abcs/reports -findings/survreports/spneu99.html. Accessed February 6, 2010.
3. CDC. *MMWR*. 1997;46(RR-8):1-24.
4. CDC. *MMWR*. 2008;57:144-148.
5. Tsai CJ, et al. *Clin Infect Dis*. 2008;46:1664-1672.
6. Grijalva CG, et al. *Lancet*. 2007;369:1179-1186.
7. Grijalva CG, et al. *Pediatrics*. 2006;118:865-873.
8. Kyaw MH, et al. *N Engl J Med*. 2006;354:1455-1463.
9. Dagan R, et al. *Lancet Infect Dis*. 2008;8:785-795.
10. Ray GT, et al. *Vaccine*. 2009;27:6483-6494.
11. O'Brien KL, et al. *J Infect Dis*. 2007;196:1211-1220.
12. Millar EV, et al. *Clin Infect Dis*. 2008;47:989-996.
13. Kaplan SL, et al. *Pediatrics*. 2010;125:429-436.
14. Lexau CA, et al. *JAMA*. 2005;294:2043-2051.
15. ACIP provisional recommendations for use of pneumococcal vaccines. Centers for Disease Control and Prevention Web site. http://www.cdc.gov/vaccines/recs/provisional/downloads/pneumo -oct-2008-508.pdf. Accessed February 6, 2010.
16. Ogilvie I, et al. *Vaccine*. 2009;27:4891-4904.
17. CDC. *MMWR*. 2008;57:343-344.
18. CDC. *MMWR*. 2010;59:258-261.
19. Farley MM, et al. *MMWR*. 2010;59:253-257.
20. Black S, et al. *Pediatr Infect Dis J*. 2000;19:187-195.
21. Eskola J, et al. *N Engl J Med*. 2001;344:403-409.
22. Pavia M, et al. *Pediatrics*. 2009;123:e1103-e1110.
23. Whitney CG, et al. *Lancet*. 2006;368:1495-1502.
24. Fine MJ, et al. *Arch Intern Med*. 1994;154:2666-2677.
25. Butler JC, et al. *JAMA*. 1993;270:1826-1831.
26. Moberley SA, et al. *Cochrane Database Syst Rev*. 2008;(1): CD000422.
27. Wise RP, et al. *JAMA*. 2004;292:1702-1710.
28. Center KJ, et al. *Vaccine*. 2009;27:3281-3284.

24 Typhoid Fever

The Pathogen

Salmonella typhi (also known as *Salmonella enterica* subspecies *enterica* serotype Typhi) is a motile, nonlactose-fermenting, gram-negative bacillus. Infection begins in the gut, where the organism invades Peyer's patches, multiplies in macrophages, and disseminates to the mesenteric lymph nodes, reticuloendothelial organs, and ultimately the bloodstream. The Vi capsular antigen interferes with complement binding and enhances virulence. *S typhi* produces a cholera-like toxin that causes efflux of electrolytes and water into the intestinal lumen.

Clinical Features

Typhoid fever refers to enteric fever caused by *S typhi*, although other salmonella species can cause a less-severe form of enteric fever.[1] The incubation period is 5 to 21 days depending on inoculum size and health of the host. The onset is insidious, with fever and abdominal pain accompanied by malaise and anorexia. Fever climbs to higher peaks each day, reaching 104°F (40°C) by the end of the first week; adults display relative bradycardia for the level of fever. Early on, up to 50% of patients have constipation and 30% diarrhea. Diarrhea is more common in infants and is typically small-volume and pea soup-like, containing red blood cells and leukocytes but not gross blood. During the first week of illness, children complain of headache and often are irritable, drowsy, or delirious. Adults may display psychosis or delirium, and arthralgia and back pain are common. Patients may appear toxic, have meningismus, a coated tongue with musty odor, and a tender doughy abdomen with slight guarding. During the second week of illness, a rash may appear on the abdomen or chest consisting of crops of 10 to 15 salmon-colored, blanching, slightly raised lesions measuring 2 to 4 mm, referred to as *rose spots*. The spleen may be palpable and tender and respiratory symptoms may develop. Untreated, the illness lasts 4 to 6 weeks.

Complications generally occur during the third or fourth week and include intestinal hemorrhage or perforation, which occurs in approximately 3% of patients. The patient's mental status may progress to coma. Additional complications include hepatitis, cholecystitis, arthritis, osteomyelitis, parotitis, endocarditis, myocarditis, pericarditis, pneumonia, meningitis, pyelonephritis, pancreatitis, and orchitis. Laboratory abnormalities include anemia, leukopenia or leukocytosis, thrombocytopenia, and elevated hepatic and muscle enzymes. Relapses occur in 5% to 20% of cases even after appropriate therapy, although they are usually milder than the initial illness. Infants are more likely than adults to develop massive hepatosplenomegaly and thrombocytopenia, and they have a higher mortality rate. However, young children may have *S typhi* bacteremia with mild disease manifestations. Typhoid fever during pregnancy increases the risk of premature labor and spontaneous abortion. Up to 4% of patients who recover from typhoid fever become chronic carriers of *S typhi* and are potential sources of infection for others.

S typhi can also cause nontyphoidal gastroenteritis, bacteremia, and extraintestinal focal infection.

Epidemiology and Transmission

There are an estimated 12 to 33 million cases of typhoid fever each year in the world, with the highest incidence in Asia (especially the Indian subcontinent), Central and South America, and Africa. In endemic areas, the annual incidence is as high as 500 to 900 cases per 100,000 people, and the peak is in school-aged children. In developed countries, the incidence is only 0.2 to 3.7 cases per 100,000. Four hundred cases are reported in the United States each year, with the highest risk among international travelers.[2]

Humans are the only reservoir of *S typhi* and transmission is by the fecal-oral route; the infectious dose is about 10^7 organisms. Patients with cholecystitis or gallstones are especially vulnerable to chronic carriage and may excrete up to 10^9 organisms per gram of stool. Direct person-to-person transmission is unusual; rather, disease spreads through feces-contaminated food or water. For this reason, countries with inadequate sanitation systems, overcrowded living conditions, and limited potable water have the highest rates of disease. Laboratory workers have acquired infection through accidents and health care personnel have acquired infection from patients because of poor handwashing. Occasionally, transplacental transmission occurs from a bacteremic mother to the fetus, and infants may be infected at the time of birth through exposure to bacteria shed in the mother's stool.

Immunization Program

Worldwide, approximately 500,000 people die each year of typhoid fever. In endemic areas, aside from the human costs, the direct medical and indirect societal costs are high. Interest in vaccination is highest in areas where antibiotic treatment is not readily available and where antibiotic-resistant strains have increased in prevalence. Outbreaks of multidrug-resistant *S typhi* infection have occurred in the Indian subcontinent, Southeast Asia, and Africa and have been associated with high rates of complications and death. Vaccination might be beneficial for persons at high risk for disease, including children, international travelers, and military personnel. Persons who travel from low-risk to high-risk areas are particularly susceptible because they have not developed immunity through repeated exposure to low doses of *S typhi* over time.

Recommendations for use of typhoid vaccine were published in 1978, 1990, and most recently in 1994.[3]

Vaccines

Characteristics of the typhoid fever vaccines licensed in the United States are given in **Table 24.1**. One of these is a parenterally administered pure polysaccharide vaccine, analogous to MPSV4 and PPSV23. The other is an orally administered live-attenuated bacterium.

Efficacy and/or Immunogenicity

In a clinical trial of TViPSV conducted in Nepal, 3454 subjects received a liquid formulation of the vaccine and 3454 controls received a pneumococcal polysaccharide vaccine.[4] Most subjects were 5 to 44 years of age; 165 children 2 to 4 years of age were included. Efficacy against blood culture-confirmed typhoid fever was 74% during the 20-month follow-up period. In a second trial conducted in South Africa, a lyophilized formulation was evaluated in school children 5 to 15 years of age who received the vaccine ($N = 5692$) or a meningococcal (serogroups A and C) polysaccharide vaccine as placebo ($N = 5692$).[5] Efficacy was 55% against blood culture-confirmed typhoid fever during a 3-year follow-up period. Four-fold or greater increases in antibody to the Vi polysaccharide were seen in 88% to 96% of US adults who received one dose of the vaccine.

A large-scale effectiveness trial was conducted in Kolkata, India from 2004 to 2006 using TViPSV manufactured by GlaxoSmithKline (Typherix).[6] Slum-dwelling residents ≥2 years of age were randomized by geographic cluster to receive TViPSV ($N = 18,869$) or HepA as control ($N = 18,804$). Vaccine effectiveness was 61% in general but as high as 80% among children 2 to 5 years of age. Effectiveness was 44% among unvaccinated persons living in TViPSV clusters, an indication of herd immunity that was achieved with only 60% vaccine coverage.

The efficacy of Ty21a was first evaluated in Egypt, where 16,486 children aged 6 to 7 years were given 3 doses of a liquid formulation on alternate days; 15,902 children were given placebo. Efficacy was 95% during a 3-year surveillance period.[7] A series of field trials were then performed in Santiago, Chile. The first one, which compared 1 or 2 doses given 1 week apart,

24

TABLE 24.1 — Typhoid Vaccines[a]

Trade name	Typhim Vi	Vivotif
Abbreviation	TViPSV	Ty21a
Manufacturer/distributor	Sanofi Pasteur	Crucell (formerly Berna Biotech)
Type of vaccine	Inactivated, purified subunit	Live-attenuated, engineered
Composition	Capsular polysaccharide Vi extracted from strain *Salmonella enterica serovar typhi*, *S typhi* Ty2	Strain *Salmonella typhi* Ty21a mutagenized and selected for attenuation
	Vi polysaccharide (25 mcg)	2 to 6.8×10^9 colony-forming units
Adjuvant	None	None
Preservative	Phenol (0.25%)	None
Excipients and contaminants	Polydimethylsiloxane (residual)	Sucrose (26 to 130 mg)
	Fatty-acid ester-based antifoam (residual)	Ascorbic acid (1 to 5 mg)
	Sodium chloride (4.15 mg)	Amino acid mixture (1.4 to 7 mg)
	Disodium phosphate (0.065 mg)	Lactose (100 to 180 mg)
	Monosodium phosphate (0.023 mg)	Magnesium stearate (3.6 to 4.4 mg)
Latex	None	None
Labeled indications	Prevention of typhoid fever	Prevention of typhoid fever
Labeled ages	≥2 years	>6 years[b]
Dose	0.5 mL	1 capsule
Route of administration	Intramuscular	PO (swallow 1 hour before meal with a cold or lukewarm drink)

Labeled schedule	1 dose	0, 2, 4, 6 days[c]
	Booster doses every 2 years (for persons with continued exposure)	Booster series of 4 doses every 5 years (for persons with continued exposure)
Recommended schedule	Same	Same
How supplied (number in package)	20-dose vial (1)	4 capsules in a single foil blister package
Storage	Refrigerate Do not freeze	Refrigerate
Cost per dose ($US, 2009):		
Public	—	—
Private	138.00	97.00
Reference package insert	December 2005	August 2006

[a] Typhoid Vaccine USP (Pfizer [formerly Wyeth]), a phenol-inactivated, whole-cell vaccine for parenteral administration, is no longer produced.
[b] The ACIP recommends use at ≥6 years of age.
[c] Some experts recommend repeating the series if all 4 doses are not given within 3 weeks.

24

involved 82,543 school-aged children. Efficacy at 24 months was 29% and 59%, respectively.[8] Another trial, which compared three doses on alternate days to three doses given 21 days apart, involved 109,594 school-aged children.[9] Efficacy was best in the group that received the shorter schedule, reaching 69% over 4 years and with persistent efficacy demonstrated at 5 years. Subsequent studies established that efficacy was best using a 4-dose, alternate-day regimen.

Safety

TViPSV causes local tenderness in 97% to 98% of vaccinees; pain is seen in 27% to 41%, induration in 5% to 15%, and erythema in 4% to 5%. Systemic signs and symptoms include malaise (4% to 24%), headache (16% to 20%), myalgia (3% to 7%), and nausea (2% to 8%). Fever $\geq 100°F$ occurs in <2% of vaccinees. Reactogenicity is similar after reimmunization but is less pronounced in children. Postmarketing surveillance in countries where >14 million doses were distributed demonstrated some systemic reactions but very few serious adverse events. From 1995 to 2002, the reporting rate to VAERS for adverse events was 4.5 per 100,000 doses distributed, and for serious adverse events, it was 0.34 per 100,000 doses distributed.

Ty21a is less reactogenic than TViPSV. Symptoms reported during clinical studies included abdominal pain (6%), nausea (6%), headache (5%), fever (3%), diarrhea (3%), vomiting (2%), and rash (1%), but only nausea occurred more frequently than in placebo groups. In field trials involving >500,000 school children, this vaccine did not cause serious adverse reactions. Postmarketing surveillance in the early 1990s, during which time 60 million doses were distributed, revealed only a handful of adverse events and only one serious allergic reaction.[10] From 1991 to 2002, the reporting rate to VAERS for adverse events was 9.7 per 100,000 doses distributed, and for serious adverse events, was 0.59 per 100,000 doses distributed.

- *Contraindications*
  - Both vaccines: allergic reaction to previous dose of vaccine or any vaccine component (risk of recurrent allergic reaction)
  - Ty21a: immune impairment (risk of disease caused by live bacterium)
- *Precautions*
  - Both vaccines: moderate or severe acute illness (difficulty distinguishing illness from vaccine reaction)
  - Ty21a: concomitant antibiotics or proguanil therapy (these may inactivate the vaccine; mefloquine and chloroquine may be given)

Routine immunization is *not* recommended in the United States, not even for sewage sanitation workers, persons attending rural summer camps, or people living in areas in which natural disasters such as floods have occurred. There is also no evidence that typhoid vaccine is useful in controlling common-source outbreaks.

Vaccination *is*, however, recommended for the following groups:

- Travelers to endemic areas (especially developing countries in Latin America, Asia, and Africa) who will have prolonged exposure to potentially contaminated food and water (people should be cautioned that vaccination is not a substitute for careful avoidance of contaminated food and drink); typhoid vaccine is not *required* for international travel, but is *recommended*.
- Persons with intimate exposure (eg, household contact) to a documented carrier of *S typhi* (the vaccine cannot be used to *treat* chronic carriers)
- Microbiology laboratory workers who are in frequent contact with *S typhi*
- Persons living in endemic areas outside the United States

There are no data on interchangeability of typhoid vaccines. However, if a booster series is necessary in a person who previously received the inactivated whole-cell vaccine, it is reasonable to give 4 doses of Ty21a or 1 dose of TViPSV. There is no evidence that concomitant administration of either vaccine with other live oral or live or inactivated parenteral vaccines impairs immune responses.

24

REFERENCES

1. Parry CM, et al. *N Engl J Med*. 2002;347:1770-1782.
2. Taylor DN, et al. *J Infect Dis*. 1983;148:599-602.
3. Cieslak PR, et al. *MMWR*. 1994;43(RR-14):1-7.
4. Acharya IL, et al. *N Engl J Med*. 1987;317:1101-1104.
5. Klugman KP, et al. *Vaccine*. 1996;14:435-438.
6. Sur D, et al. *N Engl J Med*. 2009;361:335-344.
7. Wahdan MH, et al. *J Infect Dis*. 1982;145:292-296.
8. Black RE, et al. *Vaccine*. 1990;8:81-84.
9. Levine MM, et al. *Lancet*. 1987;1:1049-1052.
10. Begier EM, et al. *Clin Infect Dis*. 2004;38:771-779.

25 Varicella

The Pathogen

VZV is a large, enveloped virus in the Herpesviridae family, subfamily Alphaherpesvirinae. It has a short reproductive cycle characterized by cellular destruction and release of free virus, as well as the ability to establish *latent infection*. After inoculation at mucosal surfaces, replication occurs in the regional lymph nodes, resulting in a primary viremia that seeds the liver and other reticuloendothelial organs. A secondary viremia then ensues, which infects epithelial cells of the skin, causing the vesicular lesions of *chickenpox*, as well as seeding of the respiratory mucosa, which facilitates contagion through respiratory droplets. Latent infection is invariably established in the dorsal root ganglia, where the linear, double-stranded DNA genome takes on a closed circular configuration. With reactivation, the genome linearizes and viral proteins are made and assembled into virions, which are then transported along sensory nerves to the skin, where replication causes *herpes zoster*, also known as *shingles*.

Cellular immunity is critical to limiting primary infection and preventing reactivation. Periodic re-exposure to exogenous natural varicella and/or subclinical reactivation of endogenous VZV may lead to boosts in immunity.

Clinical Features

The incubation period ranges from 10 to 21 days. In children, rash is often the first sign of disease, but adults may have a 1- to 2-day prodrome of fever and malaise. The rash is pruritic, usually beginning on the scalp or hairline, then moving to the trunk and the extremities.[1] Lesions are 1 to 4 mm in diameter and appear in successive crops over several days; at any given time these crops are in different stages of development. Lesions characteristically evolve from macules to papules and then to superficial, delicate vesicles containing clear fluid on an erythematous base, so-called "dew drops on rose petals." They rapidly become pustules that crust and fall off, leaving shallow ulcers. Lesions can occur on mucous membranes and on the cornea. The average patient with primary varicella has malaise and fever for 2 to 3 days and develops 200 to 500 lesions, some of which may form a scar.[2]

Varicella in vaccinated persons, termed *breakthrough* or *vaccine-modified varicella*, is generally characterized by a shorter duration of illness and the absence of systemic symptoms and complications.[3] There are usually <50 lesions, and these are often maculopapular rather than vesicular and are difficult to recognize as chickenpox. However, up to 30% of children with breakthrough disease may have an illness that is similar to mild primary varicella.

In the prevaccine era, 5% to 10% of otherwise healthy children experienced complications. One half of these were secondary bacterial infections, usually caused by *Staphylococcus aureus* or group A beta-hemolytic streptococcus (GABHS). Varicella increased the risk of severe GABHS infection among previously healthy children by 40- to 60-fold, and it was estimated that preventing varicella could prevent at least 15% of cases of severe pediatric GABHS infection. Otitis media occurred in up to 5% of cases. Serious secondary infections, such as pneumonia, bacteremia, osteomyelitis, septic arthritis, endocarditis, necrotizing fasciitis, and toxic shock syndrome, occurred much less frequently. Other complications included cerebellar ataxia, encephalitis, and Reye syndrome, which was associated with aspirin use during the illness. Although the case-fatality rate in children was very low, the absolute number of childhood deaths was high (about 50 per year in the early 1990s) because there were so many cases.[4] Ninety percent of children who died had no identifiable risk factors for severe varicella.

Adults have more severe disease and higher complication rates. Slightly >1% of all adults with varicella are admitted to the hospital, and the case-fatality rate is 25 times higher than in children.[4] In the prevaccine era, only 5% of cases, but 35% of annual deaths, occurred in adults; the majority of these had no identifiable risk factor for severe disease.

Immunocompromised individuals may develop *progressive varicella*, characterized by high fever, extensive vesicular eruption, and high complication rates. Mild hepatitis occurs in 20% to 50% of cases, but is usually asymptomatic. Similarly, 5% to 16% of patients develop thrombocytopenia, but bleeding is rare. *Hemorrhagic varicella* is characterized by thrombocytopenia and extensive purpuric lesions. Although rare, *congenital varicella syndrome*, characterized by birth defects and neurologic devastation, occurs in 1% of pregnancies complicated by varicella in the first or second trimester. Maternal varicella in the peripartum period can lead to overwhelming infection in the newborn because of a high inoculum and the absence of transplacental maternal antibody; the fatality rate is as high as 30%.

When immunity wanes (eg, as it does with aging), reactivation of latent VZV can result in herpes zoster (see *Chapter 27: Zoster*).

Epidemiology and Transmission

Humans are the only natural hosts. Transmission occurs via respiratory droplets or by direct contact with or aerosolization of virus from vesicular skin lesions. Natural chickenpox is highly contagious, with attack rates among susceptible household contacts approaching 90%; contagiousness begins 1 to 2 days before onset of rash and lasts until the last lesion has crusted. Shingles is less contagious because there is less virus in the lesions and the respiratory tract is not involved. Vaccine-modified varicella also is less contagious than primary chickenpox, unless the number of lesions is >50, in which case contagiousness approaches that of primary disease.[5]

Varicella is less common in tropical than in temperate areas. In the United States, the incidence is highest between March and May and lowest between September and November. Before universal immunization, essentially every child got chickenpox, most often by 4 years of age. Every year there were 4 million cases, 11,000 hospitalizations, and 100 deaths.[6]

Immunization Program

VAR was licensed in the United States in 1995. Initial recommendations called for universal immunization of children 12 to 18 months of age and catch-up for children 19 months to 12 years of age who had not had chickenpox.[7] Vaccination of susceptible persons ≥13 years of age (2 doses) was recommended if they were anticipated to have close contact with persons at high risk for serious complications; catch-up for other adolescents was considered desirable, but did not carry a strong recommendation. It was suggested that vaccination also be considered for certain susceptible persons at high risk for exposure. Consideration was given as well to vaccination of susceptible nonpregnant women of childbearing age, who would be at risk for complications if they became pregnant and developed varicella. In 1999, stronger recommendations for these persons were issued, essentially changing the language from "should be considered" to "recommended."[8] Vaccination of all susceptible adolescents and adults living in households with children was recommended, as was postexposure vaccination. Use of VAR for outbreak control was suggested, as was vaccination of asymptomatic or mildly symptomatic HIV-infected children without evidence of immunosuppression.

Between 1997 and 2005, vaccine uptake among 2-year-olds increased to nearly 90%. Surveillance indicated approximately 90% declines in disease incidence, and the most affected age shifted from 3 to 6 years to 9 to 11 years. Between 1995-98 and 2002-05, overall varicella-related hospitalizations declined from 2.54 per 100,000 to 0.62 per 100,000; this included a 77% decrease among persons <20 years of age and 60% decrease among those ≥20.[9] The rate of varicella-related ambulatory visits decreased 66% in the 8 years after licensure.[10] Within 5 years, the annual number of varicella-related deaths in the United

States declined from 145 to 66[11]; by 2003, the number was <20, most of those occurring in persons with immunodeficiencies. This highlights an important fact about varicella—some people cannot be protected directly because they cannot be immunized with a live-attenuated vaccine. The only way to protect them as a population is to reduce transmission of the virus in the community, although passive immunization can be used for persons after known exposure.

Despite the successes outlined above, outbreaks of varicella continued to occur, especially among elementary school students—even though the majority of them had been vaccinated. Granted, these were outbreaks of vaccine-modified varicella, which is less serious than primary disease. Nevertheless, it became clear that a 1-dose strategy would not eliminate transmission in the United States—either because a certain number of children fail to seroconvert after 1 dose or because immunity wanes with time.[12] Therefore, in 2007, a routine 2-dose strategy was adopted.[13]

At the beginning of the program in 1995, it was estimated that every dollar spent on varicella vaccination resulted in a savings of $5.40, when both direct medical and indirect societal costs were considered. For the 2006 birth cohort (4.1 million children) followed over 40 years, it was estimated that without a vaccination program there would be $333 million in direct costs from varicella and $1.5 billion in societal costs (2006 dollars).[14] A 1-dose vaccination program would prevent 3.6 million cases and result in a net savings of $1.1 billion. A 2-dose program would prevent 375,000 additional cases at an incremental cost of $104 million; the cost per quality-adjusted life year saved would be $109,000.

Vaccines

Characteristics of VAR licensed in the United States are given in **Table 25.1**. This is a single human varicella strain (originally isolated in Japan from a child named Oka) that was attenuated by serial passage in tissue culture, much the same way as was the Sabin polio vaccine. VAR is the first herpesvirus vaccine to be licensed and the first live vaccine that can establish latency.

Efficacy and/or Immunogenicity

Prelicensure studies showed seroconversion rates of 97% among children 1 to 12 years of age and 79% among adolescents after 1 dose. Adolescents and adults who received 2 doses separated by 4 to 8 weeks had seroconversion rates of 99%. In a study of children 12 months to 12 years of age conducted between 1988 and 2002, 86% of children who received 1 dose developed antibody levels ≥5 glycoprotein ELISA units/mL (this level is presumed to correlate with protection); nearly 100% achieved this level after a second dose, whether that was given 3 months or several years after the first dose. Antibodies have been detected as long as 9 years postvaccination in US studies and 20 years in Japanese studies; some studies show rising antibody levels over time, suggesting intermittent boosting by exposure to wild-type virus or perhaps reactivation of latent vaccine virus. Antibody persistence in the absence of natural boosting cannot be studied until endemic transmission is eliminated. Long-lived T-cell proliferative responses have been demonstrated in vaccinees.

In prelicensure trials, efficacy of a single dose against any disease was 70% to 90% and against severe disease was 95%. Most postlicensure studies show effectiveness of a single dose in the range of 70% to 90%, although some estimates have been lower, in the range of 44% to 56%. A case-control study set in pediatric offices from 1997-2003 demonstrated 1-dose effectiveness of 85%,[15] and a study of household exposures demonstrated 79% effectiveness at preventing secondary disease.[5] Severe varicella, characterized by >500 lesions, hospitalization, and complications, is extremely rare in vaccinees. A randomized trial in children showed 94% efficacy over 10 years of 1 dose ($N = 1104$) compared with 98% efficacy of 2 doses given 3 months apart ($N = 1017$); the breakthrough rate was reduced 3.3-fold.[16] In adults and adolescents who have seroconverted, efficacy against disease is approximately 70% after household exposure.

In three controlled trials involving a total of 110 healthy susceptible children with household varicella exposure, the attack rate among children receiving postexposure vaccination was 18% as compared to 78% among controls.[17] Most children were vaccinated within 3 days of exposure, and most breakthrough disease was mild. In a study published in 2010 involving 77 household exposures vaccinated within 5 days of exposure, effectiveness of VAR in preventing any disease was estimated at 62% and in preventing moderate to severe disease at 79%.[18] None of the breakthrough cases were severe.

Safety

Injection-site reactions are reported in about 20% of vaccinees, and 15% may have low-grade fever. About 3% of children and 1% of adults get a few vesicles at the injection site, and up to 5% may experience a generalized varicella-like rash (median of 5 lesions, mostly maculopapular). The vaccine virus establishes latency, and herpes zoster due to the vaccine virus can occur. However, the risk of herpes zoster is 4 to 12 times lower in vaccinated young children than in those with a history of natural disease.[19] Transmission of the vaccine virus from healthy vaccinees to susceptible persons is extremely rare and is only known to occur

TABLE 25.1 — Varicella Vaccine[a]

Trade name	Varivax
Abbreviation	VAR
Manufacturer/distributor	Merck
Type of vaccine	Live-attenuated, classical
Composition	Oka/Merck strain
	Propagated in human diploid (MRC-5) cells
	At least 1350 plaque-forming units
Adjuvant	None
Preservative	None
Excipients and contaminants	Sucrose (25 mg)
	Hydrolyzed gelatin (12.5 mg)
	Sodium chloride (3.2 mg)
	Monosodium L-glutamate (0.5 mg)
	Sodium phosphate dibasic (0.45 mg)
	Potassium phosphate monobasic (0.08 mg)
	Potassium chloride (0.08 mg)
	Residual components of MRC-5 cells, including DNA and protein
	Sodium phosphate monobasic (trace)
	EDTA (trace)
	Neomycin (trace)
	Fetal bovine serum (trace)
Latex	None
Labeled indications	Prevention of varicella
Labeled ages	≥12 months
Dose	0.5 mL
Route of administration	Subcutaneous
Labeled schedule	12 months to 12 years: 1 dose, with revaccination ≥3 months later
	≥13 years: 1 dose, with revaccination 4 to 8 weeks later
Recommended schedule	Same
How supplied (number in package)	1-dose vial (1, 10), lyophilized, with diluent
Storage:	
Vaccine	Freeze
	Protect from light
	Can be refrigerated for up to 72 hours before reconstitution
Diluent	Refrigerate or room temperature
	Do not freeze
Reconstituted vaccine	Use within 30 minutes

Continued

TABLE 25.1 — *Continued*

Trade name	Varivax
Abbreviation	VAR
Cost per dose ($US, 2009):	
Public	64.53
Private	80.58
Reference package insert	June 2009

[a] VAR is also available in combination with MMR (ProQuad; Merck).

when the vaccinee develops a rash after vaccination. In the few instances when transmission has occurred, mild disease has resulted and there is no evidence of reversion to virulence.

Ten years after licensure and the distribution of 55.7 million doses worldwide, 16,683 reports of adverse events (5054 of which were breakthrough disease) had been received, for a reporting rate of 3.4 per 10,000 doses distributed.[20] Vesicular rashes occurring in the first 2 weeks after vaccination were mostly due to wild-type VZV, indicating that vaccinees had been exposed to or were incubating the natural infection when they were vaccinated. Among 95 reports of herpes zoster for which specimens were available, 57 were due to the vaccine strain and 38 were wild-type VZV. There were no primary neurologic events associated with vaccination. Household transmission was reported in three instances, and in each case the vaccinee had developed a vesicular rash. Disseminated infection was seen in seven patients, all but six of whom were immunocompromised.

- *Contraindications*
  - Allergic reaction to previous dose of vaccine or any vaccine component (risk of recurrent allergic reaction; this includes reactions to gelatin and neomycin)
  - Severe immunodeficiency or immunosuppression (risk of disease caused by live virus)
  - Pregnancy (theoretic risk of live-virus vaccine to the fetus or attribution of birth defects to vaccination). ACIP recommends that vaccinated women avoid pregnancy for one month; the package insert says 3 months (ACIP recommendations are usually followed in practice).
- *Precautions*
  - Moderate or severe acute illness (difficulty distinguishing illness from vaccine reaction)
  - Recent receipt of antibody-containing blood product (risk of impaired response to vaccine)
  - Salicylate therapy in children and adolescents (theoretic risk of Reye syndrome; the manufacturer recommends withholding salicylates at least 6 weeks after administration of vaccine, but other nonsteroidal anti-inflammatory agents can be used)

25

- Active, untreated tuberculosis (risk of exacerbation of tuberculosis). Note that the package insert lists active, untreated tuberculosis as a contraindication.
- MMRV: personal, sibling or parent history of seizures (risk of febrile seizure)

Recommendations

All people without evidence of immunity to varicella should be vaccinated. The criteria for evidence of immunity are listed in **Table 25.2**; importantly, for unvaccinated children born after 1994, a reported history of chickenpox is no longer a reliable indicator of immunity.[21]

For children, the first dose is usually given at 12 to 15 months of age and the second dose at 4 to 6 years of age. The second dose may be given any time ≥3 months following the first dose. For persons ≥13 years of age, 2 doses are given 4 to 8 weeks apart. Anyone who received 1 dose in the past should receive a second dose. Evidence of immunity should be assessed in all individuals, and those without evidence of immunity should be vaccinated. Special attention should be paid to assessment of school-aged children, students in college and other postsecondary educational institutions, health care providers, household contacts of immunosuppressed persons, teachers, day care employees, residents and staff in institutional settings, inmates and staff of correctional facilities, military personnel, nonpregnant women of childbearing age, persons living in homes with children, and international travelers.

While there are no official recommendations, infants who had chickenpox before 6 months of age, and possibly before 9 months, should probably be vaccinated once they reach 12 months (there is no harm in giving the vaccine to someone who has already had chickenpox). This is because the immunity imparted by natural disease in infants who have transplacental maternal antibodies may be suboptimal. Pregnant women without evidence of immunity should be vaccinated beginning in the postpartum period. HIV-infected persons without evidence of severe immunosuppression should be vaccinated. Susceptible household and other close contacts of immunocompromised persons also should be vaccinated; if the vaccinee develops a rash, contact with an immunocompromised person at risk for severe complications of varicella should be avoided.

Vaccination of persons without evidence of immunity is recommended for outbreak control. Vaccination can also be used as postexposure prophylaxis for healthy, susceptible persons if given within 3 to 5 days of exposure, although this is not a labeled indication.

TABLE 25.2 — Evidence of Immunity to Varicella

Any one of the following criteria constitute evidence of immunity:

1. Documented age-appropriate vaccination[a]:
   – Preschool-aged children: 1 dose
   – School-aged children, adolescents, and adults: 2 doses
2. Laboratory evidence of immunity[b]
3. Laboratory confirmation of disease
4. Birth in the United States before 1980 (exception: health care personnel, pregnant women, and immunocompromised individuals)
5. Typical varicella: diagnosis or verification of history by any health care professional (eg, school or occupational clinic nurse, nurse practitioner, physician assistant, physician)[c]
6. Atypical or mild varicella: diagnosis or verification of history by a physician or physician's designee, utilizing the following information:
   – Epidemiologic link to a typical or laboratory-confirmed case
   – Laboratory confirmation performed at the time of acute disease
7. Herpes zoster: diagnosis or verification of history by any health care professional

[a] Appropriately vaccinated persons who become immunosuppressed later in life are considered immune, except for hematopoietic stem-cell transplant recipients.
[b] Serologic testing of adults before vaccination may be cost-effective since approximately 80% will be found to be seropositive. Receipt of blood products can cause false-positive serologic test results because of passive transfer of antibodies.
[c] In general, immunocompromised individuals with a verified history of varicella are considered immune. The exception is hematopoietic stem-cell transplant recipients, who are considered susceptible, regardless of their own personal history of varicella or a history of varicella in the donor. Transplant recipients who develop herpes zoster are subsequently considered immune.

Adapted from Marin M, et al; Advisory Committee on Immunization Practices, Centers for Disease Control and Prevention. *MMWR*. 2007;56 (RR-4):1-40.

Exposed persons who lack evidence of immunity (**Table 25.2**), have contraindications to vaccination, and are at high risk for complications of varicella should receive passive immunoprophylaxis with varicella zoster immune globulin (VariZIG). Exposure is constituted by living in the same household as an infectious person with either chickenpox or herpes zoster; direct, indoor, face-to-face contact with an infectious person for >5 minutes (some experts say 1 hour); or sharing the same hospital room. A special case of exposure that carries high risk is the neonate

25

whose mother develops chickenpox in the peripartum period. The following persons should receive passive immunoprophylaxis if susceptible and exposed:

- Immunocompromised patients, including those with primary and acquired immunodeficiencies, receiving immunosuppressive medications, and those with cancer. Patients who receive regular immune globulin infusions do not need prophylaxis unless the last dose was ≤3 weeks before exposure.
- Neonates whose mothers have signs and symptoms of varicella from 5 days before to 2 days after delivery.
- Preterm neonates who are exposed postnatally
  - ≥28 weeks gestation whose mothers lack evidence of immunity
  - <28 weeks gestation or birth weight ≤1000 g, regardless of maternal immunity
- Pregnant women (VariZIG is indicated to protect the mother from complications of varicella; whether it will protect the fetus is not known)

The only high-titer immune globulin product available in the United States is VariZIG, but this must be obtained under an investigational new-drug protocol (FFF Enterprises, phone number 800-843-7477; http://www.fffenterprises.com/Products/VariZIG.aspx. Accessed March 29, 2010).[22] VariZIG is supplied in 125-unit vials, and the dose is 125 units/10 kg intramuscularly; the minimum dose is 125 units and the maximum dose is 625 units. Intravenous immune globulin can be used if VariZIG is not available.

After intramuscular administration of VariZIG, varicella antibodies persist for about 6 weeks. Onset of action is very prompt, but the duration of protection is unknown. When given within 96 hours of exposure, VariZIG significantly reduces the morbidity and mortality from varicella among immunocompromised individuals. Attack rates are about one fifth as high as those in untreated, exposed persons, and the severity of disease is reduced. Receipt of VariZIG may prolong the incubation period of varicella up to 28 days. If the patient develops varicella, antiviral therapy should be instituted.

The most frequent local adverse reactions to VariZIG are pain, redness, or swelling at the injection site, occurring in about 1% of patients. Systemic reactions are less frequent and include gastrointestinal symptoms, malaise, headache, rash, and respiratory symptoms. Certain safety issues are common to all immune globulin products, including the possibility of allergic reaction to residual IgA in the product in IgA-deficient persons and the possibility of transmission of bloodborne pathogens that are not killed in the manufacturing process.

REFERENCES

1. Weller TH. *N Engl J Med*. 1983;309:1362-1368.
2. Balfour HH, et al. *J Pediatr*. 1990;116:633-639.
3. Watson BM, et al. *Pediatrics*. 1993;91:17-22.
4. Meyer PA, et al. *J Infect Dis*. 2000;182:383-390.
5. Seward JF, et al. *JAMA*. 2004;292:704-708.
6. Seward JF, et al. *JAMA*. 2002;287:606-611.
7. CDC. *MMWR*. 1996;45(RR-11):1-36.
8. CDC. *MMWR*. 1999;48(RR-6):1-5.
9. Reynolds MA, et al. *J Infect Dis*. 2008;197(suppl 2):S120-S126.
10. Shah SS, et al. *Pediatr Infect Dis J*. 2010;29:199-204.
11. Nguyen HQ, et al. *N Engl J Med*. 2005;352:450-458.
12. Chaves SS, et al. *N Engl J Med*. 2007;356:1121-1129.
13. Marin M, et al. *MMWR*. 2007;56(RR-4):1-40.
14. Zhou F, et al. *J Infect Dis*. 2008;197(suppl 2):S156-S164.
15. Vázquez M, et al. *JAMA*. 2004;291:851-855.
16. Kuter B, et al. *Pediatr Infect Dis J*. 2004;23:132-137.
17. Macartney K, et al. *Cochrane Database Syst Rev*. 2008;(3): CD001833.
18. Brotons M, et al. *Pediatr Infect Dis J*. 2010;29:10-13.
19. Civen R, et al. *Pediatr Infect Dis J*. 2009;28:954-959.
20. Galea SA, et al. *J Infect Dis*. 2008;197(suppl 2):S165-S169.
21. Perella D, et al. *Pediatrics*. 2009;123:e820-e828.
22. CDC. *MMWR*. 2006;55:209-210.

25

26
Yellow Fever

The Pathogen

Yellow fever (YF) virus (YFV) is a flavivirus with a single-stranded RNA genome surrounded by a protein nucleocapsid and a lipid envelope. After inoculation by the bite of an infected mosquito, the virus spreads through lymphatics to the viscera, and viremia ensues.[1] The liver is particularly affected, with the appearance of necrotic masses (Councilman's bodies) in hepatocytes.

Clinical Features

Infection may be asymptomatic or present as a viral syndrome of varying severity. The classic YF triad of jaundice, hemorrhage, and albuminuria occurs in 10% to 20% of patients, and the associated case fatality rate is 20% to 50%.[2] The onset of symptoms is abrupt with fever, headache, backache, malaise, myalgia, nausea, vomiting, prostration, photophobia, restlessness, irritability, and dizziness; epistaxis and bleeding from the gums may also occur. Children may experience febrile seizures. Examination reveals congestion of the skin, conjunctivae, and mucous membranes. Leukopenia, albuminuria, and elevated serum transaminase levels may be present. After about 3 days of illness, most patients experience a remission of symptoms, but this may be brief and relapse may occur with prostration, marked venous congestion, extreme bradycardia, severe nausea, vomiting, epigastric pain, jaundice, marked albuminuria and anuria, hematemesis (referred to as *vomito negro*), and melena. The hemorrhagic manifestations may be so severe as to cause hypotension, shock, acidosis, myocardial dysfunction, arrhythmias, and death, usually after 7 to 10 days. CNS signs include delirium, agitation, seizures, stupor, and coma, and complications include pneumonia, parotitis, skin infections, and renal abscesses.

Epidemiology and Transmission

Transmission of the *jungle* form of YF involves tree hole-breeding mosquitoes and nonhuman primates in the rain forests of Africa and South America. Humans exposed to the mosquitoes in this environment, such as forestry workers, soldiers, and settlers, may acquire the infection and travel to urban areas where *Aedes aegypti* mosquitoes become infected after feeding on them. These

26

mosquitoes may in turn infect other persons, leading to epidemics of *urban* YF (jungle and urban YF are clinically indistinguishable). *A aegypti* breeds in and around houses and thereby sustains interhuman transmission. YFV is also transmitted vertically from infected female mosquitoes to their offspring. This mode of transmission is important to survival of the virus during prolonged dry periods.

YF occurs throughout sub-Saharan Africa, where epidemics are common, as well as in tropical South America. Nearly 20,000 cases were reported between 1987 and 1991, with 4500 deaths.[3] After accounting for underreporting, the true number of cases is thought to be about 200,000 each year. The case-fatality rate in Africa is as high as 75% and in South America as high as 40%. Epidemics of YF have reappeared in the urban centers of West Africa and may reappear in tropical urban centers in the Americas in the near future. In South America, approximately 100 cases are reported in forested areas annually. Mass vaccination campaigns and mosquito-control programs have been instituted in South America in an attempt to prevent urban outbreaks. Interestingly, YF has never been reported in Asia.

Immunization Program

As with JE, control of mosquitoes and mosquito exposures can reduce the risk of infection, but this is not always possible. Perhaps the most important rationale for vaccination is the risk of reemergence of YF carried by *A aegypti* mosquitoes in urban areas of the Americas. This is a possibility because *A aegypti* infests many areas that are currently free of YF, including coastal regions of South America, the Caribbean, North America, the Middle East, coastal eastern Africa, the Indian subcontinent, Asia, and Australia. Travelers to and expatriates living in tropical Africa and America are candidates for vaccination as well.

YF vaccination recommendations were published in 2002[4] and updated in 2009.[5]

Vaccines

Characteristics of the YF vaccine licensed in the United States are given in **Table 26.1**. This is a live-attenuated vaccine that was attenuated by serial in vitro passage, much the same way as was the Sabin polio vaccine. Because continued serial passage can result in strains with higher rates of adverse events, vaccine lots are prepared from a large pool of secondary seed lots.

TABLE 26.1 — Yellow Fever Vaccine

Trade name	YF-Vax
Abbreviation	YF vaccine
Manufacturer/distributor	Sanofi Pasteur
Type of vaccine	Live-attenuated, classical
Composition	YFV strain 17D-204
	Propagated in chick embryos
	$\geq 4.74 \log_{10}$ plaque-forming units
Adjuvant	None
Preservative	None
Excipients and contaminants	Sorbitol
	Gelatin
	Sodium chloride
Latex	Vial stopper contains dry natural latex rubber
Labeled indications	Prevention of YF
Labeled ages	≥ 9 months[a]
Dose	0.5 mL
Route of administration	Subcutaneous
Labeled schedule	1 dose
	Booster doses every 10 years (for persons with continued exposure)
Recommended schedule	Same
How supplied (number in package)	1-dose vial (5), lyophilized, with diluent
	5-dose vial (5), lyophilized, with diluent
Storage:	
Vaccine and diluent	Refrigerate
	Do not freeze
Reconstituted vaccine	Use within 1 hour
Cost per dose ($US, 2009):	
Public	—
Private	214.00
Reference package insert	February 2008

[a] ACIP recommendations allow for immunization of infants 6 to 8 months of age under certain circumstances.

Efficacy and/or Immunogenicity

While the efficacy of YF vaccine has never been tested in a controlled clinical trial, numerous observations suggest efficacy. For example, neutralizing antibodies can be demonstrated in 90% of vaccinees in 10 days and in 99% by 30 days.[6] Infection of laboratory workers disappeared after vaccination became routine, and in Brazil and other South American countries, YF only occurs in people who have not been immunized. Immunization during outbreaks results in rapid disappearance of new cases, and high rates of coverage in endemic areas are followed by marked reduction in disease incidence. During an epidemic in Nigeria in 1986, vaccine efficacy was estimated at 85%, although there were important methodologic problems with the assessment. Immunity following vaccination persists for at least 30 to 35 years and probably for life.[7]

Safety

Reactions to YF vaccine are typically mild. Studies between 1953 and 1994 showed that <5% of vaccinees experience erythema and pain at the infection site, headaches, and fever, typically 5 to 7 days after immunization. A study in 2001 in 715 adults demonstrated mild systemic reactions such as headache, myalgia, malaise, and asthenia in 10% to 30% of subjects.[6] The rate of systemic adverse events appears to be higher in older vaccinees.

Two important serious adverse events have been seen[8,9]:

- *Vaccine-associated viscerotropic disease*: Formerly known as *febrile multiple organ-system failure*, this begins within 10 days of vaccination and is characterized by fever, nausea, vomiting, malaise, diarrhea, myalgia or dyspnea along with evidence of end-organ damage, including jaundice, hepatic dysfunction, renal impairment, myocarditis, rhabdomyolysis, and thrombocytopenia. Progression to cardiorespiratory failure and death may occur. The liver pathology resembles that seen with wild-type YF, but the disease appears to be related to host factors rather than reversion to virulence of the vaccine virus. The overall incidence of this adverse event in the United States is estimated at 1 in 250,000 doses administered, but the rate is higher in persons ≥60 years of age.[10]

- *Vaccine-associated neurotropic disease*: Formerly known as *postvaccination encephalitis*, symptoms begin within 30 days of vaccination and include fever, headache, and focal or global neurological dysfunction. Signs of inflammation or encephalopathy are seen on CSF examination, EEG, or imaging studies. The overall incidence of this adverse event in the United States is estimated at 1 in 125,000 doses administered, but the rate is higher in persons ≥60 years of age.[10]

- *Contraindications*
  - Allergic reaction to previous dose of vaccine or any vaccine component, including eggs (risk of recurrent allergic reaction). Being able to eat eggs (even in baked goods) without adverse effects is a reasonable indication of a very low risk of anaphylaxis. Mild or local manifestations of allergy to eggs or feathers are not a contraindication. Skin testing can be done and desensitization may be possible (the procedure is described in the package insert).
  - Age <6 months (risk of disease caused by live virus)
  - Immune impairment (risk of disease caused by live virus). This includes symptomatic HIV infection or CD4 count <15% or <200 cells/mcL for persons >6 years of age; thymic disorder including thymoma; primary immunodeficiencies; malignant neoplasms; transplantation; immunosuppressive or immunomodulatory therapies, including radiation). Low-dose (≤20 mg prednisone or equivalent) or short-term (<2 weeks) corticosteroid therapy or intraarticular, bursal, or tendon injections with corticosteroids should not be immunosuppressive.
- *Precautions*
  - Moderate or severe acute illness (difficulty distinguishing illness from vaccine reaction)
  - Age 6 to 8 months and ≥60 years (risk of disease caused by live virus)
  - Asymptomatic HIV infection and CD4 count 15% to 24% or 200 to 499 cells/mcL for persons >6 years of age (risk of disease caused by live virus)
  - Pregnancy (theoretic risk to the fetus or attribution of birth defects to vaccination). Vaccination may be considered if travel cannot be postponed and if exposure is very likely.
  - Breast-feeding (risk of disease caused by live virus[11])

Recommendations

The first step in prevention of YF is to avoid mosquito bites through the use of insect repellent, permethrin-impregnated clothing, and staying in screened or air-conditioned rooms.

Vaccination is *recommended* for persons ≥9 months of age who are traveling to or living in areas of South America and Africa where YF transmission is reported. Vaccination should be limited to situations where exposure to YF is likely or where vaccination is required for entry into the country. Vaccination is also recommended for those traveling to countries that do not officially report the disease but that lie in YF endemic zones. If international travel requirements are the *only* reason for vaccination of an individual at high risk for vaccine complications, consideration should be given to writing a waiver letter. Laboratory personnel

26

who might be exposed to virulent YFV or to concentrated preparations of the 17D vaccine strain should be vaccinated.

YF vaccine can only be administered at a site approved by the WHO (the CDC's Division of Global Migration and Quarantine and state and territorial health departments can designate nonfederal vaccination centers). Vaccinees must receive an *International Certificate of Vaccination or Prophylaxis* that has been completed, signed, and validated with the center's stamp. New certificates have been produced since December 15, 2007, in response to a 2005 revision of the International Health Regulations; persons vaccinated before that date may use the old certificate until it expires.[12] Certain countries in Africa require evidence of vaccination from all entering travelers. Some countries waive the requirements for travelers from areas where no evidence of substantial risk exists who will be staying <2 weeks. Certain countries require persons, even if only in transit, to have a valid certificate if they have been in countries either known or thought to have YF, or even where YF does not exist but where *A aegypti* mosquitoes are found. The CDC[13] and WHO[14] web sites contain information on YF endemic areas and countries that require certificates.

Because of the risk of vaccine-associated encephalitis, infants <6 months of age should not be vaccinated under any circumstances. Physicians considering immunization of infants between 6 and 9 months of age should contact the Division of Vector-Borne Diseases (970-221-6400) or the Division of Global Migration and Quarantine (404-498-1600) at the CDC. Vaccination of pregnant women may also be considered if travel cannot be postponed and if exposure is very likely, even though this is a live virus vaccine (data from two studies showed that only 1 of 81 infants born to mothers vaccinated during pregnancy had evidence of fetal infection and none had congenital anomalies). However, seroconversion may be markedly reduced, and the CDC should be contacted in these cases as well.

There is no evidence that concomitant administration of YF vaccine with vaccines other than cholera impairs immune responses, although all permutations have not been tested. In general, if other live vaccines are not given simultaneously, ≥ 4 weeks should elapse between them, unless time constraints do not allow. Neither immune globulin nor chloroquine therapy adversely affects antibody responses.

REFERENCES

1. Monath TP, et al. *Adv Virus Res*. 2003;60:343-395.

2. Barnett ED. *Clin Infect Dis*. 2007;44:850-856.

3. Robertson SE, et al. *JAMA*. 1996;276:1157-1162.

4. Cetron MS, et al. *MMWR*. 2002;51(RR-17):1-11.

5. ACIP provisional recommendations for the use of yellow fever vaccine. Centers for Disease Control and Prevention Web site. http://www.cdc.gov/vaccines/recs/provisional/downloads/yf-vac -dec-2009-508.pdf. Accessed February 6, 2010.

6. Monath TP, et al. *Am J Trop Med Hyg*. 2002;66:533-541.

7. Poland JD, et al. *Bull World Health Organ*. 1981;59:895-900.

8. CDC. *MMWR*. 2001;50:643-645.

9. Kitchener S. *Vaccine*. 2004;22:2103-2105.

10. Gershman M, Schroeder B, Staples JE. Yellow fever, in *Traveler's Health- Yellow Book*. Centers for Disease Control and Prevention Web site. http://wwwnc.cdc.gov/travel/yellowbook/2010/chapter-2 /yellow-fever.aspx. Accessed February 7, 2010.

11. Couto AM, et al. *MMWR*. 2010;59:130-132.

12. CDC. *MMWR*. 2008;56:1345-1346.

13. Yellow fever. Centers for Disease Control and Prevention Web site. http://www.cdc.gov/ncidod/dvbid/yellowfever/index.htm. Accessed February 6, 2010.

14. Yellow fever. World Health Organization Web site. http://www.who .int/topics/yellow_fever/en/index.html. Accessed February 6, 2010.

26

27

Zoster

The biology of VZV is described in *Chapter 25: Varicella.*
Herpes zoster, or *shingles*, results from the reactivation of latent
VZV from sensory dorsal root or cranial nerve ganglia (it has
nothing to do with herpes simplex virus, despite its name). The
virus initially reaches these ganglia by retrograde axonal transport
from the skin during an episode of chickenpox. In latency, which
may last for many decades, there is restricted gene transcription
and limited protein expression, but intact virions are not produced.
What triggers release from latency and active, lytic infection
is not clear, but it is known that reduced VZV-specific (T-cell)
responder cell frequency characterizes all conditions associated
with reactivation.

Normally there is enough constitutive immune surveillance for
antigens associated with lytic infection that when active replication begins, infected cells are destroyed or replication is otherwise
shut down. When immune surveillance wanes, lytic infection in
neuronal cell bodies can progress, and virions are transported
back along sensory nerves to the skin, where lesions much like
those of chickenpox are produced. Unlike with chickenpox,
however, the lesions are restricted to a single dermatome (more
than one dermatome may be involved in immunocompromised
individuals). Moreover, they are associated with significant pain,
the result of cell destruction and inflammation in the sensory
ganglion. Pain often persists after regression of the lesions, a
condition termed *postherpetic neuralgia* (PHN). This is associated
with degeneration of primary afferent neuronal cell bodies and
axons, scarring in the dorsal root ganglion, and *central sensitization*, which refers to changes in the dorsal horn of the spinal cord
that generalize and perpetuate pain impulses.

Zoster is a re-immunizing event—immunity to VZV is boosted,
and for this reason most people only have one lifetime episode.

Clinical Features

A prodrome of headache, photophobia, and malaise without
fever may occur.[1] Pain (often described as burning, shooting,
stabbing, or throbbing), itching, or tingling precede skin lesions
by 1 to 5 days. Lesions form over 3 to 5 days, usually in the
distribution of a single dermatome, beginning as clusters of
erythematous macules that rapidly become papules with super-

imposed clear vesicles, and—much like chickenpox—evolve to pustules and shallow ulcers with crusts that fall off within 2 to 4 weeks, often leaving scars and permanent changes in pigmentation. Thoracic, cervical, and ophthalmic dermatomes are most often involved, and the lesions do not cross the midline. Systemic symptoms occur in <20% of patients, and occasionally there are a few lesions outside the dermatome. Motor nerve involvement with associated paresis may be seen in 5% to 15% of patients (the mechanism for this is not clear). Involvement of the geniculate ganglion can lead to facial nerve paralysis (sensory and motor nerves are joined in nerve VII); the combination of lesions on the ear, hard palate, or tongue and facial paralysis is termed *Ramsay Hunt syndrome* and is associated with vertigo, hearing loss, tinnitus, and loss of taste. Occasionally, pain occurs without skin lesions, which is called *zoster sine herpete*.

Zoster tends to be more severe with advancing age. Subclinical involvement of the CNS is common in immunocompetent individuals; there may be CSF pleocytosis in up to half of patients and VZV can be detected in CSF in a third. Immunocompromised patients may experience severe localized zoster or *disseminated zoster* due to hematogenous spread of the infection outside of the original dermatome. The spectrum of illness ranges from generalized rash to life-threatening pneumonia, hepatitis, encephalitis, and disseminated intravascular coagulopathy.

PHN lasting ≥1 month occurs in 20% to 30% of patients with zoster, and about 10% have pain lasting ≥3 months. Pain may last for months or years, may be constant, intermittent, or triggered by trivial stimuli, and is described as excruciating in half of patients. The quality of life may be dramatically affected, leading to social withdrawal, depression, and even suicide. Advanced age correlates with the severity of PHN; in fact, PHN is rare in children.

Other complications of zoster include secondary bacterial infection, eye involvement with keratitis or retinitis, myelitis, and granulomatous angiitis.

Epidemiology and Transmission

Zoster only occurs in people who have had been infected with VZV; this includes >99.5% of the US population ≥40 years of age. Zoster is contagious in the sense that VZV from the lesions can cause chickenpox in a susceptible individual; however, zoster cannot directly cause zoster in another person, nor can chickenpox, because latency must first be established. Of note, the risk of contagion from zoster is less than that from chickenpox because there is less virus that can aerosolize from the lesions and there is no transmission (from respiratory sections) before the lesions erupt.

Estimates of age-adjusted incidence rates in the United States vary from 3.2 to 4.2 per 1000 population, or about 1 million cases annually.[2] The rate is much higher—about 10 per 1000—in persons ≥ 60 years of age. About one third of people in the United States will experience an episode of zoster in their lifetime. The most important risk factors are increasing age and conditions or medications that impair cell-mediated immunity; other risk factors include psychologic stress, female gender, white race, mechanical trauma, and genetic susceptibility.[3] Exposure to varicella (eg, living or working in environments with young children) appears to be protective, as one would expect since such exposures probably boost immunity.[4] Varicella vaccination is also protective—the rate of zoster is lower in vaccinated persons than in naturally infected persons, and the incidence among children has declined in the vaccine era.[5] Zoster may be up to 10 times less common in children than in adults; when it does occur, a history of maternal varicella during pregnancy or chickenpox in the first year of life is often present. These are situations that can lead to immune tolerance, ie, blunting of immune memory to VZV.

Questions have been raised about how the universal varicella vaccination program will affect the incidence of zoster. Several competing factors are involved. First, as more and more people are vaccinated, fewer and fewer will become latently infected with wild-type VZV. Because wild-type VZV reactivates more readily than the attenuated vaccine strain (which, however, *does* establish latency), this might result in fewer people developing zoster as they age. However, less circulating virus in the community means fewer opportunities for boosted immunity in those who are already infected with wild-type VZV. Therefore, episodes of zoster could increase in one generation (those who are already infected with wild-type VZV and will not have the immunologic benefit of exposure to natural virus) while they decrease in another (those who received VAR and never become latently infected with wild-type VZV). Studies done since 1995, when VAR was first licensed in the United States, have shown conflicting results regarding changes in the incidence of zoster.[6] However, a study published in 2010 showed a striking increase in incidence of zoster among veterans >40 years of age, from 3.10 episodes per 1000 in 2000 to 5.22 per 1000 in 2007.[7]

Immunization Program

It is estimated that each case of zoster results in up to three outpatient visits and from one to five medication prescriptions. Up to 4% of episodes result in hospitalization, with a mean duration of 5 days and average cost of $3221 to $7206 (2006 dollars).[2] Annualized health care costs for PHN are as high as $5000. Assuming a vaccine cost of $150, a 1-dose vaccination program for healthy persons ≥60 years of age would cost from $27,000 to $112,000 per QALY gained. This places ZOS in the intermediate-to-high end of cost-benefit when compared with other vaccination programs.

The rationale for a zoster vaccine program is simple: vaccination mimics the effect of exposure to natural varicella in people who are latently infected, boosting cellular immune responses and thereby preventing reactivation.[8] ZOS was licensed in May 2006, and recommendations for use were published in 2008.[2]

Vaccines

Characteristics of the herpes zoster vaccine licensed in the United States are given in **Table 27.1**. ZOS consists of the same live-attenuated strain of VZV that is used in VAR, only in sufficiently high titer to overcome existing antibody and replicate in previously infected persons.

Efficacy and/or Immunogenicity

ZOS was evaluated in a double-blind, randomized, placebo-controlled trial (the Shingles Prevention Study) involving 38,546 healthy adults ≥60 years of age who either had a personal history of varicella or who had resided in the United States for ≥30 years (and were therefore very likely to have been infected with VZV).[9] The majority of suspected cases were confirmed by PCR. The mean duration of follow-up was 3.1 years, and patients with confirmed zoster were followed for at least 6 months. Remarkably, 95% of those enrolled completed the study.

There were 315 cases of zoster among 19,254 vaccinees and 642 among 19,247 placebees, for a risk reduction of 51%. Overall, vaccination reduced the risk of PHN in vaccinees by 67% when defined as ≥30 days of pain and by 73% when defined as ≥182 days of pain. Among subjects who developed zoster, the risk of PHN was reduced by 39%. Other complications, such as allodynia (a painful response to a normally nonpainful stimulus), bacterial superinfection, disseminated zoster, impaired vision, peripheral motor-nerve palsies, ptosis, scarring, and sensory loss occurred with similar frequency among vaccine and placebo cases of zoster but were less common among vaccinees than placebees. These results indicate that the main benefit of ZOS is in preventing zoster rather than in modifying the severity and or complications should zoster occur. Efficacy at preventing zoster was highest among those 60 to 69 years of age, but the greatest effect in reducing the severity of illness was among persons 70 to 79 years of age. Efficacy declined during the first year following vaccination but stabilized thereafter at around 50%.

Anamnestic antibody and T-cell responses were seen in vaccinated subjects and persisted for 3 to 6 years. Immune responses were inversely related to the risk of zoster.

Safety

Erythema and pain at the injection site occur in about 35% of vaccinees; swelling occurs in 26%, and pruritus in 7%. Most of these reactions are mild and resolve within 4 days. A varicella-like rash occurs at the injection site within 3 to 4 days in 0.1% of vaccinees, and fever occurs in <1%. In the Shingles Prevention Study, serious adverse events such as death (which might be expected given the advanced age of the subjects) occurred with equal frequency among vaccines and placebees.

On rare occasion, the vaccine strain of VZV has been detected in lesions that occurred after vaccination. Horizontal transmission, while not formally evaluated, has not been reported. Standard precautions should be adequate to protect susceptible persons who are in contact with vaccinees who develop lesions.

- *Contraindications*
  - Allergic reaction to previous dose of vaccine or any vaccine component (risk of recurrent allergic reaction)
  - Immunodeficiency or immunosuppression (risk of disease caused by live virus). The following may receive ZOS: patients with leukemia in remission who have not had chemotherapy or radiation for ≥3 months; patients receiving systemic steroids for <14 days or <20 mg/day; patients receiving low doses of methotrexate (≤0.4 mg/kg/week), azathioprine (≤3 mg/kg/day), or 6-mercaptopurine (≤1.5 mg/kg/day); HIV-infected persons with CD4 count ≥200/mcL and CD4 percentage ≥15% of total lymphocytes; and persons with humoral immune deficiencies. Providers may consider immunizing hematopoietic stem-cell transplant recipients who are immunocompetent and who are ≥24 months post-transplant.
  - Pregnancy (theoretic risk of live virus vaccine to the fetus or attribution of birth defects to vaccination)
- *Precautions*
  - Moderate or severe acute illness (difficulty distinguishing illness from vaccine reaction)
  - Active, untreated tuberculosis (risk of exacerbation of tuberculosis)

27

Recommendations

All persons ≥60 years of age should be vaccinated against zoster. The usual schedule is 1 dose of ZOS at 60 years of age, but catch-up vaccination is recommended (there is no upper age

TABLE 27.1 — Zoster Vaccine

Trade name	Zostavax
Abbreviation	ZOS
Manufacturer/distributor	Merck
Type of vaccine	Live-attenuated, classical
Composition	Oka/Merck strain[a]
	Propagated in human diploid (MRC-5) cells
	19,400 plaque-forming units
Adjuvant	None
Preservative	None
Excipients and contaminants	Sucrose (31.16 mg)
	Hydrolyzed porcine gelatin (15.58 mg)
	Sodium chloride (3.99 mg)
	Monosodium L-glutamate (0.62 mg)
	Sodium phosphate dibasic (0.57 mg)
	Potassium phosphate monobasic (0.10 mg)
	Potassium chloride (0.10 mg)
	Residual components of MRC-5 cells, including DNA and protein
	Neomycin (trace)
	Bovine calf serum (trace)
Latex	None
Labeled indications	Prevention of herpes zoster (shingles)
Labeled ages	$\geq$60 years
Dose	0.65 mL
Route of administration	Subcutaneous
Labeled schedule	1 dose
Recommended schedule	Same
How supplied (number in package)	1-dose vial (1, 10), lyophylized, with diluent
Storage:	
Vaccine	Freeze
	Protect from light
	Can be refrigerated for up to 72 hours before reconstitution[b]
Diluent	Refrigerate or room temperature
	Do not freeze
Reconstituted vaccine	Use within 30 minutes
	Do not freeze

Continued

TABLE 27.1 — *Continued*

Trade name	Zostavax
Abbreviation	ZOS
Cost per dose ($US, 2009):	
Public	112.32
Private	153.93
Reference package insert	December 2009

[a] This is the same strain used in VAR (Varivax; Merck) but 14 times the amount.
[b] Vaccine stored at refrigerator temperature and not used within 72 hours should be discarded.

limit). Vaccination is recommended regardless of the personal history with respect to varicella. Patients who have had zoster should be vaccinated; while there is no minimum interval between an episode of zoster and vaccination, it would seem prudent to wait at least a year to vaccinate since immunity presumably will have been boosted by the episode. Patients with chronic medical conditions may be vaccinated, as long as those conditions are not associated with immunosuppression. ZOS is not indicated to treat acute zoster, prevent PHN in patients who already have zoster, or to treat PHN. ZOS is not recommended for persons who have received VAR, but few persons today who are ≥60 years of age will fit into that category.

If immunosuppression is anticipated, vaccination should occur at least 14 days earlier. Persons taking antiviral medications such as acyclovir, famciclovir, and valacyclovir should discontinue those medications at least 24 hours before vaccination and remain off medication for at least 14 days. Receipt of antibody-containing blood products is not a contraindication to vaccination.

The manufacturer warns against simultaneous administration of ZOS and PPSV23 because the antibody response to VZV might be impaired. Simultaneous administration is considered acceptable, however, because lower antibody levels do not necessarily mean reduced protection.

REFERENCES

1. Gnann JW Jr, et al. *N Engl J Med*. 2002;347:340-346.
2. Harpaz R, et al. *MMWR*. 2008;57(RR-5):1-30.
3. Thomas SL, et al. *Lancet Infect Dis*. 2004;4:26-33.
4. Thomas SL, et al. *Lancet*. 2002;360:678-682.
5. Civen R, et al. *Pediatr Infect Dis J*. 2009;28:954-959.
6. Reynolds MA, et al. *J Infect Dis*. 2008;197(suppl 2):S224-S227.
7. Rimland D, et al. *Clin Infect Dis*. 2010;50:1000-1005.
8. Kimberlin DW, et al. *N Engl J Med*. 2007;356:1338-1343.
9. Oxman MN, et al. *N Engl J Med*. 2005;352:2271-2284.

28

Combination Vaccines

Background

Some of the first vaccines licensed in the United States were combinations of antigens. For example, the influenza vaccine (first licensed in 1945) contains antigens from three different strains of influenza virus. Likewise, the hexavalent pneumococcal polysaccharide vaccine (1947), DTwP vaccine (1948), trivalent IPV (1955), and trivalent OPV (1963) were also combinations. Today, the term *combination vaccine* refers to a vaccine whose components could be given as separately available products (referred to herein as *component vaccines*). The modern era of combination vaccines began in the 1990s, when combinations of routinely administered childhood vaccines such as DTwP, DTaP, Hib, and HepB were developed.

As of 2010, the routine childhood schedule from birth through 18 years of age calls for 50 or more immunizations, assuming that each one is given separately. Most of these immunizations are concentrated in the first 2 years of life. Depending on how vaccine visits are scheduled, as many as 9 shots may be due on one day (eg, a 15-month-old may be due for HepB, DTaP, Hib, PCV13, IPV, influenza vaccine, MMR, VAR, and HepA). This causes distress for patients, parents, and health care professionals, enough so that compliance with universal vaccine programs may be threatened. Combination vaccines reduce the number of shots necessary without reducing the delivery of antigens and are a logical solution to this problem.

Development, Evaluation, and Licensure

Producing safe and effective combination vaccines is far more complex than simply mixing antigens together in a single vial.[1] Adjuvants, buffers, stabilizers, and excipients can have *physical or chemical interactions* with antigens that reduce immunogenicity, and many of these interactions cannot be predicted a priori. *Antigenic competition* can occur as vaccine components vie for position in binding to major histocompatibility molecules on antigen-presenting cells at the site of injection. This may explain in part the decreased anti-PRP responses that were seen with initial attempts to combine Hib with DTaP (importantly, even though the antibody titers were lower, the quality of the response in terms of avidity, opsonic activity, and memory may have been similar to the component Hib[2]). Another phenomenon, *carrier-induced epitopic suppression*, may cause decreased antibody responses to protein-polysaccharide conjugates (such as Hib) when there has been prior or simultaneous immunization with free (homologous) carrier protein.[3] Interference can be seen when different conjugates containing the same carrier protein are given at the same time, although the effects are unpredictable—for example, coadministration of Hib- and meningococcal serogroup C-tetanus toxoid conjugate vaccines results in enhanced Hib responses.[4] When live viral vaccines are given together, *viral interference* may limit responses as the replication of one virus is inhibited by the replication of the other; this is why MMRV contains 7 times the amount of VZV than does VAR—so that the VZV can replicate in the setting of measles virus replication (MMRV also contains more mumps virus than MMR, for the same reason). While these interactions are important considerations, they must be differentiated from "immune overload," a popular concept that has no scientific basis (see *Chapter 8: Addressing Concerns About Vaccines—Can Multiple Vaccines Overload the Immune System?*).

Once compatibility issues are worked out in laboratory and animal models, extensive clinical trials are required to prove that a new combination vaccine is safe and effective. FDA guidelines require that such trials compare the combination to separately but simultaneously administered component vaccines. Reactogenicity is compared with the most reactogenic of the individual components. For antigens that have an established serologic correlate of protection, it may be enough to demonstrate that the combination induces protective antibody responses. However, the FDA generally requires that *noninferiority* with component vaccines be demonstrated, generally meaning no more than a 10% reduction in seroprotection (seroprotection may be measured by a variety of ways, such as the proportion of vaccinees achieving a specific antibody titer, the proportion of vaccinees with a ≥4-fold rise in titer, the proportion of seroconverters, the geometric mean concentration of antibody, or some combination of these; the criteria are usually agreed upon before the clinical trials are performed). Efficacy against disease is inferred for most new combination vaccines rather than directly demonstrated.

Effect on Quality

The more shots that are due on a given day, the more likely it is that one or more vaccinations will be deferred to another day.[5] In recent years, it has become clear that such deferrals may lead to reduced coverage rates and poor immunization timeliness. Several studies now suggest that use of combination vaccines, by reducing the number of shots due, can lead to improvements in coverage and timeliness. A study of administrative claims from the Georgia Medicaid program demonstrated higher coverage

490

rates among children who had received a combination vaccine (either HepB-Hib-OMP or DTaP-HepB-IPV) as compared with children who had received the component vaccines, an effect that was independent of other determinants of coverage.[6] In another analysis of the same database, 2-year-olds who had received 3 doses of DTaP-HepB-IPV had markedly fewer cumulative days undervaccinated (125 days) than did control children (334 days) for the series of 4 DTaP, 3 IPV, 1 MMR, 3 Hib, 3 HepB, and 1 VAR.[7] Similar findings have been seen in managed-care populations.[8]

Barriers to the adoption of combination vaccines include cost, loss of administration fees, perceptions about adverse events, and the complexity of having so many multivalent choices.[9] More robust adoption of combination vaccines might occur if providers were incentivized through antigen-based reimbursement, rather than the current system of reimbursing for the administration of the injections per se (see *Chapter 4: Vaccine Practice—Coding, Billing and Costs*). While providers worry that fewer shots and fewer administration fees might mean less income, a 2006 study suggested that revenue loss from use of combination vaccines is minimal.[10]

Vaccines

Modern combination vaccines available in the United States that are based on DTaP are listed in **Table 28.1**; others are listed in **Table 28.2**. The following generalizations are offered:

- *Efficacy and/or immunogenicity*—Licensure by the FDA ensures that the immunogenicity (and presumably the protective efficacy) of a given combination vaccine is noninferior to that of the component vaccines given separately.
- *Safety*—Licensure by the FDA ensures that, in all clinically meaningful respects, a given combination vaccine is as safe as its separately administered components. However, a few issues are noteworthy. For example, DTaP-HepB-IPV causes higher rates of fever (when coadministered with Hib and PCV) than do the component vaccines. However, most of these fevers are low-grade (only 0.4% in one study were >103.1°F) and most (98.8% in the same study) do not result in medical attention. In a postlicensure study involving approximately 61,000 infants who received a total of 120,000 doses of DTaP-HepB-IPV, postvaccination fevers prompting medical visits occurred in <0.3% of both vaccinees and historical controls.[11] Interestingly, DTaP-IPV/Hib is not associated with increased rates of fever.[12] Another example is the occurrence of febrile seizures after MMRV. Prelicensure clinical trials demonstrated higher rates of fever following MMRV than MMR plus VAR.[13] Postlicensure studies showed

28

TABLE 28.1 — DTaP-Based Combination Vaccines

	Kinrix	Pediarix	Pentacel	TriHIBit
Trade name	Kinrix	Pediarix	Pentacel	TriHIBit
Abbreviation	DTaP-IPV	DTaP-HepB-IPV	DTaP-IPV/Hib-T	DTaP/Hib-T
Manufacturer/distributor	GlaxoSmithKline	GlaxoSmithKline	Sanofi Pasteur	Sanofi Pasteur
Diseases prevented:				
Diphtheria	√	√	√	√
Tetanus	√	√	√	√
Pertussis	√	√	√	√
Hepatitis B	—	√	—	—
H influenzae type b	—	—	√	√
Polio	√	√	√	—
Type of vaccine	Inactivated, purified subunits, toxoids, and whole agent	Inactivated, purified subunits, toxoids, engineered subunit, and whole agent	Inactivated, purified subunits, toxoids, engineered subunit, and whole agent	Inactivated, purified subunits, toxoids, and engineered subunit
Component vaccines[a]:				
DTaP	Infanrix	Infanrix	Similar to Daptacel	Tripedia
HepB	—	Engerix-B	—	—
Hib	—	—	ActHIB[b]	ActHIB[c]
IPV	IPV[d]	IPV[d]	Poliovax[d]	—
Composition:				
Diphtheria toxoid	25 Lf units	25 Lf units	15 Lf units	6.7 Lf units
Tetanus toxoid	10 Lf units	10 Lf units	5 Lf units	5 Lf units

Inactivated pertussis toxin	25 mcg	25 mcg	20 mcg	23.4 mcg
Filamentous hemagglutinin	25 mcg	25 mcg	20 mcg	23.4 mcg
Pertactin	8 mcg	8 mcg	3 mcg	—
Fimbriae types 2 and 3	—	—	5 mcg	—
HBsAg	—	—	Expressed in yeast (*S cerevisiae*) (10 mcg)	—
Polyribosylribitol phosphate	—	—	10 mcg conjugated to tetanus toxoid (24 mcg)	10 mcg conjugated to tetanus toxoid (24 mcg)
Poliovirus type 1 (Mahoney)	40 D antigen units	40 D antigen units	40 D antigen units	—
Poliovirus type 2 (MEF-1)	8 D antigen units	8 D antigen units	8 D antigen units	—
Poliovirus type 3 (Saukett)	32 D antigen units	32 D antigen units	32 D antigen units	—
Poliovirus propagation	Vero (African Green Monkey kidney) cells	Vero (African Green Monkey kidney) cells	Human diploid (MRC-5) cells	—
Poliovirus inactivation	Formaldehyde	Formaldehyde	Formaldehyde	—
Adjuvant	Aluminum hydroxide Aluminum phosphate (≤0.6 mg aluminum)	Aluminum hydroxide Aluminum phosphate (≤0.85 mg aluminum)	Aluminum phosphate (0.33 mg aluminum)	Aluminum phosphate (≤0.17 mg aluminum)
Preservative	None	None	None	Nonc

Continued

28

TABLE 28.1 — *Continued*

Trade name	Kinrix	Pediarix	Pentacel	TriHIBit
Abbreviation	DTaP-IPV	DTaP-HepB-IPV	DTaP-IPV/Hib-T	DTaP/Hib-T
Excipients and contaminants	Sodium chloride (4.5 mg)	Sodium chloride (4.5 mg)	Polysorbate 80 (10 ppm)	Gelatin
	Formaldehyde ($\leq$100 mcg)	Formaldehyde ($\leq$100 mcg)	Formaldehyde ($\leq$5 ng)	Formaldehyde ($\leq$100 mcg)
	Polysorbate 80 ($\leq$100 mcg)	Polysorbate 80 ($\leq$100 mcg)	Glutaraldehyde (<50 ng)	Polysorbate 80
	Neomycin sulfate ($\leq$0.05 ng)	Neomycin sulfate ($\leq$0.05 ng)	Bovine serum albumin ($\leq$50 ng)	Thimerosal ($\leq$0.3 mcg mercury)
	Polymyxin B ($\leq$0.01 ng)	Polymyxin B ($\leq$0.01 ng)	2-phenoxyethanol (3.3 mg)	Sucrose (8.5%)
		Yeast protein ($\leq$5%)	Neomycin (<4 pg)	
			Polymyxin B sulfate (<4 pg)	
Latex	Tip cap and plunger of prefilled syringe contain dry natural rubber	Tip cap and plunger of prefilled syringe contain dry natural rubber	None	Vial stopper contains dry natural rubber
Labeled ages	4 to 6 years	6 weeks to 6 years[e]	6 weeks to 4 years	15 to 18 months
Dose	0.5 mL	0.5 mL	0.5 mL	0.5 mL
Route of administration	Intramuscular	Intramuscular	Intramuscular	Intramuscular

Labeled schedule	Dose 5 of DTaP and Dose 4 of IPV in previous recipients of Pediarix and Infanrix	2, 4, 6 months of age[f]	2, 4, 6, 15 to 18 months of age[g]	Dose 4 of DTaP and Dose 4 of Hib
Recommended schedule	Same[h]	Same	Same	Same[h]
Total reduction in shots[i]	1	5	6 or 7[j]	1
How supplied (number in package)	1-dose vial (10) Prefilled syringe (5)	1-dose vial (10) Prefilled syringe (5)	1-dose vial (5) of ActHIB, lyophilized, with 1-dose vial (5) of DTaP-IPV as diluent	1-dose vial (5) of Act-HIB, lyophilized (5) with 1-dose vial (5) of as Tripedia as diluent
Storage	Refrigerate Do not freeze	Refrigerate Do not freeze	Vaccines: Refrigerate Do not freeze Reconstituted vaccine: use immediately	Vaccines: Refrigerate Do not freeze Reconstituted vaccine: use within 30 minutes
Cost per dose ($US, 2009):				
Public	32.35	48.75	51.49	27.31
Private	48.00	70.72	72.91	44.88
Reference package insert	March 2009	July 2009	June 2008	December 2003

Continued

28

TABLE 28.1 — *Continued*

a The combination vaccines may not be strict mixtures of the component vaccines. In some cases, the amount of antigen or the method of production may be different than the separate components.

b The liquid DTaP-IPV combination is used to reconstitute the lyophilized ActHIB.

c The liquid Tripedia is used to reconstitute the lyophilized ActHIB.

d Not licensed or distributed separately in the United States.

e Only labeled for the primary series (not booster doses). Not labeled for use in infants of HBsAg-positive or -unknown mothers, but use in these infants is considered acceptable.

f With the birth dose of HepB, use of this combination vaccine will result in four total doses of HepB. This does not increase reactogenicity or compromise immunogenicity. Patients who receive Pediarix according to this schedule will need DTaP boosters at 15 to 18 months and 4 to 6 years of age, as well as an IPV booster at 4 to 6 years of age.

g Patients who receive Pentacel according to this schedule do not need further doses of Hib but they *do* need DTaP and IPV boosters at 4 to 6 years of age.

h ACIP expresses a preference for the same DTaP product for the entire series, but vaccination should not be deferred if the same product is not immediately available or if the previous products are not known.

i Reduction in shots across the complete routine immunization schedule if the practice uses component vaccines and switches to the combination.

j The lower number applies if the office uses PedvaxHIB (Hib-OMP), because a dose of that vaccine is not given at 6 months (there is one less shot saved).

that the rate of febrile seizures after the first dose of MMRV was approximately twice as high (about 7 per 10,000) as after the separate vaccines in the 5 to 12 days following vaccination (there is no increased risk after the second dose of MMRV).[14] This amounts to about one febrile seizure attributable to the vaccine for every 2600 children vaccinated.

• *Contraindications and precautions*—Contraindications and precautions for combination vaccines are the same as for the individual components. One exception is MMRV, where there is the additional precaution about febrile seizures after the first dose.

Recommendations

In 1999, recognizing the potential advantages (**Table 28.3**), the ACIP, AAP, and AAFP issued a statement expressing a clear preference for combination vaccines over separate injections of the component vaccines.[15] The preference for combination vaccines was reiterated annually in the routine childhood schedule and in the *General Recommendations on Immunization*. In 2009, ACIP reworded the preference for combination vaccines, stating that combination vaccines are "generally" preferred, and that the following factors should be considered in deciding whether or not to use them: patient preference, potential for adverse events, number of injections, vaccine availability, likelihood of improved coverage, likelihood of patient return, storage, and costs.[16] ACIP has also offered guidance for integrating particular combination vaccines into the schedule (see **Table 8.2**).[17,18]

One exception to the preference for combination vaccines is MMRV. For the first dose in children <4 years of age, either MMRV or separate MMR and VAR may be used. However, MMRV is generally preferred for the first dose in children 4 through 12 years of age as well as for second doses.

Use of combination vaccines may result in *overimmunization* because unnecessary doses of an antigen may be given. For example, an infant who receives the birth dose of HepB and then receives DTaP-HepB-IPV at 2, 4, and 6 months of age will receive 4 total doses of HepB, when only 3 doses are required. As another example, a child who receives DTaP-IPV/Hib at 2, 4, 6, and 15 months of age will need DTaP and IPV at 4 to 6 years of age—a total of 5 doses of IPV will be given, when only 4 are required. These extra doses are not harmful and are an accepted consequence of using combination vaccines.

Providers are warned not to combine vaccines in the same syringe unless the products are specifically labeled for this purpose.

28

497

TABLE 28.2 — Other Combination Vaccines

Trade name	Comvax	ProQuad	Twinrix
Abbreviation	HepB-Hib-OMP	MMRV	HepA-HepB
Manufacturer/distributor	Merck	Merck	GlaxoSmithKline
Diseases prevented	Hepatitis B Invasive *H influenzae* type b	Measles Mumps Rubella Varicella	Hepatitis A Hepatitis B
Type of vaccine	Inactivated, engineered subunits	Live-attenuated, classical	Inactivated, whole agent, and engineered subunit
Component vaccines[a]	Recombivax HB (HepB) PedvaxHIB (Hib-OMP)	Similar to M-M-R$_{II}$ (MMR)[b] Varivax (VAR)[c]	Havrix (HepA) Engerix-B (HepB)
Composition	HBsAg expressed in yeast (*S cerevisiae*) (5 mcg) Polyribosylribitol phosphate (7.5 mcg) conjugated to *N meningitidis* serogroup B (strain B11) outer membrane protein (125 mcg)	Measles virus, Moraten strain (derived from the Edmonston B strain), propagated in chick embryo cells, at least 1000 TCID$_{50}$ Mumps virus, Jeryl Lynn strain (actually consists of two distinct strains), propagated in chick embryo cells, at least 19,950 TCID$_{50}$	HAV, HM175 strain, propagated in human diploid (MRC-5) cells and inactivated with formalin (720 ELISA units) HBsAg expressed in yeast (*S cerevisiae*) (20 mcg)

		Rubella virus, RA 27/3 strain, propagated in human diploid lung fibroblast (WI-38) cells, at least 1000 TCID$_{50}$ Varicella virus, Oka/Merck strain, propagated in human diploid (MRC-5) cells, at least 9770 plaque-forming units	
Adjuvant	Aluminum hydroxide (0.225 mg aluminum)	None	Aluminum phosphate Aluminum hydroxide (0.45 mg aluminum)
Preservative	None	None	None
Excipients and contaminants	Yeast protein (≤5%) Sodium borate decahydrate (35 mcg) Sodium chloride (0.9%) Formaldehyde (≤0.0004%)	Sucrose (21 mg) Hydrolyzed gelatin (11 mg) Sodium chloride (2.4 mg) Sorbitol (1.8 mg) Monosodium L-glutamate (0.40 mg) Sodium phosphate dibasic (0.34 mg) Human albumin (0.31 mg) Sodium bicarbonate (0.17 mg) Potassium phosphate monobasic (72 mcg)	Amino acids Sodium chloride Phosphate buffer Polysorbate 20 Formalin (≤0.1 mg) Residual MRC-5 proteins (≤2.5 mcg) Neomycin sulfate (≤20 ng) Yeast protein (≤5%)

Continued

28

TABLE 28.2 — *Continued*

	Comvax	ProQuad	Twinrix
Trade name			
Abbreviation	HepB-Hib-OMP	MMRV	HepA-HepB
Excipients and contaminants (*continued*)		Potassium chloride (60 mcg) Potassium phosphate dibasic (36 mcg) Residual components of MRC-5 cells, including DNA and protein Neomycin (<16 mcg) Bovine calf serum (0.5 mcg) Other buffer and media ingredients	
Latex	Vial stopper contains dry natural rubber	None	Tip cap and plunger of prefilled syringe contain dry natural rubber
Labeled ages	6 weeks to 15 months[d]	12 months to 12 years	≥18 years
Dose	0.5 mL	0.5 mL	1 mL
Route of administration	Intramuscular	Subcutaneous	Intramuscular
Labeled schedule	2, 4, 12 to 15 months of age[e]	12 to 15 months of age Revaccination at 4 to 6 years of age	0, 1, 6 months Alternative schedule: 0, 7, 21 to 30 days; booster at 12 months

Recommended schedule[f]	Same	Same	Same
Total reduction in shots	2 or 3[g]	2	2 (alternative schedule:1)
How supplied (number in package)	1-dose vial (10)	1-dose vial (10), lyophilized with diluent	1-dose vial (10) Prefilled syringe (5)
Storage	Refrigerate Do not freeze	Vaccine: Freeze Can be refrigerated for up to 72 hours before reconstitution Protect from light Diluent: Refrigerate or room temperature Do not freeze Reconstituted vaccine: use within 30 minutes	Refrigerate Do not freeze
Cost per dose ($US, 2009):			
Public	28.80	82.67	41.50
Private	43.56	128.90	89.85
Reference package insert	August 2004	October 2009	May 2009

Continued

[a] The combination vaccines may not be strict mixtures of the component vaccines. In some cases, the amount of antigen or the method of production may be different than the separate components.

[b] The amount of mumps virus in MMRV is 1.6-times higher than in MMR (M-M-R$_{II}$; Merck).

[c] The amount of varicella virus in MMRV is 7-times higher than in VAR (Varivax; Merck).

28

501

TABLE 28.2 — *Continued*

[d] Not labeled for use in infants of HBsAg-positive or -unknown mothers, but use in these infants is considered acceptable.

[e] With the birth dose of HepB, use of this combination vaccine will result in four total doses of HepB. This does not increase reactogenicity or compromise immunogenicity. Patients who receive Comvax according to this schedule do not need further doses of HepB or Hib.

[f] Reduction in shots across the complete routine immunization schedule if the practice uses component vaccines and switches to the combination.

[g] The higher number applies if ActHIB is currently in use, because switching to Comvax reduces the total number of Hib doses needed to complete the primary series from 3 to 2.

TABLE 28.3 — Potential Advantages and Disadvantages of Combination Vaccines

Potential Advantages

- Fewer injections
- Decreased pain and anxiety
- Decreased injection risk
- Fewer sharps injuries
- Simplified schedule
- Decreased administration costs and overhead
- Improved billing efficiency
- Improved record-keeping and tracking
- Improved coverage rates
- Improved timeliness
- Decreased preparation time
- More efficient well-child visits
- Easier storage and inventory management
- Less vaccine wastage
- More efficient federal documentation
- Introduction of new vaccines without additional visits

Potential Disadvantages

- Increased reactogenicity
- Difficulty attributing adverse events to specific antigens
- Confusion over antigen content and errors in record-keeping
- Extraimmunization
- Decreased flexibility
- Increased cost of vaccines
- Loss of revenue from administration fees

28

REFERENCES

1. International Symposium on Combination Vaccines. *Clin Infect Dis.* 2001;33(suppl 4):S261-S375.

2. Poolman J, et al. *Vaccine.* 2001;19:2280-2285.

3. Dagan R, et al. *Infect Immun.* 1998;66:2093-2098.

4. Pöllabauer EM, et al. *Vaccine.* 2009;27:1674-1679.

5. Meyerhoff AS, et al. *Prevent Med.* 2005;41:540-544.

6. Marshall GS, et al. *Pediatr Infect Dis J.* 2007;26:496-500.

7. Happe LE, et al. *Pediatr Infect Dis J.* 2009;28:98-101.

8. Happe LE, et al. *Am J Manag Care.* 2007;13:506-512.

9. Gidengil CA, et al. *Clin Pediatr.* 2009;48:539-547.

10. Freed GL, et al. *Pediatrics.* 2006;118:e251-e257.

11. Zangwill KM, et al. *Pediatrics.* 2008;122:e1179-e1185.

12. Black S, et al. *Expert Rev Vaccines.* 2005;4:793-805.

13. Kuter BJ, et al. *Hum Vaccine.* 2006;2:205-214.

14. Jacobsen SJ, et al. *Vaccine.* 2009;27:4656-4661.

15. Advisory Committee on Immunization Practices (ACIP), et al. *Pediatrics.* 1999;103:1064-1077.

16. ACIP provisional recommendations for the use of combination vaccines. Centers for Disease Control and Prevention Web site. http://www.cdc.gov/vaccines/recs/provisional/default.htm#acip. Accessed February 7, 2010.

17. CDC. *MMWR.* 2008;57:1078-1079.

18. CDC. *MMWR.* 2008;57:1079-1080.

Appendix

(All web sites accessed March 31, 2010)

Governmental Agencies

Centers for Medicare & Medicaid Services (CMS)
http://www.cms.hhs.gov

Department of Defense (DOD)
http://www.defenselink.mil

Department of Health and Human Services
- National Institutes of Health (NIH):
  - National Institute of Allergy and Infectious Diseases (NIAID)
    http://www3.niaid.nih.gov
  - Division of Microbiology and Infectious Diseases (DMID)
    http://www3.niaid.nih.gov/about/organization/dmid
  - Vaccine Research Center (VRC)
    http://www.niaid.nih.gov/vrc/default.htm
  - Vaccine and Treatment Evaluation Units (VTEU)
    http://www3.niaid.nih.gov/LabsAndResources/resources/vteu/
- Food and Drug Administration (FDA):
  - Center for Biologics Evaluation and Research (CBER)
    http://www.fda.gov/AboutFDA/CentersOffices/CBER/default.htm
  - Vaccines and Related Biological Products Advisory Committee (VRBPAC)
    http://www.fda.gov/CBER/advisory/vrbp/vrbpmain.htm
  - Vaccine Adverse Events Reporting System (VAERS, cosponsored by CDC)
    http://vaers.hhs.gov
- Centers for Disease Control and Prevention (CDC):
  - National Center for Immunization and Respiratory Diseases (NCIRD)
    http://www.cdc.gov/vaccines
  - Advisory Committee on Immunization Practices (ACIP)
    http://www.cdc.gov/vaccines/recs/ACIP/default.htm
  - Vaccines for Children Program (VFC)
    http://www.cdc.gov/vaccines/programs/vfc/default.htm
- Health Resources and Services Administration (HRSA):
  - National Vaccine Injury Compensation Program (VICP)
    http://www.hrsa.gov/vaccinecompensation
  - Advisory Commission on Childhood Vaccines (ACCV)
    http://www.hrsa.gov/vaccinecompensation/accv.htm

- National Vaccine Program Office (NVPO)
  http://www.hhs.gov/nvpo
  – National Vaccine Advisory Committee (NVAC)
    http://www.hhs.gov/nvpo/nvac

US Agency for International Development (USAID)
http://www.usaid.gov

International Agencies

Pan American Health Organization (PAHO)
http://www.paho.org/english/ad/fch/im/Vaccines.htm

World Health Organization (WHO)
http://www.who.int/immunization/en

Professional Associations

American Academy of Family Physicians (AAFP)
http://www.aafp.org

American Academy of Pediatrics (AAP)
http://www.aap.org/immunization/

American College Health Association (ACHA)
www.acha.org

American Nurses Association (ANA)
http://nursingworld.org

American Pharmacists Association (APhA)
http://www.pharmacist.com

American Public Health Association (APHA)
http://www.apha.org

Association for Prevention Teaching and Research (APTR)
(formerly the Association of Teachers of Preventive Medicine)
http://www.atpm.org

Infectious Diseases Society of America (IDSA)
http://www.idsociety.org

Pediatric Infectious Diseases Society (PIDS)
http://www.pids.org

Advocacy, Implementation, and Safety

All Kids Count
http://www.allkidscount.org

Allied Vaccine Group
http://www.vaccine.org

Brighton Collaboration
http://www.brightoncollaboration.org

Children's Hospital of Philadelphia Vaccine Education Center
http://www.vaccine.chop.edu

Children's Vaccine Program at PATH
http://www.path.org/vaccineresources/

Clinical Immunization Safety Assessment Network (CISA)
http://www.vaccinesafety.org

Every Child by Two (ECBT)
http://www.ecbt.org

Global Alliance for Vaccines and Immunization (GAVI)
http://www.gavialliance.org

Immunization Action Coalition (IAC)
http://www.immunize.org

Institute for Vaccine Safety, Johns Hopkins Bloomberg School of Public Health
http://www.vaccinesafety.edu

National Foundation for Infectious Diseases (NFID)
http://www.nfid.org

National Network for Immunization Information (NNii)
http://www.immunizationinfo.org

Parents of Kids With Infectious Diseases (PKIDs)
http://www.pkids.org

Sabin Vaccine Institute (SVI)
http://www.sabin.org

Vaccinate Your Baby
http://www.vaccinateyourbaby.org

Voices for Vaccines
http://www.voicesforvaccines.org

Coverage and Assessment

Behavioral Risk Factor Surveillance System (BRFSS)
http://www.cdc.gov/brfss

Comprehensive Clinic Assessment Software Application (CoCASA)
http://www.cdc.gov/vaccines/programs/cocasa

Healthcare Effectiveness Data and Information Set (HEDIS)
http://web.ncqa.org/tabid/59/Default.aspx

National Health Interview Survey (NHIS)
http://www.cdc.gov/nchs/nhis.htm

29

National Immunization Survey (NIS)
http://www.cdc.gov/nis

National Notifiable Diseases Surveillance System (NNDSS)
http://www.cdc.gov/ncphi/disss/nndss/nndsshis.htm

Books

Allen A. *Vaccine: The Controversial Story of Medicine's Greatest Lifesaver*. New York, NY: WW Norton; 2008.

Atkinson W, Wolfe C, Hamborsky J, McIntyre L. *Epidemiology and Prevention of Vaccine-Preventable Diseases*. 11th ed. Washington, DC: Public Health Foundation; 2009.

Brunette GW, Kozarsky PE, Magill AJ, Shlim DR. *CDC Health Information for International Travel 2010*. St Louis, MO: Elsevier; 2009.

Colgrove J. *State of Immunity: The Politics of Vaccination in Twentieth-Century America*. Berkeley, CA: University of California Press; 2006.

Cunningham RM, Boom JA, Baker CJ. *Vaccine-Preventable Disease: The Forgotten Story*. Houston, TX: Texas Children's Hospital; 2009.

Gold R. *Your Child's Best Shot: A Parent's Guide to Vaccination*. Ottawa, Ontario; Canadian Paediatric Society; 2006.

Myers MG, Pineda D. *Do Vaccines Cause That?! A Guide for Evaluating Vaccine Safety Concerns*. Galveston, TX: Immunizations for Public Health; 2008.

Offit PA. *The Cutter Incident: How America's First Polio Vaccine Led to the Growing Vaccine Crisis*. New Haven, CT: Yale University Press; 2007.

Offit PA. *Vaccinated: One Man's Quest to Defeat the World's Deadliest Diseases*. New York, NY: Harper Collins Publishers; 2007.

Offit PA. *Autism's False Prophets: Bad Science, Risky Medicine, and the Search for a Cure*. New York, NY: Columbia University Press; 2008.

Offit PA. *Deadly Choices: How the Anti-Vaccine Movement Threatens Our Children*. New York, NY; Basic Books; 2011.

Oshinsky DM. *Polio: An American Story*. New York; Oxford University Press; 2006.

Pickering, LK, ed. *Red Book: 2009 Report of the Committee on Infectious Diseases*. 28th ed. Elk Grove Village, IL: American Academy of Pediatrics; 2009.

Plotkin SA, Orenstein WA, Offit PA. *Vaccines.* 5th ed. St Louis, MO: Elsevier; 2008.

Smith MJ, Bouck L. *The Complete Idiot's Guide to Vaccinations: A Balanced Look at the Pros and Cons.* Indianapolis, IN; Alpha Books; 2009.

Manufacturers and Distributors

Bioport (Emergent BioDefense Operations Lansing)
http://www.bioport.com

Crucell (acquired Berna Biotech in 2006)
http://www.crucell.com/

CSL Biotherapies
http://www.cslbiotherapies-us.com

GlaxoSmithKline
http://www.gsk.com

Massbiologics (University of Massachusetts Medical School, formerly Massachusetts Public Health Biologic Laboratories)
http://www.umassmed.edu

MedImmune (acquired by AstraZeneca in 2007)
http://www.medimmune.com

Merck
http://www.merck.com

Novartis
http://www.novartis.com

Pfizer *(acquired Wyeth in 2009)*
http://www.pfizer.com

Sanofi Pasteur *(acquired Acambis in 2008)*
http://www.sanofipasteur.com

State Health Department Immunization Programs

State health department web sites can be accessed through the following URL: http://www.cdc.gov/mmwr/international/relres .html.

29

AAFP ....American Academy of Family Physicians
AAP ....American Academy of Pediatrics
ACCV.................Advisory Commission on Childhood Vaccines
ACHA ....American College Health Association
ACIP...................Advisory Committee on Immunization Practices
AIDS ....acquired immune deficiency syndrome
AOM ....acute otitis media
ANA...................American Nurses Association
APC ....antigen-presenting cell
APhA.................American Pharmaceutical Association
APHA.................American Public Health Association
ASD ....autistic-spectrum disorder
ATPM.................Association of Teachers of Preventive Medicine
AVG ....Allied Vaccine Group
BCG ....Bacille Calmette-Guérin (tuberculosis vaccine)
BLA ....Biologics License Application
BRFSS.................Behavioral Risk Factor Surveillance System
CASA.................Clinical Assessment Software Application
CBER.................Center for Biologics Evaluation and Research
CDC ....Centers for Disease Control and Prevention
CHD ....congenital heart disease
CI ....confidence interval
CISA...................Clinical Immunization Safety Assessment (Network)
CLD ....chronic lung disease (bronchopulmonary dysplasia)
CMS ....Centers for Medicare and Medicaid Services, formerly
                     known as the Health Care Financing Administration
                     (HCFA)
CMV...................cytomegalovirus
CMV-IGIV ....cytomegalovirus immune globulin, intravenous
CNS ....central nervous system
CPT ....Current Procedural Terminology
CRM_{197} ....cross-reactive material (a mutant diphtheria toxin)
CSF ....cerebrospinal fluid
CTL ....cytotoxic T lymphocyte
DHHS.................Department of Health and Human Services
DMARD.............disease-modifying antirheumatic drug
DMEM ....Dulbecco's Modified Eagle Medium
DMID.................Division of Microbiology and Infectious Diseases
DNA...................deoxyribonucleic acid
DOD...................Department of Defense
DT ....diphtheria, tetanus vaccine (infant/child formulation)
DTaP...................diphtheria, tetanus, acellular pertussis vaccine (infant/
                     child formulation)
DTwP.................diphtheria, tetanus, whole-cell pertussis vaccine
EDTA ....ethylene diamine tetraacetic acid

EMLA	eutectic mixture of local anesthetic
EMT	emergency medical technician
EPA	Environmental Protection Agency
FDA	(US) Food and Drug Administration
FHA	filamentous hemagglutinin
FIM	fimbriae (also known as agglutinogens)
FQHC	federally qualified health center
GABHS	group A beta-hemolytic streptococcus
GCP	Good Clinical Practices
GLP	Good Laboratory Practices
GMP	Good Manufacturing Practices
GVHD	graft-versus-host disease
H	hemagglutinin
HAV	hepatitis A virus
HBIG	hepatitis B immune globulin
HbOC	polyribosylribotol phosphate (the capsular polysaccharide of *H influenzae* type b) conjugated to mutant diphtheria toxin CRM_{197}
HBsAb	antibody to hepatitis B surface antigen
HBsAg	hepatitis B surface antigen
HBV	hepatitis B virus
HCFA	Health Care Financing Administration, now known as the Centers for Medicare and Medicaid Services (CMS)
HCP	health care personnel
HEDIS	Healthcare Effectiveness Data and Information Set
HepA	hepatitis A vaccine
HepB	hepatitis B vaccine
HEPES	N-2-hydroxyethylpiperazine-N'2-ethanesulfonic acid
HHS	(Department of) Health and Human Services
Hib	*Haemophilus influenzae* type b conjugate vaccine
Hib-CRM	*Haemophilus influenzae* type b vaccine, CRM_{197} conjugate
Hib-D	*Haemophilus influenzae* type b vaccine, diphtheria toxoid conjugate
Hib-OMP	*Haemophilus influenzae* type b vaccine, (*N meningitidis*) outer membrane protein conjugate
Hib-T	*Haemophilus influenzae* type b vaccine, tetanus toxoid conjugate
HICPAC	Healthcare Infection Control Practices Advisory Committee
HIV	human immunodeficiency virus
HPV	human papillomavirus
HPV2	human papillomavirus vaccine, 2-valent
HPV4	human papillomavirus vaccine, 4-valent
HRIG	human rabies immune globulin
HSCT	hematopoietic stem-cell transplant
IAC	Immunization Action Coalition

IBD ....inflammatory bowel disease
ICD-9-CM...........International Classification of Diseases, 9th Revision, Clinical Modification
IDSA ....Infectious Diseases Society of America
IG ....immune globulin
IgE ....immunoglobulin E
IgG ....immunoglobulin G
IGIM ....(polyclonal) immune globulin, intramuscular
IGIV ....(polyclonal) immune globulin, intravenous
IgM ....immunoglobulin M
IIV ....inactivated influenza vaccine
IIV-seasonal ....inactivated influenza vaccine, seasonal (3-valent)
IIV-2009 H1N1 ...inactivated influenza vaccine, 2009 H1N1 strain (monovalent)
IIS ....Immunization Information Systems (also known as registries)
IM ....intramuscular
IN ....intranasal
IOM ....Institute of Medicine
IPD ....invasive pneumococcal disease
IPV ....inactivated poliovirus vaccine
ISRC....................Immunization Safety Review Committee
ITP ....immune thrombocytopenic purpura
IU ....international unit
IV ....intravenous
JE ....Japanese encephalitis
JE-MB ....Japanese encephalitis vaccine, mouse brain-derived
JE-VC..................Japanese encephalitis vaccine, Vero cell-derived
JEV ....Japanese encephalitis virus
LAIV ....live-attenuated influenza vaccine
LAIV-seasonal ....live-attenuated influenza vaccine, seasonal (3-valent)
LAIV-2009 H1N1 ..live-attenuated influenza vaccine, 2009 H1N1 strain (monovalent)
LEP ....low egg passage
LRI ....lower respiratory infection
MCD ....mad cow disease
MCV.....................meningococcal conjugate vaccine
MCV4 ....meningococcal conjugate vaccine, 4-valent
MCV4-CRM ....meningococcal vaccine, 4-valent, CRM_{197} conjugate
MCV4-D ....meningococcal vaccine, 4-valent, diphtheria toxoid conjugate
MHC ....major histocompatibility complex
MMR...................measles, mumps, rubella vaccine
MMRV ....measles, mumps, rubella, varicella vaccine
MPSV..................meningococcal polysaccharide vaccine
MPSV4...............meningococcal polysaccharide vaccine, 4-valent
MRI ....magnetic resonance imaging
MS ....multiple sclerosis

NCES	National Childhood Encephalopathy Study
NCIRD	National Center for Immunization and Respiratory Diseases
NCQA	National Committee on Quality Assurance
NCVIA	National Childhood Vaccine Injury Act
NDC	National Drug Code
NHIS	National Health Interview Survey
NIAID	National Institute of Allergy and Infectious Diseases
NIH	National Institutes of Health
NIP	National Immunization Program
NIS	National Immunization Survey
NNDSS	National Notifiable Disease Surveillance System
NNii	National Network for Immunization Information
NREVSS	National Respiratory and Enteric Surveillance System
NRSSS	National Rotavirus Strain Surveillance System
NVAC	National Vaccine Advisory Committee
NVPO	National Vaccine Program Office
NVSN	New Vaccine Surveillance Network
OMP	(*N meningitidis*) outer membrane protein
OPV	oral polio vaccine
OSHA	Occupational Safety and Health Administration
PAHO	Pan American Health Organization
PCV	pneumococcal conjugate vaccine
PCV7	pneumococcal conjugate vaccine, 7-valent
PCV13	pneumococcal conjugate vaccine, 13-valent
PCV7-CRM	pneumococcal vaccine, 7-valent, CRM_{197} conjugate
PCV13-CRM	pneumococcal vaccine, 13-valent, CRM_{197} conjugate
PDD	pervasive developmental disorder
PDUFA	Prescription Drug User Fee Act
PFU	plaque-forming units
PHN	postherpetic neuralgia
PHS	(US) Public Health Service
PI	package insert (also known as product information)
PO	per os (orally by mouth)
PPSV	pneumococcal polysaccharide vaccine
PPSV23	pneumococcal polysaccharide vaccine, 23-valent
PRN	pertactin
PRP	polyribosylribitol phosphate
PS	(capsular) polysaccharide
PT	pertussis toxin
QALY	quality-adjusted life year
RAB	rabies vaccine
RAB-HDC	rabies vaccine, human diploid cell
RAB-PCEC	rabies vaccine, purified chick embryo cell
RET	Reportable Events Table
RHC	rural health clinic
RhoGAM	Rho(D) immune globulin
RIG	rabies immune globulin

RNA ....ribose nucleic acid
RR ....relative risk
RRV-TV ....rhesus-human reassortant rotavirus vaccine, tetravalent
RSV ....respiratory syncytial virus
RSV-IGIV ....respiratory syncytial virus immune globulin, intravenous
RSVmAB ....respiratory syncytial virus monoclonal antibody
RV ....rotavirus vaccine
RV1 ....rotavirus vaccine, monovalent (live-attenuated human rotavirus vaccine)
RV5 ....rotavirus vaccine, 5-valent (pentavalent bovine rotavirus vaccine)
RVU ....relative value unit
SC ....subcutaneous
SCHIP ....State Children's Health Insurance Program
SIDS.....................sudden infant death syndrome
SIV ....simian immunodeficiency virus
sp ....species
Tc ....cytotoxic T-cells
TCID$_{50}$ ....median tissue culture infective dose
TCR ....T-cell receptor
Td ....tetanus, diphtheria vaccine (adolescent/adult formulation)
Tdap ....tetanus, diphtheria, acellular pertussis vaccine (adolescent/adult formulation)
TIG ....tetanus immune globulin
tRNA....................transfer ribonucleic acid
TST ....tuberculin skin test, formerly referred to as PPD (purified protein derivative)
TT ....tetanus toxoid
TViPSV ....typhoid Vi polysaccharide vaccine
Ty21a...................(oral) typhoid vaccine
URI ....upper respiratory infection
US$ ....United States currency
USAID ....US Agency for International Development
USAMRIID.........US Army Medical Research Institute of Infectious Diseases
USP ....United States Pharmacopoeial Convention
v/v ....percent by volume in volume (mL per 100 mL of solution)
VAERS................Vaccine Adverse Event Reporting System
VAR ....varicella vaccine
VariZIG ....varicella-zoster immune globulin
VFC ....Vaccines for Children (Program)
VICP....................(National) Vaccine Injury Compensation Program
VIG ....vaccinia immune globulin
VIS ....Vaccine Information Statement
VIT ....Vaccine Injury Table
VLP ....virus-like particle
VRBPAC.............Vaccines and Related Biological Products Advisory Committee
VRC ....(Dale and Betty Bumpers) Vaccine Research Center

VSD .... .Vaccine Safety Datalink
VTEU................_.Vaccine and Treatment Evaluation Unit
VZV ....varicella-zoster virus
WHO................ ..World Health Organization
WIC ....(US Department of Agriculture's Special Supplemental
                      Nutrition Program for) Women, Infants and Children
YF   ....yellow fever
YFV ....yellow fever virus
ZOS ....zoster vaccine

Nomenclature

(See *Appendix Table*, next page)

29

APPENDIX TABLE — Vaccine and Infectious Agent Nomenclature

Disease	Infectious Agents Name	Abbreviation	Vaccine Designation(s)[a]
Anthrax	*Bacillus anthracis*	*B anthracis*	Anthrax vaccine
Diphtheria, tetanus (lockjaw), pertussis (whooping cough)	*Corynebacterium diphtheriae*	*C diphtheriae*	DTwP, DTaP, Tdap, DT, Td, TT
	Clostridium tetani	*C tetani*	
	Bordetella pertussis	*B pertussis*	
H influenzae type b (invasive)	*Haemophilus influenzae* type b	*H influenzae* type b	Hib (Hib-OMP, Hib-T)
Hepatitis A	Hepatitis A virus	HAV	HepA
Hepatitis B	Hepatitis B virus	HBV	HepB
Human papillomavirus-induced cervical cancer and genital warts	Human papillomavirus	HPV	HPV vaccine (HPV2, HPV4)
Influenza	Influenza virus	—	IIV-seasonal, LAIV-seasonal, IIV-2009 H1N1, LAIV-2009 H1N1
Japanese encephalitis	Japanese encephalitis virus	JEV	JE vaccine (JE-MB, JE-VC)
Measles, mumps, rubella	Measles virus, mumps virus, rubella virus	—	MMR
N meningitidis (invasive)	*Neisseria meningitidis*	*N meningitidis*	MCV (MCV4-CRM, MCV4-D), MPSV4
Polio	Poliovirus	—	IPV
Rabies	Rabies virus	—	RAB
Rotavirus gastroenteritis	Rotavirus	—	RV (RV1, RV5)

S pneumoniae (invasive, otitis media)	S pneumoniae	S pneumoniae	PCV (PCV7-CRM, PCV13-CRM), PPSV23
Smallpox	Variola virus	—	Smallpox vaccine (vaccinia)
Typhoid fever	Salmonella typhi	S typhi	TViPSV, Ty21a
Varicella (chickenpox)	Varicella zoster virus	VZV	VAR
Yellow fever	Yellow fever virus	YFV	YF vaccine
Zoster (shingles)	Varicella zoster virus	VZV	ZOS
Modern combination vaccines			HepB-Hib-OMP
			DTaP/Hib-T
			DTaP-IPV/Hib-T
			DTaP-IPV
			DTaP HepB-IPV
			MMRV
			HepA-HepB

[a] For conjugate vaccines, "CRM," "-D," "-OMP," and "-T," indicate the protein carrier to which the polysaccharide is conjugated (respectively, CRM[197] [a mutant diphtheria toxin]; diphtheria toxoid; N meningitidis outer membrane protein; and tetanus toxoid). Numbers following the abbreviations indicate the valency of the vaccine (eg, HPV2 contains two serotypes whereas HPV4 contains four serotypes). For combination vaccines, dashes indicate that the components are premixed (eg, DTaP-HepB-IPV); slash marks indicate that the components must be combined prior to administration (eg, DTaP/Hib-T, where liquid DTaP is used to reconstitute the lyophilized Hib-T).

29

Note: Page numbers in *italics* indicate figures.
Page numbers followed by a "t" indicate tables.

Abbreviations, 510-515
ACAM2000 (smallpox vaccine), 431, 431t, 433-435
  CPT and ICD-9-CM codes, 127t
Acetaminophen, 117
ACIP. See *Advisory Committee on Immunization Practices.*
ActHIB (Hib-T), 289, 290t-292t
  CPT and ICD-9-CM codes, 125t
  efficacy/immunogenicity, 289
  recommendations, 289-293
Active Bacterial Core surveillance, 64
Active immunization, 11-16
Acute disseminated encephalomyelitis (ADEM), 358
Acute illness, as precaution, 156. See also *specific vaccines.*
Acute otitis media (AOM), 440, 442
Ad-hoc committees and task forces, 68-69
Adacel (Tdap), 252, 272t-275t. See also *Tdap vaccine.*
  CPT and ICD-9-CM codes, 128t
Adaptive immune system, 17-21
Additives in vaccines, 213-214, 489
Adenocarcinomas, HPV and, 319
Adenovirus vaccine, 15
Adenylate cyclase toxin, 267
Adjuvants, 27. See also *specific vaccines.*
  aluminum salts, 212-213
  AS04, 213, 324t
  interactions of, 489
  safety concerns, 212-213
Administration of vaccines, 113-117. See also *Delivery of vaccines.*
  anxiety, pain, and fever, dealing with, 117
  CPT codes for, 130t-133t
  emergencies following, 117-122
  errors in, and remedies, 149, 152t-154t
  general rules for, 139-155
  intervals between vaccines, 139-141, 142t-146t
    live vaccines and antibody-containing products, 148-149, 150t-151t
  intramuscular, 116, *118*, 120t-121t
  intranasal, 116-117
  multiple vaccines, simultaneous administration of, 70t, 113-116, 139
  oral, 115
  preferred sites and needle length, 120t-121t
  schedules for, 241-256
  subcutaneous, 116, *118*, 120t-121t
Adolescent immunization
  coverage, 62, 91
  hepatitis B vaccine, 242, 312
  HPV vaccine, 255
  mandates for, 102

Adolescent immunization *(continued)*
  schedules
    catch-up, 248t
    routine, 245t
  syncope and, 119
  Tdap vaccine for, 271
  waning immunity and, 209
Adolescents, sexual activity among, 321
Adoptees, international, 178-179
Adult immunization
  financing of, 78-79
  mandates/legislation on, 102-103
  schedules. See also *specific vaccines.*
    by age group, 249t
    by medical condition, 250t-251t
  standards for, 91, 92t
Adverse events, 43, 191-192. See also *Vaccine Safety Net; specific vaccines.*
  emergencies following vaccine administration, 117-122
  package insert information, 55-56
  Reportable Events Table, 94t-95t
  reporting system (VAERS), 66-67, 96
Advertising claims, package insert and, 56
Advisory Commission on Childhood Vaccines, 93-96, 505
Advisory Committee on Immunization Practices (ACIP), 56-58, *57,* 497, 505
  recommendations, 55, 58-59
  working groups, 58
Advocacy organizations, 506-507
Aedes aegypti mosquitoes, 473-474, 478
Afluria (IIV, influenza), 340t-342t
  CPT and ICD-9-CM codes, 125t-126t
Age. See also *Schedules for immunizations.*
  adult immunization schedule by, 249t
  grace period for immunizations, 103
  minimum ages for routine vaccines, 141, 142t-146t
Agenticity, 194-195
Agriflu (IIV, influenza), 340t-342t
AIDS, polio vaccine and, concerns about, 234-235. See also *HIV.*
Alastrim (variola minor), 426
Alcoholism, vaccination recommendations, 250t-251t
All Kids Count, 506
Allergies. See also *specific vaccines.*
  concern about vaccines causing, 215-217
  delayed-type hypersensitivity, 155
  to eggs, 338, 351, 352
  to gelatin, 214
  severe, to vaccine/components, 155, 213-214
Allied Vaccine Group, 506
Aluminum salts, 212-213
American Academy of Family Physicians (AAFP), 506
American Academy of Pediatrics (AAP), 506
  Red Book, iv, 59

30

American College Health Association (ACHA), 506
American Immunization Registry Association, 111
American Nurses Association (ANA), 506
American Pharmacists Association (APA), 506
American Public Health Association (APHA), 506
Anal cancers, 320
Anamnestic response, 26
Anaphylaxis/anaphylactic shock, 94t, 119-122
  symptoms, 119
  treatment, 119-122
Anesthetics, topical, 117
Animal viruses, natural attenuation for humans, 14
Animal workers, vaccination of, 188t
Anogenital warts, 320
Anthrax, 257-265, 516t
  antibiotic therapy for, 259
  as bioterrorism agent, 258
  clinical features, 257
  cutaneous, gastrointestinal, inhalational, and oropharyngeal
    anthrax, 257
  epidemiology and transmission, 257-258
  immunization program, 258-259
  pathogen, 257
  vaccines for, 259, 260t
    civilian use, 258-259, 264t-265t
    contraindications/precautions, 147, 261-262
    CPT and ICD-9-CM codes, 124t
    efficacy/immunogenicity, 259
    military use, 259, 262
    pre-exposure vaccination, 259
    recommendations/schedule, 260t, 262, 264t-265t
    safety, 261-262
    storage, 260t
Antibodies, 21-30. See also *Immune globulin.*
  action mechanisms and sites, 21
  engineered, 17
  germline, 23
  inactivation of live vaccines by, 148
  measurement of, 37-39
  passive immunization with, 16-17
  persistence of, 29-30
  production of, 21-30
    extrafollicular reaction, 22-23, *22*
    germinal center reaction, 23-30, *25*
  specificity of, 28-29
  testing for, 149
  time course of responses, *28*
Antibody-containing blood products
  intervals for live vaccines and, 148-149, 150t-151t
  recent receipt of, as precaution, 467
Antibody-dependent cell-mediated cytotoxicity, 21
Antigen-presenting cells (APCs), 24-26, *25*
Antigen-sparing, 27

Antigens, 21. See also *Antibodies.*
  antigenic competition, 489
  antigenic drift/antigenic shift, 333
  number of, in routine vaccines, 211t
  reassortment, 333
  T-cell independent, 23
Antihistamine, 122
Antitoxins, in passive immunization, 17
Antivaccinationism, 200-204, 201t-203t, 205t-207t
Anxiety, dealing with, 117
AOM. See *Acute otitis media.*
APCs. See *Antigen-presenting cells.*
Apoptosis, 34
Arthritis, Hib and, 287
Arthus-type reaction, 280, 281
AS04, 213, 324t
Aspirin use, 188t, 354, 467
  Reye syndrome and, 462, 467
Asplenia, 164-165, 440
  vaccination recommendations, 250t-251t, 388, 451t
Association for Prevention Teaching and Research (APTR), 506
Association for Professionals in Infection Control
    and Epidemiology, 102
Asthma
  as contraindication, 353-354
  as indication for PPSV23, 253
  pneumonia risk and, 450
  vaccine concerns and, 216
Attenuation of vaccines, 11-15
  engineered, 14-15
  heterologous host, 14
  route of inoculation, 15
  serial passage, 11-14
Autism, 219-229
  MMR vaccine and, 70t, 219-222, *221, 223,* 225-226
  Omnibus Autism Proceedings, 225-226
  safety review findings, 71t
  thimerosol and, 224-229, *227, 228*
Autoimmune disease, vaccines and, 215-217
Avian flu. See *Bird flu.*

B cells, 21-23, *22, 25*
  memory, *25,* 26, 29
Bacille Calmette-Guérin (BCG), 14
Bacillus anthracis, 257. See also *Anthrax.*
Bacteremia, 287, 439, 454, 462
Bacteria. See also *specific bacteria.*
  attenuation of, 14
  lysis/opsonization of, 21
  vaccines against, 34
BCG. See *Bacille Calmette-Guérin.*
Behavioral Risk Factor Surveillance System (BRFSS), 62, *63,* 507
Billing. See *Coding and billing.*

30

Biohazard labels, 101
Biologics License Application (BLA), 54
Bioterrorism
  anthrax and, 257, 258, 262
  polio and, 353
  smallpox and, 44, 426
BioThrax, 124t, 260t, 261
Bird flu (influenza A; H5N1), 334, 335, 336
  vaccine for, 339
BLA (Biologics License Application), 54
Bleeding diathesis, 188t
Blood products, intervals for live vaccines and, 148-149, 150t-151t
Blood transfusion, interval for live vaccines and, 150t
Bloodborne Pathogens Standard, 97-102
Bone marrow transplantation. See *Hematopoietic stem cell transplantation.*
Books on vaccines, iv, 508-509
Booster vaccination, 27-28, *28*
Boostrix (Tdap), 252, 272t-275t. See also *Tdap vaccine.*
  CPT and ICD-9-CM codes, 128t
Bordetella pertussis, 15, 267, 269. See also *Pertussis.*
Brain damage, pertussis vaccine concerns, 229-231
Breast-feeding, 175, 421. See also *Pregnancy.*
  as contraindication, 264t, 436, 477
BRFSS. See *Behavioral Risk Factor Surveillance System.*
Brighton Collaboration, 67-68, 507
Buccal cellulitis, 287
Buffers, 155, 489
Butte County, California, HepA in, 301

Cancer
  chemotherapy for, 165-167
  HPV and, 319-320
  vaccines and, 70t, 234
Carrier-induced epitopic suppression, 489-490
Catch-up immunization schedules
  children, age 4 months-6 years, 246t-247t
  children, age 7-18 years, 248t
CBER. See *Centers for Biologics Evaluation and Research.*
CDC. See *Centers for Disease Control and Prevention.*
Cell-mediated immunity defects, 163
Cellulitis, Hib and, 287
Centers for Biologics Evaluation and Research (CBER), 49-51, *50*, 505
Centers for Disease Control and Prevention (CDC), 505
  monitoring and surveillance, 64
  vaccine policy and, 56, *57*
Centers for Medicare & Medicaid Services (CMS), 505
Cervarix (HPV2), 27, 324t-326t. See also *Human papillomavirus.*
  efficacy/immunogenicity, 323-327
  recommendations, 329-330
  safety, 329
  schedule, 125t, 255, 325t
Cervical cancer, 255, 319-320, 321

Cervical intraepithelial neoplasia (CIA) grades, 320
Cervical transformation zone, 319
Chemotherapy
  impaired immunity and, 165-167
  pneumonia vaccination and, 450
Chickenpox. See *Varicella.*
Childhood Immunization Support Program, 59
Children. See also *Infants.*
  anxiety and pain, dealing with, 117
  cocoon strategy, 110
  costs of immunization, 72-73, 72t, 88-89
  coverage rates, 60-63, *61*, 111
  CPT codes, 130t-131t
  HIV-exposed/infected, vaccination issues, 167-169
  immunization schedules
    catch-up, age 4 months-6 years, 246t-247t
    catch-up, age 7-18 years, 248t
    combination vaccines in, 255-256
    exemptions, 103
    financing for, *73*, 74-78
    grace period for, 103
    hepatitis A, 297, 302
    hepatitis B, 312
    pneumonia, 447, 448t
    routine, age 0-6 years, 243t-244t
    routine, age 7-18 years, 245t
    school mandates and state legislation, 102-103
    travel and, 182
  routine health care recommendations, 91
  Vaccines for Children (VFC) Program, 74-78
Children's Hospital of Philadelphia Vaccine Education Center, 507
Children's Vaccine Program at PATH, 507
Chronic disease, impaired immunity and, 165
Chronic liver disease, vaccination recommendations, 250t-251t, 302,
  313, 354
Chronic lung disease, vaccination recommendations, 250t-251t
Chronic meningococcemia, 379-380
Cidofovir, 436
CISA. See *Clinical Immunization Safety Assessment (CISA) Network.*
Civic duty, immunization as, 198
Classification of vaccines, 12t-13t
Clinical Immunization Safety Assessment (CISA) Network, 67, 507
Clinical trials, 51-54, *51*
  numbers of subjects required, *51*, 52, 53t
Clinically preventable burden, 47
Clonal expansion, 22
Clostridium tetani, 267, 269. See also *Tetanus.*
Clotting-factor disorders, 302
CoCASA (Comprehensive Clinic Assessment Software Application),
  113, 507
Cochlear implants
  pneumonia risk and, 448
  pneumonia vaccination and, 450
  vaccination and, 188t

Cocoon strategy, 110
Coding and billing, 122-136
  CPT (Current Procedural Terminology) codes, 122-134
    immune globulin administration, 128t-129t
    preventive medicine services, 122, 123t
    vaccine administration, 122, 130t-133t
    vaccines and immune globulins, 122, 124t-129t
  ICD-9-CM (International Classification of Diseases, Ninth Revision,
    Clinical Modification) codes, 122-134
    preventive medicine services, 123t
    vaccines and immune globulins, 124t-129t
  National Drug Codes (NDCs), 134
  routine office visit, example, 134, 135t
College students, vaccination of, 188t, 355, 388
Combination vaccines, 489-504, 517t
  advantages of, 489, 490-491, 497, 503t
  background on, 489
  barriers to adoption of, 491
  contraindications/precautions, 497
  development, evaluation, and licensure of, 489-490
  disadvantages of, 497, 503t
  DTap-based, 242, 492t-496t
  efficacy/immunogenicity, 491
  incorporating in pediatric schedule, 244t, 255-256
  noninferiority standard, 490
  other, 498t-502t
  overimmunization and, 497
  preference for, 497
  production of, 489-490
  quality, effect on, 490-491
  recommendations on, 497
  safety, 491-497
  schedule, 497
Communicating about vaccines, 191-240. See also *Concerns about
  vaccines, addressing.*
  communicating risks and benefits, 191-197, 208-236
  specific concerns and questions, 208-236
  strategies for, 195-197
  tips for, 195-196
  vaccine refusal, 197-200
Complement assays, 383-387
Complement deficiencies, 159-160, 163-164
  vaccination recommendations, 250t-251t, 388
Complement-mediated lysis, 21
Component vaccines, 12t-13t, 15-16. See also *specific combination
  vaccines.*
Comprehensive Clinic Assessment Software Application (CoCASA),
  113, 507
Comvax (HepB-Hib-OMP), 242, 252, 498t-502t
  component vaccines/composition, 498t
  CPT and ICD-9-CM codes, 125t
  schedule, 500t-501t

Concerns about vaccines, addressing, 191-240
  antivaccinationism, 200-204, 201t-203t
    flawed thinking, 205t
    public harm from, 206t-207t
  communicating risks and benefits, 191-197
    communication strategies, 195-197
    probabilistic and heuristic thinking, 192-195
  costs of public concern, 204-208, 206t-207t
  specific concerns, 208-236
    additives, safety of, 213-214
    adjuvants, danger of, 212-213
    AIDS, polio vaccine and, 234-235
    allergies and autoimmune disease causation, 215-217
    alternative schedules, 214-215
    autism, MMR vaccine and, 219-222, 221, 223
    autism, thimerosol and, 224-229, 227, 228
    brain damage, pertussis vaccine and, 229-231
    cancer, vaccines and, 234
    fetal tissue in vaccine manufacture, 217-219
    Guillain-Barré syndrome, vaccines and, 231-232
    Kawasaki disease, vaccines and, 236
    mad cow disease, vaccines and, 233-234
    multiple sclerosis, vaccines and, 232
    multiple vaccines, immune overload and, 70t, 210-212, 211t
    natural infection vs immunization, 209-210
    necessity for vaccines, 208-209
    SIDS, vaccines and, 235
  vaccine refusal, 197-200
Condyloma acuminata, HPV and, 320
Confidentiality, protecting, 111-112
Confirmation bias, 194
Contaminants, 213-214. See also *specific vaccines.*
Contraindications and precautions, 155-156. See also *specific vaccines.*
  distinguishing, 156
  erroneous contraindications, 156, 157t-158t
  impaired immunity and, 250t, 255
  screening for, 113, 114t-115t
Correctional facility staff/inmates, vaccination of, 189t, 297,
    302, 313, 355
Correlates of protection, 36-39, 38t
Corynebacterium diphtheriae, 267, 269. See also *Diphtheria.*
Costs, 72-79
  cost-benefit analysis, 47
    influenza vaccination, 338
    N meningitidis vaccination, 381-382
    pneumococcal vaccination, 441
    rotavirus vaccination, 415
    varicella vaccination, 464
    zoster (shingles) vaccination, 483-484
  financing methods, 72-79
  provider costs for vaccination services, 136t
  of public concern about vaccines, 204-208
  public/private sector participation in, 72-79, 73

30

Costs *(continued)*
  of registry maintenance, 112
  of routine childhood vaccinations, 72t
  of vaccine development, 49
  of vaccines (purchase price), 134-136. See also *specific vaccines.*
Coverage, 60-64, 109-111
Coverage and assessment groups, 507-508
Cowpox, 14. See also *Smallpox.*
Cows, mad cow disease and, 233-234
CPT (Current Procedural Terminology) codes, 122-134
  for immune globulin administration, 132t
  pediatric-specific, 130t-131t
  for preventive medicine services, 123t
  for routine office visit at 6 months, 135t
  for vaccine administration, 130t-133t
  for vaccines and immune globulins, 124t-129t
Creutzfeldt-Jakob disease, variant (vCJD), 233-234
Criteria for immunity, 374t-375t
-CRM suffix, 517t (footnote)
Cross-protection, 29, 35
Culex mosquitoes, 358
Current Procedural Terminology codes. See *CPT codes.*
Cytokines, 24, 33, *33*
Cytomegalovirus immune globulin intravenous (CMV-IGIV), 150t
Cytotoxic T cells (Tc cells), 30-35, *33*, 305
  implications for vaccination, 34-35
  Th1-cells and, 26, 33, *33*
Cytotoxicity, antibody-dependent cell-mediated, 21
Cytotoxins, 34

Danish Cohort Study
  Hib vaccine and diabetes, 217, *218*
  MMR and autism, 222, *223*
  thimerosol and autism, 226-229, *228*
Daptacel (DTaP), 272t-275t
  CPT and ICD-9-CM codes, 124t
  efficacy, 279
Day care center staff, vaccination of, 189t, 355
Decavac (Td, preservative-free), 276t-278t
  CPT and ICD-9-CM codes, 127t
Delayed-type hypersensitivity, 155
Delivery of vaccines
  improving, 108-113
    expanding access, 109-110
    Immunization Information Systems (IISs), 111-112
    missed opportunities, 109
    other strategies, 112-113
    reminder, recall, and tracking systems, 108-109
    standing orders, 110-111
  monitoring, 60-64
Dendritic cells, 24-26, *25*
Department of Defense (DOD), 505
Department of Health and Human Services, 56, *57*, 505-506

Development. See *Vaccine development and licensure*.
Developmentally disabled, vaccination of staff for, 189t, 313
Diabetes, 217, *218*
  vaccination recommendations, 250t-251t
DiGeorge syndrome, 155-156, 160, 163
Diphenhydramine, 122
Diphtheria, 267-286, 516t. See also *Pertussis; Tetanus*.
  clinical features, 268
  epidemiology and transmission, 269
  immunization program, 270
  infection vs disease, 269
  morbidity and mortality from, 46t
  pathogen, 267
  toxoid, 276t-278t
  vaccines for, 272t-278t. See also *DT; DTaP vaccine; Tdap vaccine*.
    adult. See *Tdap vaccine*.
    children/infants. See *DTaP vaccine*.
    combination vaccines, 492t-496t
    contraindications/precautions, 279-281
    CPT and ICD-9-CM codes, 124t
    efficacy/immunogenicity, 271-279
    indications, 273t, 277t
    recommendations, 281-283
    safety, 279-281
    schedule, 274t, 277t
    storage, 274t, 277t
Diphtheria and Tetanus Toxoids Adsorbed USP (for Pediatric Use; DT),
    276t-278t
Disease-modifying antirheumatic drugs (DMARDs), 167
Diseases. See also *specific diseases*.
  chronic, 165
  vaccinating patients who have already had, 147-148
  vaccination goals for, 44-45
  vaccine-preventable, monitoring, 64-65
Do no harm, 193
Doses of vaccine
  administration errors, and remedies, 152t-154t
  multidose series, administration of, 141
  partial or fractional, 141
Dryvax (smallpox vaccine), 430, 433-434
  CPT and ICD-9-CM codes, 127t
DT (diphtheria, tetanus toxoids), 276t-278t
  contraindications/precautions, 280-281
  recommendations, 281
DTaP vaccine, 272t-275t. See also *Daptacel; Infanrix; Tripedia*.
  combination vaccines, 242, 492t-496t
    component vaccines/composition, 492t-493t
    safety, 491
    schedule, 244t, 495t
  contraindications/precautions, 279-280
  coverage, 61, *61*
  CPT and ICD-9-CM codes, 124t, 130t
  efficacy/immunogenicity, 279

DTaP vaccine *(continued)*
  recommendations, 281
  safety, 279-280
  schedule, 242, 274t
    administration errors, and remedies, 152t-153t
    catch-up, children age 4 months-6 years, 246t
    children, age 0-6 years, 243t, 244t
    minimum ages and intervals, 140-141, 142t
  shortages of, *84*
  vs Tdap, 147
DTwP vaccine, 489

Eczema, as contraindication for vaccination, 435
Education on immunizations, 112-113
Effectiveness, monitoring, 64-65
Efficacy
  correlates of protection, 36-39, 38t
  efficacy/immunogenicity. See *specific vaccines.*
Eggs, allergy to, 338, 351, 352
Elimination of disease, 44-45
Embryonic cells, use in vaccine production, 217-219
Emergencies following vaccine administration, 117-122
  anaphylaxis, 119-122
  preparation for, 117-119
  standing orders for, 119
  syncope, 119
Emergencies, vaccine storage and handling during, 107t
Emerging Infections Program Network (CDC), 64
EMLA cream, 117
Encephalitis
  Japanese, 357-364
  postvaccination (yellow fever vaccine), 476, 478
Encephalopathy
  acute, as vaccine contraindication, 155, 280
  concerns about, 204
End stage renal disease (ESRD), vaccination recommendations,
    250t-251t, 313
Engerix-B (HepB), 241-242, 308t-310t
  CPT and ICD-9-CM codes, 125t
  dosing, 309t, 312
  efficacy/immunogenicity, 311
  schedule, 309t
Engineered agent vaccines, 12t-13t
Engineered attenuation, 14-15
Engineered subunits, 16
Epidemiology and Prevention of Vaccine-Preventable Diseases.
    See *"Pink Book".*
Epiglottitis, 287
Epilepsy, as vaccination contraindication/precaution, 280
Epitopes, 21
  epitope spreading, 27
  epitopic suppression, carrier-induced, 489-490
Eradication of disease, 44-45

Erythema, 279, 434, 484
Every Child by Two (ECBT), 507
Excipients and contaminants, 155, 213-214. See also *specific vaccines.*
    interactions of, 489
Exemptions from school immunization requirements, 103
Exposure-control plan, 97-100
Extinction of disease, 44-45
Extrafollicular reaction, 22-23, *22*

FDA. See *Food and Drug Administration (FDA).*
Fear of vaccines, harm from, 204-208, 206t-207t
Febrile multiple organ-system failure, 476
Febrile seizures, 191, 369, 491-497
Federal requirements regarding vaccination, 98t-99t
Fetal tissue in vaccine manufacture, 217-219
Fever, dealing with, 117
Filamentous hemagglutinin (FHA), 267, 272t, 493t
Fimbriae (FIM), 267, 272t, 493t
Financing of immunization, 72-79, *73*
    adults, 78-79
    children, 74-78
    cost of vaccines, 72-73, 72t
    future of, 79
    NVAC recommendations, 80t-81t
    public/private sector participation, 72-79, *73*
Flu. See *Influenza.*
Fluarix (IIV, influenza), 340t-342t
    CPT and ICD-9-CM codes, 125t-126t
Flulaval (IIV, influenza), 125t, 340t-342t
Flumist (LAIV, live influenza), 127t, 254, 343t-346t
Fluvirin (IIV, influenza), 343t-346t
    CPT and ICD-9-CM codes, 125t-126t
Fluzone (IIV, influenza), 343t-346t
    CPT and ICD-9-CM codes, 125t-126t
Fluzone-High Dose (IIV, influenza), 343t-346t, 351
Folk numeracy, 194
Food and Drug Administration (FDA), 49, *57*, 505
Food handlers, vaccination of, 188t, 303-304
Foresters, vaccination of, 188t
Formaldehyde, 213-214
Freeloading, 193-194
Freezers, 105-106, 107t
FUTURE (Females United To Unilaterally Reduce Endo/Ectocervical
    Disease) I and II, 322-323

GABHS (group A beta-hemolytic streptococcus), 462
GamaSTAN S/D (immune globulin, human, IM), 128t
Gardasil (HPV4), 255, 324t-326t. See also *Human papillomavirus.*
    CPT and ICD-9-CM codes, 125t
    efficacy/immunogenicity, 322-323
    recommendations, 329-330
    safety, 328-329
Gastroenteritis. See *Rotavirus.*

30

Gelatin, 214, 233. See also *specific vaccines.*
Genetics of vaccine responses and adverse events, 43
Genital warts, 319, 329-330
Germinal center reaction, 23-30, *25*
  implications for vaccination, 26-30
Germline antibodies, 23
Global Alliance for Vaccines and Immunization (GAVI), 507
Gloves, 100-101, 116
  not routinely needed, 149
Good Clinical Practices (GCPs), 51
Good Laboratory Practices (GLPs), 49
Good Manufacturing Practices (GMPs), 49, 52
Governmental agencies and committees, 56-60, *57*, 505-506
Grace period, 103, 140-141
Group A beta-hemolytic streptococcus (GABHS), 462
Guillain-Barré syndrome, 68, 231-232
  as contraindication/precaution
    for diphtheria/tetanus/pertussis vaccines, 280, 281
    for influenza vaccines, 351, 352, 353
    for MCV4, 156, 388
Gulf War Syndrome, 261

H1N1 influenza, 68, 231
  vaccine, 181, 231
    administration, 131t, 139
    mandates and, 102
Haemophilus influenzae type b (Hib), 287-293, 516t. See also *Influenza.*
  clinical features, 287
  diabetes and, 217, *218*
  epidemiology and transmission, 287-288
  herd immunity and, 40, 288
  immunization program, 288
  morbidity and mortality from, 46t
  newborn protection against, 16
  pathogen, 287
  vaccines for, 288, 290t-292t
    combination vaccines, 252-253, 492t-496t, 498t-502t
    contraindications/precautions, 289
    correlates of protection, 37, 38t
    coverage, 61, *61*
    CPT and ICD-9-CM codes, 124t, 125t, 130t
    efficacy/immunogenicity, 288-289
    minimum ages and intervals, 142t
    recommendations, 289-293
    safety, 95t, 289
    schedule, 252-253, 291t
      administration errors, and remedies, 153t
      catch-up, children age 4 months-6 years, 246t
      children, age 0-6 years, 243t
      combination vaccines, 244t
    shortages of, *84*
Handling, storage, and transport of vaccines, 105-108
Harm, from fear of vaccines, 204-208, 206t-207t

Harmless, definition of, 191

HAV. See *Hepatitis A.*

Havrix (HepA), 255, 298t-300t
  CPT and ICD-9-CM codes, 124t
  efficacy/immunogenicity, 297-301

HBIG. See *Hepatitis B immune globulin (HBIG).*

HCP. See *Health care personnel.*

HDVC. See *Imovax Rabies.*

Health care personnel, 179-181
  needlestick injuries/blood exposure, 97-102
  vaccination recommendations, 101, 102, 180-181, 250t-251t, 313,
      355, 427, 437
    contraindications/precautions, 355

Healthcare Effectiveness Data and Information Set (HEDIS), 507

Healthy People 2010, 87, 111
  vaccine coverage goals, 62, 63

Healthy People 2020, 87

Heart disease, vaccination recommendations, 250t-251t

HEDIS. See *Healthcare Effectiveness Data and Information Set.*

Helper T lymphocytes (Th cells), 24-26, *25*

Hemagglutinin, 340t, 343t

Hematopoietic stem cell transplantation (HSCT), 169, 170t-172t

Hemodialysis, vaccination recommendations, 250t-251t

HepaGam B (hepatitis B immune globulin), 307
  CPT and ICD-9-CM codes, 128t

Hepatitis A, 295-304
  in Butte County, California, 301
  clinical features, 295
  disease vs infection, 296
  epidemiology and transmission, 295-296
    endemic regions of world, 185t-187t
  herd immunity and, 40-43, *41*
  immunization program, 46, 296-297
  morbidity and mortality from, 46t
  pathogen, 295
  vaccines for, 297, 298t-300t
    combination vaccines, 498t-502t
    contraindications/precautions, 301
    CPT and ICD-9-CM codes, 124t-125t
    efficacy/immunogenicity, 297-301
    minimum ages and intervals, 142t
    preferred over immune globulin, 302-303
    recommendations, 255, 297, 302-304
      postexposure prophylaxis, 297, 302-304
      pre-exposure prophylaxis, 297, 302
      for travel, 183, 297, 302
      universal childhood immunization, 46, 302
    safety, 95t, 301
    schedule, 255, 299t
      adults, by age, 249t
      adults, by medical condition/indication, 250t
      catch-up, children age 4 months-6 years, 247t
      catch-up, children age 7-18 years, 248t

Hepatitis A, schedule *(continued)*
    children, age 0-6 years, 243t
    children, age 7-18 years, 245t
    shortages of, *84*
Hepatitis B, 305-318
  chronic carriers, 305
  clinical features, 305-306
  epidemiology and transmission, 306
  HBsAg/HBsAb status and, 242, 306-308, 316t-318t
    testing for, 313-314
  immunization program, 306-307
  incidence, 307
  morbidity and mortality from, 46t
  pathogen, 305
  vaccines for, 15, 307-311, 308t-310t. See also *Hepatitis B immune globulin.*
    combination, 242, 244t, 492t-496t, 498t-502t
    contraindications/precautions, 312
    correlates of protection, 37, 38t
    coverage, 61-62, *61*
    CPT and ICD-9-CM codes, 125t
    efficacy/immunogenicity, 311
    minimum ages and intervals, 142t
    recommendations, 312-315
      adult vaccination, 312-314
      during pregnancy, 306-307
      for health care personnel, 101, 102, 180, 313
      for nonoccupational exposures, 318t
      for occupational exposures, 316t-317t
      postexposure prophylaxis, 314-315, 316t-318t
      preterm and low birth weight infants, 175
      for travel, 183
      universal infant, child and adolescent immunization, 312
    reportable events, 95t
    safety, 70t, 311-312
      MS concern, 232, 310-311
      SIDS concern, 235
    schedule, 241-242, 309t
      administration errors, and remedies, 153t
      adults, by age, 249t
      adults, by medical condition/indication, 251t
      birth dose, 241-242, 312
        deferral of, 312
      catch-up, children age 4 months-6 years, 246t
      catch-up, children age 7-18 years, 248t
      children, age 0-6 years, 243t
      children, age 7-18 years, 245t
    standing orders for, 312, 313
    waning immunity and, 311
Hepatitis B immune globulin (HBIG), 307
  contraindications, 307-311
  interval for receipt of live vaccines, 151t
  recommendations
    for exposed neonates, 314-315

Hepatitis B immune globulin (HBIG), recommendations *(continued)*
    for nonoccupational exposures, 318t
    for occupational exposures, 316t-317t
  safety, 307-311
Hepatitis B surface antigen/antibody. See *Hepatitis B, HBsAg/HBsAb status.*
Herd immunity, 39-43, *41-42*
  threshold, 40
Herpes zoster (shingles). See *Zoster (herpes zoster; shingles).*
Heterologous host, 14
Heterologous hyperimmune sera, 17
Heterologous infections, 212
Heterotypic responses, 29
Heuristic thinking about vaccines, 192-195
Hib. See *Haemophilus influenzae type b.*
Hib-OMP. See *PedvaxHIB.*
Hib-T. See *ActHIB.*
Hiberix (HibT), 252, 289, 290t-292t
  efficacy/immunogenicity, 289
  recommendations, 289-293
HIV (human immunodeficiency virus) infection, 167-169
  in children/adolescents, MMR vaccination and, 376
  immunoprophylaxis and, 162
  live vaccines and, 160
  pneumonia and, 440, 450
  polio vaccine, concerns, 234-235
  universal precautions, 101-102
  vaccination recommendations, 250t-251t, 313-314, 354, 376, 389,
    451t, 468
    contraindications/precautions, 477
Home visits for vaccination, 110
Homotypic responses, 29
Hooper, Edward, 234
Household contacts, immunization of, 160-161, 161t, 313, 355, 376,
    459, 468
  contraindications/precautions, 353
HPV. See *Human papillomavirus (HPV).*
HPV2. See *Human papillomavirus (HPV), vaccines for.*
HPV4. See *Human papillomavirus (HPV), vaccines for.*
HRV. See *Rotavirus, vaccines for, human (HRV).*
HSCT. See *Hematopoietic stem cell transplantation.*
Human complement assay, 383-387
Human embryo cell lines, 217-219
Human immunodeficiency virus. See *HIV.*
Human leukocyte antigens (HLAs), 24, 43
Human papillomavirus (HPV), 319-331, 516t
  clinical features, 319-320
  epidemiology and transmission, 320-321
  immunization program, 321-322
  pathogen, 319
  vaccines for, 322, 324t-326t
    contraindications/precautions, 329
    cross-protection from, 323

30

Human papillomavirus (HPV), vaccines for *(continued)*
  efficacy/immunogenicity, 322-327
  HPV2 (Cervarix), 27, 324t-326t
    CPT and ICD-9-CM codes, 125t
    efficacy/immunogenicity, 323-327
  HPV4 (Gardasil), 322-323, 324t-326t
    CPT and ICD-9-CM codes, 125t
    efficacy/immunogenicity, 322-323
    immunization program, 321-322
    schedule, 255, 325t
      adults, by age, 249t
      adults, by medical condition/indication, 250t
      catch-up, children age 7-18 years, 248t
      females age 7-18 years, 245t
      minimum ages and intervals, 142t-143t
  recommendations, 255, 329-330
  safety, 95t, 328-329
Human rabies immune globulin (HRIG). See *Rabies immune globulin, human.*
Human rotavirus vaccine. See *Rotavirus, vaccines for, human (HRV).*
Humoral immune deficiencies, 159, 163
Hundred-day cough, 268. See also *Pertussis.*
Hydroxyzine, 122
Hygiene hypothesis, 215-216
HyperHEP B S/D (hepatitis B immune globulin, human), 128t, 307
Hyperimmune globulins, in passive immunization, 16-17
HyperRAB S/D (rabies immune globulin), 128t, 400
Hypersensitivity, delayed-type, 155
HyperTET (tetanus immune globulin), 129t
Hyporesponsiveness, 23

ICD-9-CM (International Classification of Diseases, Ninth Revision, Clinical Modification) codes, 122, 134
  for preventive medicine services, 123t
  routine office visit, example, 135t
  for vaccines and immune globulins, 124t-129t
ICD-10-CM, compliance date, 134
IgA deficiency, selective, 401
IGIM (intramuscular immune globulin), 17, 150t
IGIV (immune globulin, intravenous), 17, 150t, 169
Illegal drug users, vaccination of, 188t, 302, 303, 306, 313
Immigrants, vaccination policies on, 178-179
Immune deficiency. See *Impaired immunity.*
Immune globulin, 16-17. See also *Antibodies; specific immune globulins.*
  administration procedure, 116
  CPT and ICD-9-CM codes, 128t-129t, 132t
  intervals for vaccination with live vaccines, 149, 150t-151t
  intramuscular (IGIM), 17, 150t
  intravenous (IGIV), 17, 150t, 169
  isotypes, 21
  vaccination preferred over, 302-303
Immune memory, 26, 29

Immune overload, concerns about, 210-212, 211t, 214
Immune response, 17-35
  adaptive immune system, 17-21
  anamnestic response, 26
  antibodies, 21-30
    persistence of, 29-30
  antigens, 21
  cytotoxic T cells, 30-35
  extrafollicular reaction, 22-23, *22*
  germinal center reaction, 23-30, *25*
  homotypic vs heterotypic, 29
  hygiene hypothesis, 215-216
  innate immune system, 23-24
    stimulating, 26-27
  multiple immunizations and, 70t, 210-212, 211t
  priming and boosting, 27-28
Immune thrombocytopenic purpura, 371
Immunity
  criteria for (specific diseases), 374t-375t
  impaired. See *Impaired immunity.*
  surrogates of, 36-39, 38t
  testing for, 149
  waning, 209
Immunization, 11-17
  active, 11-16
  booster, 27-28
  correlates of protection, 36-39
  definition of, 11
  education on, 112-113
  herd immunity, 39-43, *41-42*
  mandates and legislation regarding, 102-103
  passive, 16-17
  primary, 27-28, *28*
  reactions to. See *Adverse events.*
  schedules. See *Schedules for immunizations.*
  screening for, 113, 114t-115t
  standards. See *Standards, principles, and regulations.*
Immunization Action Coalition (IAC), 113, 507
Immunization Information Systems (IISs), 111-112
Immunization programs. See also *specific vaccines.*
  impact of, 45-47, 46t, 191
Immunization Safety Review Committee (ISRC), 69, 70t-71t
Immunocompromised states. See *Impaired immunity.*
Immunogenicity, 30, *31*, 36. See also *specific vaccines.*
Immunogenicity bridging studies, 52
Immunoglobulins, transfer in pregnancy, 16
Immunosuppression, 165-167, 212. See also *Impaired immunity.*
Imogam Rabies-HT (rabies immune globulin), 128t, 400
Imovax Rabies (RAB-HDC), 402t-404t
  CPT and ICD-9-CM codes, 127t
  safety, 400-401
Impact of vaccines/vaccination programs, 45-47, 46t, 191

30

Impaired immunity, 159-173
  close contacts, immunization of, 160-161, 161t
  general considerations, 159-162
  HIV infection, 167-169
  live vaccines, contraindications/precautions for, 160, 435
  medication-induced immunosuppression, 165-167
  official recommendations vs product labeling, 161-162
  passive immunoprophylaxis, 162
  pneumonia risk and, 450
  risk-benefit balance of vaccination, 159
  specific states other than HIV infection, 162-165
  vaccine contraindications/precautions, 250t, 255, 371, 401, 421, 435,
      477, 484
  vaccine recommendations, 250t-251t, 255, 313-314, 354, 450
Inactivated vaccines, 12t-13t, 15
  characteristics of, 18t-20t
  intervals for vaccination, 140
  vs live vaccines, 18t-20t, 35
Infanrix (DTaP), 272t-275t
  CPT and ICD-9-CM codes, 124t
  efficacy, 279
Infants. See also *Children.*
  hepatitis B vaccination, 175, 241-242, 314-315
  HIV-exposed/infected, 167-168
  pneumonia vaccination, 447, 448t
  preterm and low birth weight, 175
  rotavirus vaccination, 242, 421-422
  smallpox vaccination, precautions, 436
  varicella vaccination, 468
Infection
  control/elimination/eradication/extinction of agents, 44-45
  preventing, 21, 34-35
Infectious Diseases Society of America (IDSA), 88, 102, 506
Influenza, 333-356, 516t
  clinical features, 335
  epidemics and pandemics, 333-334, 336-337
    Spanish flu (1918), 333-334
  epidemiology and transmission, 335-337
  immunization program, 337-338
  mortality from, annual, 209, 336
  pathogen, 333-334
  strains, 333-337
    A(H1N1), 333, 339
      2009, 68, 334
        in 2010-2011 seasonal vaccine, 338
    A(H3N2), 333, 334, 339, 350
    A(H5N1), bird flu, 334, 335, 336
      vaccine for, 339
    B, 339
  vaccines for, 338-339, 340t-346t, 516t
    contraindications/precautions, 352-353
    cost-benefit analysis, 338
    coverage, 62, *63*

Influenza, vaccines for *(continued)*
   CPT and ICD-9-CM codes, 125t-126t, 127t, 131t-132t
   efficacy/immunogenicity, 339-347
   egg protein allergy and, 213-214, 338, 339, 351, 352
   Guillain-Barré syndrome and, 231, 351
   health care workers, vaccination of, 102, 181, 353
   IIV (inactivated), 340t-346t
     contraindications/precautions, 351
     differences from LAIV, 348t-349t
     efficacy/immunogenicity, 347-350
     high-dose, 343t-346t, 351
     production of, 338
     safety, 351
     TIV (trivalent inactivated influenza virus vaccine), 346t
   LAIV (live-attenuated), 343t-346t
     attenuation of, 14-15
     contraindications/precautions, 351-352, 353-354
     CPT and ICD-9-CM codes, 127t, 131t-132t
     differences from IIV, 348t-349t
     efficacy/immunogenicity, 350
     production of, 338-339
     safety, 352-353
   minimum ages and intervals, 143t
   in pregnancy, 173
   production of, 338-339
   recommendations, 254, 337-338, 353-355
     live vs inactivated vaccines, 348t-349t
     priority groups, 254, 354-355
     for travel, 183
     universal immunization, 353-354
   safety, 71t, 95t, 351-353
   schedule 255, 341t, 344t
     administration errors, and remedies, 153t
     adults, by age, 249t
     adults, by medical condition or indication, 250t
     children, age 0-6 years, 243t
     children, age 7-18 years, 245t
   shortages of, *84*
   swine flu, 68, 71t, 231
Injection techniques and sites, 116, *118*, 120t-121t
Injury. See *National Childhood Vaccine Injury Act; Vaccine Injury
    Compensation Program.*
Innate immune system, 23-24
Innate immunity, stimulating, 26-27
Institute for Vaccine Safety, Johns Hopkins Bloomberg School of
   Public Health, 507
Institute of Medicine (IOM)
  Immunization Safety Review Committee, 69, 70t-71t
  report on vaccine financing, 80t-81t
Intention-to-treat, 323
International adoptees, refugees, and immigrants, 178-179
International agencies, 506

30

Intervals for vaccinations
  grace period, 140-141
  inactivated vaccines, 140
  live vaccines, 139-140
  between live vaccines and antibody-containing blood products,
    148-149, 150t-151t
  minimum acceptable, 140-141, 142t-146t
  simultaneous administration, 139
Intramuscular (IM) administration of vaccines, 116, *118*, 120t-121t
Intramuscular (IM) immune globulin (IGIM), 17, 150t
Intranasal administration of vaccines, 116-117
Intravenous immune globulin (IGIV), 17, 150t, 169
Intussusception, 415, 421
Invasive pneumococcal disease (IPD), 439, 440. See also *Streptococcus pneumoniae.*
IOM. See *Institute of Medicine.*
IPOL (IPV), 253, 394t. See also *Polio, vaccines for.*
  CPT and ICD-9-CM codes, 126t
IPV. See *Polio, vaccines for.*
Isotype switching, 26
ISRC. See *Immunization Safety Review Committee.*
Ixiaro (JE-VC), 360t-361t
  CPT and ICD-9-CM codes, 126t

Japanese encephalitis, 357-364, 516t
  clinical features, 357
  epidemiology and transmission, 357-358
    endemic regions of world, 185t-187t
  immunization program, 358-359
  pathogen (Japanese encephalitis virus; JEV), 357
  vaccines for, 359, 360t-361t
    contraindications/precautions, 362
    CPT and ICD-9-CM codes, 126t
    efficacy/immunogenicity, 359
    JE-MB, 358, 359, 360t-361t
    JE-VC, 358-359, 360t-361t
    recommendations, 363
    safety, 362
    schedule/storage, 361t
JE-Vax (JE-MB), 126t, 360t-361t
Jenner, Edward, 14, 44
JEV (Japanese encephalitis virus). See *Japanese encephalitis.*

Kawasaki disease, 55-56, 236
Kidney failure, vaccination recommendations, 250t-251t, 354
Kinrix (DTaP-IPV), 242, 254, 492t-496t
  component vaccines/composition, 492t-493t
  CPT and ICD-9-CM codes, 124t
  schedule, 495t
Koplik's spots, 366

Laboratory workers, vaccination of, 188t, 302, 363, 388, 427, 437, 458, 477-478

LAIV (live-attenuated influenza vaccine), 343t-346t. See also *Influenza, vaccines for, LAIV (live-attenuated)*.

Langerhans cells, 24

Latex. See *specific vaccines.*

Leukemia, impaired immunity and. 169

Liability issues. See *National Childhood Vaccine Injury Act; National Vaccine Injury Compensation Program.*

Licensure. See *Vaccine development and licensure.*

Live-attenuated influenza vaccine. See *LAIV.*

Live-attenuated vaccines, 12t-13t

Live vaccines, 11, 12t-13t
  characteristics of, 18t-20t
  contraindications, 155, 160, 166
  impaired immunity and, 160, 166
  intervals for receipt of antibody-containing products, 148-149, 150t-151t
  intervals for vaccinations, 139-140
  live-attenuated, 12t-13t
  pregnancy and, 155, 174
  vs inactivated vaccines, 18t-20t, 35

Liver disease, vaccination recommendations, 250t-251t, 302, 313, 354

Local anesthetics, 117

Lockjaw, 268

Long-term care facilities, 189t, 355

Low birth weight infants, 175

Lung disease, vaccination recommendations, 250t-251t

Lyssavirus, 397. See also *Rabies.*

Mad cow disease (MCD), vaccines and, 233-234

Major histocompatibility complex (MHC)
  class I molecules (MHC-I), 30-33, 34
  class II molecules (MHC-II), 24, *31*
  genes for, 43

Mandates for vaccination, 102-103

Manufacturers of vaccines, 508
  different, interchangeability of vaccines, 147
  number of, 82

Marketing claims, package insert and, 56

MCV4, 381, 384t-386t. See also *Neisseria meningitidis.*
  contraindications/precautions, 156, 388
  coverage, 62
  efficacy/immunogenicity, 382-387
  Guillain-Barré syndrome and, 231-232, 388
  licensure of, 39, 382, 383, 387
  MCV4-CRM, 382, 384t-386t, 388
  MCV4-D, 383-387, 384t-386t, 388
  recommendations, 255, 382, 388-389
  safety, 387-388
  schedule, 255, 385t
    administration errors, and remedies, 153t
    adults, by age, 249t
    adults, by medical condition/indication, 251t
    children, age 0-6 years, 243t

30

MCV4, schedule *(continued)*
  children, age 7-18 years, 245t
  minimum ages and intervals, 143t
shortages of, *84*
vs MPSV, 147, 384t-386t
Measles, Mumps, Rubella, 365-377, 516t
  clinical features, 366-367
  criteria for immunity, 373, 374t-375t
  epidemiology and transmission, 367-369
  immunization program, 369
  measles immune globulin, 376
  measles outbreak in Indiana, 204-208
  morbidity and mortality from, 46t, 209
  pathogens, 365
  vaccines for (MMR), 370, 372t-373t
    combination. See *MMRV.*
    contraindications/precautions, 371-373, 435-436
    coverage, 61, *61*
    CPT and ICD-9-CM codes, 127t, 131t
    efficacy/immunogenicity, 370-371
    impact of vaccine refusal, 204-208
    interval for receipt of antibody-containing products, 150t-151t
    recommendations, 373-376
    reportable events, 94t
    safety, 217, 371-373
      autism concerns, 219-222, *221*, *223*, 225-226
      fear of MMR, public harm from, 204-208, 206t
      thimerosol concerns, 208, 225-229
    schedule, 254, 372t
      adults, by age, 249t
      adults, by medical condition/indication, 250t
      catch-up, children age 4 months-6 years, 247t
      catch-up, children age 7-18 years, 248t
      children, age 0-6 years, 243t
      children, age 7-18 years, 245t
      minimum ages and intervals, 143t
    vs MMRV, 369
Medicaid, 63, 79, 80t, 505
Medicare, 78, 505
Medication-induced immunosuppression, 165-167
Membrane attack complex, 21
Membranous nasopharyngitis, 268
Memory B-cells, *25*, 26, 29
Men who have sex with men, vaccination of, 188t, 302, 313
Menactra (MCV4), 255, 384t-386t
  CPT and ICD-9-CM codes, 127t
MenHibrix, CPT and ICD-9-CM codes, 125t
Meningitis, 379-380. See also *Neisseria meningitidis.*
  bacterial, 439
  Hib and, 288
Meningococcal disease, vaccines for, 147. See also *Neisseria meningitidis.*
Meningococcal polysaccharide conjugate vaccine, 4-valent. See *MPSV4.*

Meningococcemia, 379

Meningococcemia, chronic, 379-380

Meningococcus, endemic regions of world, 185t-187t

Meningococcus. See *Neisseria meningitidis.*

Menomune-A/C/Y/W-135 (MPSV4), 255, 384t-386t
  CPT and ICD-9-CM codes, 127t

Menveo (MCV4-CRM), 255, 384t-386t
  CPT and ICD-9-CM codes, 127t

Mercury in vaccines/thimerosol, 224

MHC, MHC-I, MHC-II. See *Major histocompatibility complex.*

Military personnel, vaccination of, 338
  anthrax vaccination, 259, 262
  smallpox vaccination, 434-435

Minimum acceptable intervals for vaccinations, 140-141, 142t-146t

Minimum age for vaccination, 141, 142t-146t

Misinformation, 200-204

Missed opportunities, 109

MMR vaccine. See *Measles, Mumps, Rubella, vaccines for.*

MMRV vaccine, 254, 369
  combination vaccines, 498t-502t
  contraindications/precautions, 373, 468, 497
  interval for receipt of antibody-containing products, 150t-151t
  in pediatric schedule, 244t
  safety issues, 491-497
  schedule/recommendations, 497
  shortages of, *84*
  vs MMR, 369

Monitoring
  for adverse events. See *Vaccine Adverse Event Reporting System.*
  for vaccine delivery, 60-64
  for vaccine effectiveness, 64-65

Morbidity and mortality, from vaccine-preventable diseases, 46t

Morbidity and Mortality Weekly Report, 58-59

Mortality, from vaccine-preventable diseases, 46t

Morticians, vaccination of, 188t

Mosquitoes
  Aedes aegypti, yellow fever and, 473-474, 478
  control/avoidance of, 474, 477
  Culex, Japanese encephalitis and, 358

MPSV4 (meningococcal polysaccharide conjugate vaccine, 4-valent),
    381, 384t-386t, 387. See also *Neisseria meningitidis.*
  CPT and ICD-9-CM codes, 127t
  minimum ages and intervals, 143t
  recommendations, 255
  safety, 387
  schedule
    adults, by age, 249t
    adults, by medical condition/indication, 251t
  vs MCV, 147

Multidose vaccine series, dosing intervals, 141

Multiple sclerosis, vaccines and, 232, 310-311

Multiple vaccines, simultaneous administration of, 70t, 113-116, 139
  immune overload concerns, 210-212, 211t
  number of antigens, 211t

Mumps, 365-377. See also *Measles, Mumps, Rubella.*
  clinical features, 366-367
  criteria for immunity, 373, 374t-375t
  epidemiology and transmission, 368
  immunization program, 369
  pathogen, 365
  resurgence of, 46, *46*
  vaccines for, 370, 372t-373t
    contraindications/precautions, 371-373
    efficacy/immunogenicity, 370
    recommendations, 373-376
    safety, 371-373
Mycobacterium bovis, 14

Nabi-HB (hepatitis B immune globulin), 307
  CPT and ICD-9-CM codes, 128t
National Center for Immunization and Respiratory Diseases (NCIRD), 56, 505
National Childhood Vaccine Injury Act, 66, 68, 91-97
National Committee for Quality Assurance, 64
National Drug Codes (NDCs), 134
National Foundation for Infectious Diseases (NFID), 507
National Health Interview Survey (NHIS), 62, 507
National Immunization Survey (NIS), 60-62, *61*, 508
National Institutes of Health (NIH), *57*, 505
National Network for Immunization Information (NNii), 507
National Notifiable Disease Surveillance System (NNDSS), 64, 508
National Nursing Home Survey, 63
National Respiratory and Enteric Surveillance System (NREVSS), 64-65
National Vaccine Advisory Committee (NVAC), 60, 506
  financing recommendations, 80t-81t
  pediatric immunization standards, 88-91
National Vaccine Injury Compensation Program (VICP), 90, 505
National Vaccine Plan, 59-60
National Vaccine Program Office (NVPO), *57*, 59, 506
Native Americans and Alaskans
  Hib infection and, 287, 288
  pneumonia and, 440
  vaccination of, 188t
Natural infection, vs immunization, 209-210
NCIRD. See *National Center for Immunization and Respiratory Diseases.*
Necessity for vaccines, 208-209
Necrotizing fasciitis, 212
Needle length, 116, *118*
Needlestick injuries, 97-102
Needlestick Safety and Prevention Act, 97
Negri bodies, 397
Neisseria meningitidis, 379-390, 516t
  clinical features, 379-380
  epidemiology and transmission, 380
  immunization program, 381-382
  pathogen, 379

Neisseria meningitidis (continued)
  vaccines for, 382, 384t-386t, 516t. See also *MCV4; MPSV4.*
    contraindications/precautions, 388
    cost-benefit analysis, 381-382
    efficacy/immunogenicity, 382-387
    herd effects, 381
    MCV4-CRM, 382, 387
    MCV4-D, 383-387, 384t-386t
    MPSV4, 381, 384t-386t, 387
    recommendations, 388-389
    safety, 387-388
    schedule, 385t
Neomycin, allergy to, 214
Nephrotic syndrome, pneumonia vaccination in, 451t
Neurotropic disease, vaccine-associated, 476
Neutralization of viruses/toxins, 21
New Vaccine Surveillance Network (NVSN), 64
Nomenclature, 516t-517t
Noninferiority, 52, 490
NVAC. See *National Vaccine Advisory Committee.*
NVPO. See *National Vaccine Program Office.*
NVSN. See *New Vaccine Surveillance Network.*

Observation period after vaccination, 117-119
Obstructive laryngotracheitis, 268
Occupational Safety and Health Administration (OSHA), 97-102
Office visit
  coding for, example, 134, 135t
  communicating about vaccines in, 195-197
Omnibus Autism Proceedings, 225-226
-OMP suffix, 517t (footnote)
Opsonization, 21
OPV. See *Polio, vaccines for.*
Oral administration of vaccines, 116
Original polysaccharide sin, 23
Oropharyngeal cancers, 320
OSHA. See *Occupational Safety and Health Administration.*
Otitis media, 440, 442, 462

Package insert (PI), 54-56
Pain, dealing with, 117
Palivizumab (RSV-mAb), 131t
Pan American Health Organization (PAHO), 506
Pap test, 320
Parents of Kids With Infectious Diseases (PKID), 507
PARSIFAL study, 217
Partial doses, 141
Passive immunization, 16-17
Passive immunoprophylaxis, 162
Pasteur, Louis, 14, 15
Pathogen-specific molecular patterns, 24
PATRICIA (Papilloma Trial Against Cancer In Young Adults), 3
Patternicity, 194

30

PCECV. See *RabAvert.*

PCV7. See *Pneumococcal vaccines, PCV7.*

PCV13. See *Pneumococcal vaccines, PCV13.*

Pediarix (DTaP-HepB-IPV), 242, 253, 492t-496t
  component vaccines/composition, 492t-493t
  CPT and ICD-9-CM codes, 124t
  schedule, 495t

Pediatric immunization practices. See also *Children.*
  CPT codes for, 130t-131t
  standards for, 88-91

Pediatric Infectious Diseases Society (PIDS), 506

PedvaxHIB (Hib-OMP), 252, 288-289, 290t-292t
  CPT and ICD-9-CM codes, 125t
  efficacy/immunogenicity, 288-289
  recommendations, 289-293

Penile cancers, 320

Pentacel (DTaP-IPV/Hib), 242, 252-253, 492t-496t
  component vaccines/composition, 492t-493t
  CPT and ICD-9-CM codes, 124t

Pentavalent rotavirus vaccine (PRV). See *RotaTeq (rotavirus, RV5).*

Periorbital cellulitis, 287

Permissive statements, 59

Pertactin (PRN), 267, 272t, 493t

Pertussis, 267-286, 516t
  catarrhal, paroxysmal, and convalescent stages, 268
  clinical features, 268-269
  epidemiology and transmission, 269-270
  immunity from natural infection, 281
  immunization program, 271
  incidence, 270
  morbidity and mortality from, 46t
  pathogen, 267
  resurgence of, 46t
  toxin (PT), 267
  vaccines for, 15, 272t-275t
    acellular, 271
    adult. See *Tdap vaccine.*
    children/infants. See *DTaP vaccine.*
    combination vaccines, 492t-496t
    contraindications/precautions, 279-281
    correlates of protection, 39
    efficacy/immunogenicity, 271-279
    encephalopathy and, 155, 204
    recommendations, 281-283
    safety, 94t, 279-281
    safety fears, 216
      brain damage, 229-231
      public cost of, 204, 206t
    schedule, 274t
    whole-cell, 271
  waning immunity and, 271

Phagocyte disorders, 163

Phase 1, 2, 3, and 4 trials, 51-54, *51*

Physical examination, no requirement for, 149

PI. See *Package insert*.

"Pink Book" (*Epidemiology and Prevention of Vaccine-Preventable Diseases*), iv, 59

Plasma cells, 21-23, *22*, 29

Pneumococcal vaccines, 440-452, 444t-446t, 517t. See also *Streptococcus pneumoniae*.
  contraindications/precautions, 447
  cost-benefit analysis, 441
  efficacy/immunogenicity, 442-443
  immunization program, 440-442
  minimum ages and intervals, 143t-144t
  PCV7 (pneumococcal conjugate vaccine, 7-valent), 442, 442t-446t
    contraindications/precautions, 447
    coverage, 61, *61*, *63*
    CPT and ICD-9-CM codes, 127t
    efficacy/immunogenicity, 442-443
    herd immunity and, *42*, 43
    recommendations, 441, 447, 449t
    replacement with PCV13, 441-442, 449t
    safety, 443-447
    schedule, 253, 445t, 451t
      catch-up, children age 4 months-6 years, 246t-247t
      children, age 0-6 years, 243t
    shortages of, *84*
  PCV13, 47, 442, 444t-446t
    CPT and ICD-9-CM codes, 127t
    efficacy/immunogenicity, 442-443
    recommendations, 447-448, 448t, 449t
    replacement of PCV7 with, 441-442, 449t
    safety, 447
    schedule, 253, 445t, 448t, 451t
  Pnu-Immune 23, 440
  PPSV23, 440-441, 442, 444t-446t
    CPT and ICD-9-CM codes, 127t
    efficacy/immunogenicity, 443, 450
    number of doses, reactogenicity and, 147
    recommendations, 183, 448-450
    safety, 447, 487
    schedule, 253, 445t, 451t
      administration errors, and remedies, 154t
      adults, by age, 249t
      adults, by medical condition/indication, 250t
      children, age 7-18 years, 245t
  recommendations, 447-450, 448t, 449t, 451t
  risk categories for IPD, 448-450
  safety, 95t, 443-447
  scenarios for/optimizing use of, 451t
  schedule, 445t, 449t, 451t

Pneumonia, 439-440. See also *Pneumococcal vaccines; Streptococcus pneumoniae*
  from Hib, 287

30

Pneumovax 23 (PPSV23), 440-441, 442, 444t-446t. See also *Pneumococcal vaccines, PPSV23.*
  CPT and ICD-9-CM codes, 127t
  recommendations, 448-450
  safety, 447, 487
Pnu-Immune 23, 440
Policy. See *Vaccine policy.*
Polio, 391-396, 516t
  clinical features, 391
  eliminated from United States, 45, 392
  epidemiology and transmission, 391-392
    endemic regions of world, 185t-187t
  eradication initiative, 392-393
  immunization program, 392-393
  morbidity and mortality from, 46t
  pathogen, 391
  vaccines for, 393, 394t
    AIDS pandemic, concerns about, 234-235
    cancer and, concerns about, 234
    contraindications/precautions, 395
    inactivated (IPV), 15, 393, 394t
      combination vaccines, 253-254, 492t-496t
      contraindications/precautions, 395
      efficacy/immunogenicity, 393
      minimum ages and intervals for, 143t
      recommendations, 395
      safety, 94t, 395
      schedule, 253-254, 394t, 395
        catch-up, children 7-18 years, 248t
        catch-up, children age 4 months-6 years, 247t
        children, age 0-6 years, 243t
        children, age 7-18 years, 245t
    oral (OPV), 393
      efficacy/immunogenicity, 393
      reportable events, 94t, 191
    recommendations, 393, 395
      travel in endemic areas, 183
    safety, 191, 395
    SV40 contamination and, 70t, 234
Poliomyelitis. See *Polio.*
Polyclonal immune globulins, 16, 17
Polysaccharide vaccines, 16, 30
  hyporesponsiveness and, 23
  protein-polysaccharide vaccines, 16, 30, *31*
    advantages of, 32t
  pure, 16, 23
Postherpetic neuralgia (PHN), 481, 484
Postpartum women, vaccinations for, 110, 148, 252, 271, 282
Power outages, 107t
PPSV23. See *Pneumococcal vaccines, PPSV23.*
Precautions. See *Contraindications and precautions.*
Pregnancy, 173-175
  FDA Pregnancy Categories, 173-174

Pregnancy *(continued)*
  natural immunization of fetus during, 16
  rubella in, effects on fetus, 367
  typhoid, transplacental transmission of, 454
  vaccination during, 173-175, 176t-177t, 250t-251t
    contraindications/precautions, 155, 255, 264t, 301, 329, 353, 371,
      395, 435, 467, 468, 477
    hepatitis B, 306-307
    influenza vaccines, 173, 176t, 354
    live vaccines, 174
    MMR, 373
    pertussis, 271
    pneumonia vaccination, 450
    Tdap and Td vaccines, 176t, 250t, 252, 282-283
    tetanus and diphtheria boosters, 174, 282-283
    VariZIG, 174-175
    yellow fever vaccination, 155, 478
Prescription Drug User Fee Act (PDUFA), 54
Preservative-free vaccines, 229. See also *specific vaccines.*
Preservatives, 224-229. See also *specific vaccines.*
Preterm and low birth weight infants, 175, 314, 421
Prevention of infection. See *Infection, preventing.*
Prevnar (PCV7-CRM), 253, 442, 444t-446t. See also *Pneumococcal
  vaccines, PCV7.*
  CPT and ICD-9-CM codes, 127t
  replacement with Prevnar 13 (PCV13), 441-442, 449t
  safety, 443-447
  schedule/recommendations, 441, 445t, 447, 449t, 451t
Prevnar 13 (PCV13-CRM), 442, 444t-446t. See also *Pneumococcal
  vaccines, PCV13.*
  replacement of Prevnar (PCV7) with, 441-442, 449t
  safety, 447
  schedule/recommendations, 445t, 447-448, 449t, 451t
Primary immunization, 27-28, *28*
Primary vaccine failures, 29
Prions, 233-234
Probabilistic thinking, 192-195
Production problems, 82
Professional associations, 506
Proguanil therapy, 458
ProQuad (MMRV), 254, 498t-502t
  component vaccines/composition, 498t-499t
  CPT and ICD-9-CM codes, 127t
Protein-polysaccharide vaccines, 30, *31*. See also *specific vaccines.*
  advantages of, 32t
Protest organizations (antivaccination), 201-204, 201t-203t
Pseudomembranes, 267
Public health, 44-47. See also *Concerns about vaccines, addressing.*
  immunization programs, goals of, 44-45
  impact of vaccines/vaccination programs, 45-47, 46t, 191
  risks of refusal of vaccination, 197-200
Public Health Service Act, 78
Public safety workers, vaccination of, 189t

30

Purified subunits, 12t-13t, 15
Purpura fulminans, 379. See also *Neisseria meningitidis.*

Questions about vaccines. See *Concerns about vaccines, addressing.*

RAB-HDC. See *Imovax Rabies.*
RAB-PCEC. See *RabAvert.*
RabAvert (RAB-PCEC), 402t-404t
  CPT and ICD-9-CM codes, 127t
  safety, 401
Rabbit complement assay, 383
Rabies, 397-411, 516t
  clinical features, 397-398
  death from, 398
  epidemiology and transmission, 398
  immune globulin (HRIG), 399, 400, 410t
  immunization program, 399
  pathogen, 397
  vaccines for, 400, 402t-404t. See also *Rabies immune globulin,
    human (HRIG).*
    administration errors, and remedies, 154t
    for animal handlers, 102
    contraindications/precautions, 401
    CPT and ICD-9-CM codes, 127t
    efficacy/immunogenicity, 400
    postexposure prophylaxis, 399, 400, 408t-409t
      regimens, 410t-411t
    pre-exposure prophylaxis, 399, 406t-407t
    recommendations, 401, 406t-409t
    safety, 400-401
    schedule/regimens, 403t, 410t-411t
    vaccination of wildlife, 398
Rabies immune globulin, human (HRIG), 399, 400, 410t
  contraindications/precautions, 401
  efficacy/immunogenicity, 400
  interval for receipt of live vaccines, 151t
  regimens, 410t
  safety, 401
Ramsay Hunt syndrome, 482
Reactions. See *Adverse events.*
Reassortment, 14, 333
Recall and tracking systems, 108-109
Recombinant DNA technology, 16
Recombinant subunit vaccines, 12t-13t
Recombivax HB (HepB), 241-242, 308t-310t
  CPT and ICD-9-CM codes, 125t
  dosing, 309t, 312
  efficacy/immunogenicity, 311
Recommendations, 139-158. See also *specific vaccines.*
  ACIP, 58-59
  agencies involved with, 56-60, 57
  contraindications and precautions, 155-156
  general rules for vaccination, 139-155

Recommendations *(continued)*
  permissive statements, 59
  risk-based immunization, 59
  routine immunization, 59
  schedules for routine vaccinations, 241-256
  vaccine handling, storage, and transport, 105-108
  vs package insert information, 55, 156
Reconstitution of vaccine, 113
Recurrent respiratory papillomatosis, 320
"Red Book" (Report of the Committee on Infectious Diseases), iv, 59
Refrigerators and freezers, 105-106, 107t
Refugees, international, 178-179
Refusal of vaccination, 197-200
  impact of, examples, 204-208, 206t-207t
  Refusal to Vaccinate form, 198-199
Registries. See *Immunization Information Systems (IISs).*
Regulations. See *Standards, principles, and regulations.*
Religious exemptions, 103
Reminder, recall, and tracking systems, 108-109
Report of the Committee on Infectious Diseases. See *"Red Book".*
Reportable Events Table, 94t-95t
Respiratory syncytial virus (RSV), monoclonal antibody to (RSVmAB),
    17, 131t, 150t
Respiratory syncytial virus (RSV) immune globulins, 129t
REST (Rotavirus Efficacy and Safety Trial), 416, 417
Reverse genetics, 338
Reye syndrome, 353, 354, 462, 467
Rhesus rotavirus vaccine, tetravalent. See *RRV-TV.*
RhoGAM (IM), 151t
Risks
  of daily activities, 191-192
  of delayed vaccination, 215
  known vs unknown, 193
  perceived, 193
Risks and benefits of vaccines
  communicating about, 191-197, 208-236
  in impaired immunity, 159
  public health risk of vaccine refusals, 197-200
  safety and utility of vaccines, 191-197
  thought processes about, 192-195
  weighing, 155-156, 173, 191-192, 210
The River: A Journey to the Source of HIV and AIDS (Hooper), 234
Rose spots, 453
Rotarix (rotavirus, RV1), 242, 416, 418t-420t
  composition, 416, 418t
  CPT and ICD-9-CM codes, 127t
  efficacy/immunogenicity, 417
  safety, 417-421
RotaShield (RRV-TV), 69-72, 415
RotaTeq (rotavirus, RV5), 242, 415, 418t-420t. See also *Rotavirus, vaccines for.*
  composition, 416, 418t
  cost of development of, 49

30

RotaTeq (rotavirus, RV5) *(continued)*
  CPT and ICD-9-CM codes, 127t
  efficacy/immunogenicity, 416
  safety, 55-56, 417
Rotavirus, 413-423, 516t
  clinical features, 413-414
  epidemics, 414
  epidemiology and transmission, 414
  immunization program, 415-416
  office visits, hospitalizations, and deaths, annual, 414
  pathogen, 413
  Rotavirus Efficacy and Safety Trial (REST), 416, 417
  vaccines for, 14, 416, 418t-420t
    composition, 416, 418t
    contraindications/precautions, 421
    cost-benefit analysis, 415
    CPT and ICD-9-CM codes, 127t, 130t-131t
    efficacy/immunogenicity, 416-417
    minimum ages and intervals, 144t
    monitoring, 64-65
    recommendations, 421-422
    RRV-TV, 415
    RV-1, 416, 418t-420t
    RV-5, 415, 418t-420t
    safety, 95t, 417-421
      Kawasaki disease concerns, 236
    schedule, 242, 419t
      catch-up, children, 4 months-6 years, 246t
      children, age 0-6 years, 243t
Routes of inoculation, 15
RRV-TV (rhesus rotavirus vaccine; RotaShield), 69-72, 415
RSV. See *Respiratory syncytial virus (RSV).*
Rubella, 365-377, 516t. See also *Measles, Mumps, Rubella.*
  clinical features, 367
  criteria for immunity, 373, 374t-375t
  eliminated from United States, 45
  epidemiology and transmission, 368-369
  immunization program, 369
  morbidity and mortality from, 46t
  pathogen, 365
  in pregnant women, 367
  vaccines for, 370, 372t-373t
    contraindications/precautions, 371-373
    CPT and ICD-9-CM codes, 127t, 131t
    efficacy/immunogenicity, 370-371
    recommendations, 373-376
    safety, 94t, 371-373
Rubeola. See *Measles.*
Rules for vaccination. See *Recommendations.*

Sabin, Albert, 11
Sabin Vaccine Institute (SVI), 507
Safety net. See *Vaccine Safety Net.*

Safety of vaccines. See also *Vaccine Safety Net; And specific vaccines.*
  communicating about, 191-197, 208-236
  definitions of, 191-192
  ISRC findings, 70t-71t
  specific concerns, 208-236
Salicylate use. See *Aspirin use.*
Salk, Jonas, 15
Salmonella enterica. See *Salmonella typhi.*
Salmonella typhi, 14, 453. See also *Typhoid fever.*
Schedules for immunizations, 241-256. See also *specific vaccines.*
  adults, by age group, 249t
  adults, by medical condition, 250t-251t
  catch-up schedule, children age 4 months-6 years, 246t-247t
  catch-up schedule, children age 7-18 years, 248t
  children, age 0-6 years, 243t-244t
  children, age 7-18 years, 245t
  modified/alternative, 199, 214-215
  specific vaccines,, s for, 241-256
SCHIP (State Children's Health Insurance Program), 78
School mandates, 102-103
School surveys, 62-63
Screening for contraindications/precautions/other problems,
    113, 114t-115t
Section 317 Funds, *73,* 78, 111
Serial passage, 11-14
Seroconversion, testing for, 149
Serology, 149
Serotype replacement, 43
Sewage workers, 189t
Sharps use and precautions, 100-101
Shingles. See *Zoster (herpes zoster; shingles).*
Shortages of vaccines, 79-83, 84
Sickle cell disease, 164
  pneumonia and, 440
  pneumonia vaccination, 451t
Side effects. See *Adverse events.*
SIDS. See *Sudden infant death syndrome.*
Simian immunodeficiency virus (SIV), 234-235
Simian virus 40 (SV40), 70t, 234
Smallpox, 425-438, 517t
  bioterrorism potential of, 44, 426
  clinical features, 425-426
  diagnosis of, 426, 428t-429t
  eradication of, 44-45, 426
  immunization program, 427-430
  morbidity and mortality from, 46t
  pathogen, 425
  Smallpox Health Care Teams, 437
  Smallpox Response Teams, 430
  vaccines for, 430-433, 431t
    ACAM2000, 431t, 433-434
    amount available, 430
    contraindications/precautions, 435-436

Smallpox, vaccines for *(continued)*
    CPT and ICD-9-CM codes, 127t
    Dryvax, 430, 433
       vs ACAM2000, 433-434
    efficacy/immunogenicity, 433-434
    handling and administration, 116, 430-433
    injury compensation program, 436
    postevent vaccination, 427, 436-437
    pre-event vaccination, 427, 436
    recommendations, 427-430, 436-438
    ring vaccination (surveillance and containment), 427
    safety, 434-436
    schedule, 139, 431t
    vaccinia immune globulin (VIG), 436
    variola major and minor, 425-426
    variola virus, 425-426
    vs chickenpox, 428t-429t
Special circumstances, 159-190
    health care personnel, 179-181
    impaired immunity, 159-173
      general considerations, 159-162
      hematopoietic stem cell transplantation and leukemia, 169, 170t-172t
      HIV infection, 167-169
      medication-induced immunosuppression, 165-167
      specific states other than HIV infection, 162-165
    international adoptees, refugees, and immigrants, 178-179
    other special circumstances, 184, 188t-189t
    pregnancy and breast-feeding, 173-175, 176t-177t
    preterm and low birth weight infants, 175
    travel, 182-184, 185t-187t
Spelunkers, 189t
Split doses, 141
Squamous cell carcinoma of the cervix, 319
Standards, principles, and regulations, 87-104
    Bloodborne Pathogens Standard, 97-102
    CBER, for vaccine development, 49-51
    federal requirements regarding vaccination, 98t-99t
    Healthy People 2010 and 2020, 87
    immunization practices, standards, 88-91
      adult, 91, 92t
      pediatric, 88-91
    National Childhood Vaccine Injury Act, 91-97
    Occupational Safety and Health Administration, 97-102
    school mandates and state legislation, 102-103
Standing orders, 110-111
    for birth dose, HepB vaccination, 312
    for emergencies, 119
Staphylococcus aureus, secondary infections in varicella, 462
State and local funds for vaccination, *73,* 78
State Children's Health Insurance Program (SCHIP), 78
State health department immunization program web sites, 508
State legislation on vaccinations, 102-103
Status quo, maintaining, 194

Steroids, impaired immunity and, 166-167
Storage of vaccines, 105-108. See also *specific vaccines.*
  during emergencies, 107t
Streptococcus pneumoniae, 439-452, 517t
  clinical features, 439-440
    invasive pneumococcal disease (IPD), 439, 440
  epidemiology and transmission, 440
  immunization program, 440-442
  morbidity and mortality from, 46t, 440
  newborn protection against, 16
  pathogen, 439
  replacement disease, 441
  risk categories for IPD, 448-450
  vaccines for, 442, 444t-446t. See also *Pneumococcal vaccines.*
    cost-benefit analysis, 441
    efficacy/immunogenicity, 442-443
    recommendations, 447-450
    safety, 443-447
    scenarios for/optimizing use of, 451t
    schedule, 447-448, 448t, 449t
Students. See *College students.*
Subcutaneous (SC) administration of vaccines, 116, *118*, 120t-121t
Subunits
  engineered, 12t-13t, 16
  purified, 12t-13t, 15
  recombinant, 12t-13t
Sudden infant death syndrome (SIDS), vaccinations and, 71t, 235
Supply of vaccines, 79-83, *84*
Surrogates of protection, 36-39, 38t
Surveillance, 64-72
SV40 contamination of polio vaccine, 70t, 234
Swine flu vaccine, 68, 71t, 231
Synagis (RSV immune globulin, monoclonal, IM), 129t
Syncope, 119

T-cell dependent response, 30
T-cell independent antigens and responses, 23, 30
T-cell receptor (TCR), 24, *25*, 30
T cells, cytotoxic. See *Cytotoxic T cells.*
T lymphocytes, helper (Th-cells), 24-26, *25*, 33
Task Force on Safer Childhood Vaccines (TFSCV), 68-69
TB. See *Tuberculosis.*
Tc cells. See *Cytotoxic T cells.*
Td (tetanus, diphtheria) vaccine, 276t-278t
  contraindications/precautions, 280-281
  CPT and ICD-9-CM codes, 127t
  indications, 277t
  minimum ages and intervals for, 144t
  recommendations
    boosters, 252
    pregnancy, 176t
    travel, 183-184

30

Td (tetanus, diphtheria) vaccine *(continued)*
  schedule, 252, 277t
    adults, by age, 249t
    adults, by medical condition/indication, 250t
    catch-up, children age 7-18 years, 248t
  shortages of, *84*
Tdap vaccine, 39, 252, 272t-275t. See also *Adacel; Boostrix; DTaP.*
  adolescent immunization, 271
  contraindications/precautions, 279-280
  CPT and ICD-9-CM codes, 128t
  efficacy/immunogenicity, 279
  health care workers, vaccination of, 102, 181
  intervals for vaccination, 144t
  minimum ages and intervals, 144t
  in pregnancy, 176t
  recommendations, 252, 281-283
  safety, 279-281
  schedule, 252, 274t
    administration errors, and remedies, 154t
    adults, by age, 249t
    adults, by medical condition/indication, 250t
    catch-up, children, age 7-18 years, 248t
    children, age 7-18 years, 245t
Terrorism. See *Bioterrorism.*
Tetanospasmin, 267
Tetanus, 267-286, 516t
  clinical features, 268
  epidemiology and transmission, 269
  immunization program, 270
  morbidity and mortality from, 46t
  pathogen, 267
  toxin, 267, 272t
  toxoid. See *Tetanus toxoid (TT).*
  vaccination for travel, 183-184
  vaccines for, 252, 272t-278t, 516t. See also *DT; Tetanus toxoid (TT).*
    adult. See *Tdap vaccine.*
    children/infants. See *DTaP vaccine.*
    combination vaccines, 492t-496t
    contraindications/precautions, 279-281
    CPT and ICD-9-CM codes, 127t-128t
    efficacy/immunogenicity, 271-279
    indications, 273t, 277t
    minimum ages and intervals, 144t
    recommendations
      general use, 281-283
      wound management, 284t-285t
    safety, 94t, 279-281
    schedule, 274t, 277t
Tetanus immune globulin (TIG)
  for at-risk HIV-infected children, 162
  CPT and ICD-9-CM codes, 129t
  interval for receipt of live vaccines, 151t

Tetanus Toxoid Adsorbed (TT), 276t-278t
  CPT and ICD-9-CM codes, 124t, 127t
Tetanus toxoid (TT), 276t-278t
  contraindications/precautions, 147, 280-281
  CPT and ICD-9-CM codes, 124t, 127t-128t
  recommendations, 284t-285t
Th-cells (helper T lymphocytes), 24-26, *25*, 33, *33*
Th1-cells, 26, 33, *33*
Thimerosal, 224-229. See also *specific vaccines.*
  autism and, 224-229, *227*, *228*
  in MMR, concerns about, 208
  safety findings, 70t
Thrombocytopenia/thrombocytopenic purpura, 371
TIG. See *Tetanus immune globulin.*
Timeliness, 60-64
TIV, 346t
TLRs. See *Toll-like receptors (TLRs).*
Toll-like receptors (TLRs), 24
Topical anesthetics, 117
Toxins
  concerns about, 213
  diphtheria, tetanus, and pertussis, 267, 272t
  enterotoxin, rotavirus, 413
  neutralization of, 21
  typhoid, 453
Toxoid vaccines, 12t-13t, 15, 276t-278t
Tracheal cytotoxin, 267
Tracking systems, 108-109
Transplantation, impaired immunity and, 165-166, 169, 170t-172t
Transportation of vaccines, 106-108
Travel, vaccination for, 182-184, 185t-187t, 297, 302, 355, 363, 388, 459, 477
Trials, clinical, 51-54, *51*
TriHIBit (DTaP/Hib), 242, 252, 492t-496t
  component vaccines/composition, 492t-493t
  CPT and ICD-9-CM codes, 124t
Tripedia (DTaP), 272t-275t
  CPT and ICD-9-CM codes, 124t
  efficacy, 271-279
TT. See *Tetanus toxoid (TT).*
Tuberculosis (TB), untreated, as precaution for vaccination, 468, 484
TViPSV. See *Typhim Vi.*
Twinrix (HepA-HepB), 242, 255, 498t-502t
  component vaccines/composition, 498t
  CPT and ICD-9-CM codes, 125t
Typhim Vi (TViPSV, pure polysaccharide vaccine), 445, 456t-457t
  CPT and ICD-9-CM codes, 128t
  efficacy/immunogenicity, 455
  safety, 458
Typhoid fever, 453-460, 517t
  clinical features, 453-454
  epidemiology and transmission, 454
    endemic regions of world, 185t-187t

30

Typhoid fever *(continued)*
  immunization program, 454-455
  multidrug-resistant infection, 454-455
  pathogen, 453
  vaccines for, 445, 456t-457t
    contraindications/precautions, 458
    CPT and ICD-9-CM codes, 128t
    efficacy/immunogenicity, 455-458
    engineered attenuation of, 14-15
    interval for other live vaccine, 139-140
    recommendations, 459
    safety, 458

Universal precautions, 100-101
US Agency for International Development (USAID), 506
US Food and Drug Administration. See *Food and Drug Administration
  (FDA)*.
Utility of vaccines, 192

Vaccinate Your Baby, 507
Vaccination. See also *Immunization; Vaccinology*.
  basic concepts, 11-48
  costs-benefit analysis of, 47
  goals of, 44-45
  public health impact, 45-47, 46t, 191
  reduction in morbidity/mortality from, 46t
Vaccination programs, 44-47, 46t. See also *Immunization programs*.
Vaccination refusal. See *Refusal of vaccination*.
Vaccine Adverse Event Reporting System (VAERS), 66-67, 90,
  96, 98t, 505
Vaccine and Treatment Evaluation Unit (VTEU), *57*
Vaccine court, 225-226
Vaccine development and licensure, 49-56. See also *Vaccine
  infrastructure*.
  agencies involved with, 56-60, *57*
  Biologics License Application (BLA), 54
  clinical trials, 51-54
  financial risk in, 49
  package insert (PI), 54-56
  process of, *50*
Vaccine immunology, 17-35. See also *Immune response*.
Vaccine Information Statements (VISs), 89, 97, 98t
Vaccine infrastructure in the United States, 49-86
  financing, 72-79
  monitoring delivery, 60-64
  monitoring effectiveness, 64-65
  policy and recommendations, 56-60
  supply, 79-83, *84*
  vaccine development and licensure, 49-56
  Vaccine Safety Net, 65-72
Vaccine Injury Compensation Program (VICP), 92-96, 505
  covered vaccines, 99t
  important point, 96
  Reportable Events Table, 94t-95t

Vaccine policy and recommendations, 56-60. See also
   Recommendations.
   agencies involved with, 56, *57*
Vaccine practice, 105-138
   administration, 113-117
   coding, billing, and vaccine costs, 122-136
   delivery, improving, 108-113
   emergencies, 117-122
   handling, storage, and transport, 105-108
   screening, 113, 114t-115t
Vaccine-preventable diseases, 64-65
   morbidity and mortality from, 45, 46t
Vaccine protest organizations, 201-204, 201t-203t
Vaccine recommendations. See *Recommendations.*
Vaccine registries. See *Immunization Information Systems (IISs).*
Vaccine Research Center (VRC), 505
Vaccine Safety DataLink (VSD), 67, 220
Vaccine Safety Net, 65-72, 65t
   safety findings, ISRC, 70t-71t
Vaccine(s). See also *Immunization; specific vaccines.*
   classification, 12t-13t
   communicating about, 191-240
   concerns about, addressing, 191-240
   costs/cost-benefit analyses. See *Costs.*
   delivery. See *Delivery of vaccines.*
   development. See *Vaccine development and licensure.*
   equivalence of different manufacturers, 147
   funding for. See *Financing.*
   inactivated, 15, 18t-20t
   licensure. See *Vaccine development and licensure.*
   live, 11-16, 12t-13t
      vs inactivated, 18t-20t
   necessity for, 208-209
   recommendations regarding. See *Recommendations.*
   schedules for. See *Schedules for immunizations.*
   specificity of, 28-29
   supply/shortages, 79-83, *84*
   types of, 12t-13t
Vaccines and Related Biological Products Advisory Committee
   (VRBPAC), 54, 505
Vaccines for Children (VFC) Program, 56, 74-78, 505
   actions required under, 75t
   common questions about, 76t-77t
   potential expansion of, 80t
Vaccinia immune globulin (VIG), 436
Vaccinia virus. See also *Smallpox.*
Vaccinology, 11-48. See also *Immunization.*
   basic vaccine immunology, 17-35
   correlates of protection, 36-39, 38t
   genetics of vaccine responses/adverse events, 43
   herd immunity, 39-43
   immunization, 11-16
   public health and vaccines, 44-47, 46t, 191

Vaccinomics, 43

VAERS. See *Vaccine Adverse Event Reporting System.*

Vaginal intraepithelial neoplasia (VaIN), 320

Vapocoolant sprays, 117

Vaqta (HepA), 255, 298t-300t
  CPT and ICD-9-CM codes, 124t
  efficacy/immunogenicity, 301

Varicella, 461-471, 517t
  breakthrough/vaccine-modified, 461-462
  chickenpox and, 461
  clinical features, 461-462
  congenital, 462
  criteria for immunity, 469t
  epidemiology and transmission, 462-463
  herpes zoster (shingles) and, 462. See also *Zoster.*
  immunization program, 463-464
  latent infection, 461
    reactivation of, 462, 481
  morbidity and mortality from, 46t
  passive immunoprophylaxis (VariZIG), 469-470
  pathogen, 461
  progressive, 462
  vaccines for, 464, 466t-467t
    contraindications/precautions, 160, 467-468
    cost-benefit of vaccination, 464
    coverage, *61*
    CPT and ICD-9-CM codes, 128t, 131t
    efficacy/immunogenicity, 464-465
    interval for receipt of antibody-containing products, 150t-151t
    minimum ages and intervals, 144t
    recommendations, 468-470
    safety, 95t, 465-468
    schedule, 47, 254, 466t
      administration errors, and remedies, 154t
      adults, by age, 249t
      adults, by medical condition/indication, 250t
      catch-up, children age 4 months-6 years, 247t
      catch-up, children age 7-18 years, 248t
      children, age 0-6 years, 243t
      children, age 7-18 years, 245t
      interval for smallpox and, 139
    shortages of, *84*
    vs zoster (shingles) vaccine, 35, 147
  vs smallpox, 428t-429t
  waning immunity and, 462

Varicella-zoster immune globulin (VariZIG), 469-470
  adverse reactions, 470
  CPT and ICD-9-CM codes, 129t, 131t
  interval for receipt of live vaccines, 151t
  investigational new drug protocol, obtaining under, 470
  post-exposure, 162, 469-470
  recommendations, 469-470
  safety, 470

Varicella-zoster virus (VZV), 461. See also *Varicella.*
  reactivation of latent, 462, 481. See also *Zoster (herpes zoster; shingles).*
Variola, 425-426. See also *Smallpox.*
Varivax (varicella vaccine), 254, 466t-467t. See also *Varicella, vaccines for.*
  CPT and ICD-9-CM codes, 128t
  efficacy/immunogenicity, 464-465
  recommendations, 468-470
  safety, 465-468
VariZIG, 174-175, 469-470
VFC. See *Vaccines for Children (VFC) Program.*
VICP. See *Vaccine Injury Compensation Program.*
Viscerotopic disease, vaccine-associated, 476
VISs. See *Vaccine Information Statements.*
Vivotif (Ty21a, live-attenuated typhoid vaccine), 445-448, 456t-457t
  CPT and ICD-9-CM codes, 128t
Voices for Vaccines, 507
Vomito negro, 473
VRBPAC. See *Vaccines and Related Biological Products Advisory Committee.*
VSD. See *Vaccine Safety DataLink.*
VTEU. See *Vaccine and Treatment Evaluation Unit.*
Vulvar intraepithelial neoplasia (VIN), 320

Waning immunity, 209, 271, 462
Warnings, 156. See also *Contraindications and precautions.*
Whole agent vaccines, 12t-13t, 15
Whooping cough, 268-269. See also *Pertussis.*
Woolsorter's disease, 257
World Health Organization (WHO), 49, 506
Wound management, tetanus prophylaxis for, 284t-285t
Wounds, contamination of. See *Tetanus.*

X-linked agammaglobulinemia, 163

Yellow fever, 473-479, 517t
  certificates of vaccination, 478
  clinical features, 473
  epidemiology and transmission, 473-474
    endemic regions of world, 185t-187t
  immunization program, 474
  pathogen, 473
  vaccine for, 11, 474, 475t
    adverse events, serious, 476
    contraindications/precautions, 162, 477
    CPT and ICD-9-CM codes, 128t
    efficacy/immunogenicity, 476
    intervals for vaccination, 139
    polyclonal immune globulin and, 17
    recommendations, 485-487
      mandatory for some travel, 184
    safety, 476-477
    schedule, 475t

30

Yellow fever virus (YFV), 473
YF-Vax (yellow fever vaccine), 474, 475t. See also *Yellow fever.*
  CPT and ICD-9-CM codes, 128t
Youth Risk Behavior Study, 321

Zostavax (ZOS, zoster vaccine), 474, 476t-477t
  CPT and ICD-9-CM codes, 128t
  recommendations, 486-487
Zoster (herpes zoster; shingles), 461, 481-488, 517t. See also *Varicella.*
  clinical features, 481-482
  epidemiology and transmission, 482-483
  immunization program, 483-484
  incidence, 483
  pathogen, 481
  postherpetic neuralgia (PHN) and, 481, 484
  vaccine for, 474, 476t-477t
    contraindications/precautions, 484, 487
    cost-benefit of vaccination, 483-484
    CPT and ICD-9-CM codes, 128t
    efficacy/immunogenicity, 484-485
    minimum ages and intervals, 144t
    recommendations, 255, 485-487
    safety, 484
    schedule, 255, 486t, 487
      administration errors, and remedies, 154t
      adults, by age, 249t
      adults, by medical condition/indication, 250t
    vs varicella vaccine, 35, 147